Guide to Ruminant Anatomy

Guide to Ruminant Anatomy

Dissection and Clinical Aspects

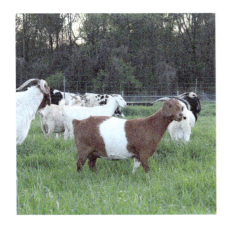

Second Edition

Mahmoud Mansour, DVM, PhD
Professor of Anatomy, Auburn University, Auburn, AL, USA

Ray Wilhite, MS, PhD
Anatomy Laboratory Coordinator, Auburn University, Auburn, AL, USA

Joe Rowe, DVM
Anatomy Instructor, Auburn University, Auburn, AL, USA

Saly Hafiz, DVM, MS, PhD
Research Assistant, Auburn University, AL, USA

WILEY Blackwell

This edition first published 2023
© 2023 John Wiley & Sons, Inc.

Edition History
John Wiley & Sons (1e, 2018)

All rights reserved. No part of this publication may be reproduced, stored in a retrieval system, or transmitted, in any form or by any means, electronic, mechanical, photocopying, recording or otherwise, except as permitted by law. Advice on how to obtain permission to reuse material from this title is available at http://www.wiley.com/go/permissions.

The right of Mahmoud Mansour, Ray Wilhite, Joe Rowe, and Saly Hafiz to be identified as the authors of the material in this work has been asserted in accordance with law.

Registered Office
John Wiley & Sons, Inc., 111 River Street, Hoboken, NJ 07030, USA

For details of our global editorial offices, customer services, and more information about Wiley products visit us at www.wiley.com.

Wiley also publishes its books in a variety of electronic formats and by print-on-demand. Some content that appears in standard print versions of this book may not be available in other formats.

Trademarks: Wiley and the Wiley logo are trademarks or registered trademarks of John Wiley & Sons, Inc. and/or its affiliates in the United States and other countries and may not be used without written permission. All other trademarks are the property of their respective owners. John Wiley & Sons, Inc. is not associated with any product or vendor mentioned in this book.

Limit of Liability/Disclaimer of Warranty
The contents of this work are intended to further general scientific research, understanding, and discussion only and are not intended and should not be relied upon as recommending or promoting scientific method, diagnosis, or treatment by physicians for any particular patient. In view of ongoing research, equipment modifications, changes in governmental regulations, and the constant flow of information relating to the use of medicines, equipment, and devices, the reader is urged to review and evaluate the information provided in the package insert or instructions for each medicine, equipment, or device for, among other things, any changes in the instructions or indication of usage and for added warnings and precautions. While the publisher and authors have used their best efforts in preparing this work, they make no representations or warranties with respect to the accuracy or completeness of the contents of this work and specifically disclaim all warranties, including without limitation any implied warranties of merchantability or fitness for a particular purpose. No warranty may be created or extended by sales representatives, written sales materials or promotional statements for this work. This work is sold with the understanding that the publisher is not engaged in rendering professional services. The advice and strategies contained herein may not be suitable for your situation. You should consult with a specialist where appropriate. The fact that an organization, website, or product is referred to in this work as a citation and/or potential source of further information does not mean that the publisher and authors endorse the information or services the organization, website, or product may provide or recommendations it may make. Further, readers should be aware that websites listed in this work may have changed or disappeared between when this work was written and when it is read. Neither the publisher nor authors shall be liable for any loss of profit or any other commercial damages, including but not limited to special, incidental, consequential, or other damages.

Library of Congress Cataloging-in-Publication Data applied for
Paperback ISBN: 9781119800835

Cover Images: Mahmoud Mansour
Cover Design by Wiley

Set in 10/12pt Warnock by Straive, Pondicherry, India

SKY10043385_022223

Contents

Contributor xv
Preface xvii
Acknowledgments xix
About the Companion Website xxi

1	**The Head, Neck, and Vertebral Column** *1*	
1.1	Skull *2*	
1.2	Mandible *9*	
1.3	Paranasal Sinuses *9*	
1.4	Vertebral Column *14*	
1.5	Teeth and Age Estimation of Cattle and Small Ruminants (Goats and Sheep) *15*	
1.5.1	Definitions and Criteria for Estimating the Age of Ruminants *21*	
1.5.2	Steps for Estimating the Age of Cattle *22*	
1.6	Joints of the Head *24*	
1.6.1	Temporomandibular Joint *24*	
1.6.2	Atlantooccipital Joint *24*	
1.6.3	Mandibular Symphysis *24*	
1.6.4	Vertebral Joints *25*	
1.7	Muscles of the Head *25*	
1.7.1	Cutaneous Muscles *27*	
1.7.2	Muscles of Facial Expression *27*	
1.7.3	Muscles of Mastication *28*	
1.7.4	Pharyngeal Muscles *28*	
1.7.4.1	Nomenclature of Pharyngeal Muscles *28*	
1.7.5	Laryngeal Muscles *28*	
1.7.6	Hyoid Muscles *29*	
1.7.7	Lingual Muscles *29*	
1.7.8	Extraocular Muscles *29*	
1.8	Blood Vessels, Lymph Nodes, and Nerves of the Head *30*	
1.8.1	Blood Vessels (Arteries and Veins) *30*	
1.8.1.1	Arteries of the Head *30*	
1.8.1.2	Veins of the Head *32*	
1.8.2	Lymph Nodes of the Head and Neck *33*	
1.8.3	Nerves of the Head *35*	
1.8.3.1	Summary of Cranial Nerves and Their Functions *35*	

1.9	Salivary Glands	39
1.10	The Pharynx	40
1.10.1	Oropharynx	40
1.10.2	Nasopharynx	40
1.10.3	Laryngopharynx	40
1.11	Tongue	40
1.12	The Larynx and Hyoid Apparatus	42
1.12.1	Larynx	42
1.12.2	Hyoid Apparatus	43
1.13	The Eye	43
1.13.1	Superficial Features of the Eye	44
1.13.2	Layers of the Eye	46
1.13.3	Sectioning of the Eyeball	48
1.13.3.1	Chambers of the Eye	48
1.13.4	Drainage Pathway of the Aqueous Humor	48
1.14	Neck Skeleton	48
1.15	Neck Muscles, Nerves, and Vessels	50
1.15.1	Neck Muscles	50
1.15.1.1	Superficial Neck Muscles	50
1.15.1.1.1	Brachiocephalicus Muscle	50
1.15.1.1.2	Omotransversarius Muscle	53
1.15.1.1.3	Trapezius Muscle	53
1.15.1.1.4	Sternocephalicus Muscle	53
1.15.1.1.5	Sternothyroideus and Sternohyoideus Muscles	54
1.15.1.2	Deep Neck Muscles	54
1.15.2	Nerves of the Neck	54
1.15.3	Blood Vessels of the Neck	55
1.16	Nuchal Ligament	56
1.17	Surface Topography (Head and Neck)	57
1.18	Lab ID List for the Head and Neck	60
2	**The Thorax**	**63**
2.1	Introduction	64
2.2	Bones of the Thorax	64
2.3	Thoracic Inlet	65
2.4	Basal Border of the Lung and Area for Lung Auscultation	66
2.5	Diaphragmatic Line of Pleural Reflection	66
2.6	Muscles of the Thoracic Wall	68
2.7	Pleura	71
2.7.1	Parietal Pleura	71
2.7.2	Visceral Pleura	72
2.7.3	Connecting Pleura	72
2.7.4	Content of the Pleural Cavity	72
2.7.5	Lung Lobes	72
2.7.6	Mediastinum	74
2.8	Vessels (Arteries and Veins)	74
2.8.1	Blood Circulation: An Overview	75

2.9	Major Veins of the Thorax	76
2.9.1	Cranial Vena Cava	76
2.9.2	Caudal Vena Cava	76
2.9.3	Azygos Veins (Left and Right)	77
2.10	Major Arteries of the Thorax	77
2.10.1	Brachiocephalic Trunk	77
2.10.2	Costocervical Trunk	78
2.10.3	Vertebral Artery	78
2.10.4	Superficial Cervical Artery	78
2.10.5	Internal Thoracic Artery	78
2.11	Lymphatic Structures	78
2.11.1	Thymus	79
2.11.2	Thoracic Duct	79
2.11.3	Mediastinal and Tracheobronchial Lymph Nodes	79
2.12	Nerves (Motor Somatic, Sympathetic, and Parasympathetic)	80
2.12.1	Phrenic Nerve	81
2.12.2	Autonomic Nerves in the Thorax	81
2.12.3	Vagus Nerve	81
2.12.4	Sympathetic Trunk and Sympathetic Ganglia	82
2.13	Heart (Cor)	82
2.13.1	Pericardium	82
2.13.2	External Features of the Heart	82
2.13.3	Interior of the Heart	85
2.13.3.1	Structures of the Right Atrium	86
2.13.3.2	Structures of the Right Ventricle	86
2.13.3.2.1	Right Atrioventricular Valve	87
2.13.3.2.2	Chordae Tendineae, Papillary Muscles, and Cusps of the Right Atrioventricular Valve	87
2.13.3.2.3	Trabecula Septomarginalis	87
2.13.3.2.4	Ossa Cordis	87
2.13.3.2.5	Coronary Arteries	87
2.14	Point of Maximum Intensity or Puncta Maxima	88
2.15	Lab ID List for the Thorax	88
3	**The Abdomen**	*91*
3.1	Lumbar Vertebrae	92
3.1.1	Bovine Lumbar Vertebrae	92
3.1.2	Goat and Sheep Lumbar Vertebrae	92
3.2	Ligaments of Lumbar Vertebrae	93
3.2.1	Supraspinous Ligament	93
3.2.2	Interspinous Ligaments	94
3.2.3	Intertransverse Ligaments	94
3.2.4	Yellow Ligaments (Interarcuate or Ligament Flava)	94
3.2.5	Dorsal and Ventral Longitudinal Ligaments	94
3.2.6	Intervertebral Disc	94
3.3	Abdominal Wall	94
3.3.1	Paralumbar Fossa	94
3.3.2	Nerves of the Paralumbar Fossa (Flank Anesthesia)	95

3.3.3	Cutaneus Trunci and Omobrachialis Muscles	98
3.3.4	Tunica Flava Abdominis	98
3.3.5	External Abdominal Oblique Muscle	98
3.3.6	Internal Abdominal Oblique Muscle	101
3.3.7	Transversus Abdominis Muscle	102
3.3.8	Rectus Abdominis Muscle	102
3.3.9	Rectus Sheath	102
3.4	Abdominal Cavity	105
3.4.1	Dissection Plan	105
3.4.2	Peritoneum	105
3.4.3	Omentum	107
3.4.4	Ruminant Stomach	111
3.4.4.1	Reticulum	111
3.4.4.1.1	Cardia	118
3.4.4.2	Rumen	118
3.4.4.3	Omasum	120
3.4.4.4	Abomasum	121
3.5	Intestines	123
3.5.1	Small Intestine	123
3.5.1.1	Duodenum	123
3.5.1.2	Mesoduodenum	125
3.5.1.3	Duodenocolic Fold	125
3.5.1.4	Jejunum	125
3.5.1.5	Ileum	126
3.5.1.6	Ileal Orifice	126
3.5.1.7	Ileocecal Fold	126
3.5.2	Large Intestine	126
3.5.2.1	Cecum and Cecocolic Orifice	126
3.5.2.2	Ascending Colon	129
3.5.2.2.1	Proximal Loop	129
3.5.2.2.2	Spiral Loop	129
3.5.2.2.3	Distal Loop	129
3.6	Other Abdominal Organs	130
3.6.1	Liver	130
3.6.2	Spleen	130
3.6.3	Pancreas	130
3.6.4	Kidney	130
3.7	Vessels	134
3.7.1	Arteries	134
3.7.2	Veins	136
3.7.3	Lymphatics	136
3.8	Palpation of the Live Animal	136
3.9	Lab ID List for the Abdomen	137
4	**The Pelvis and Reproductive Organs**	**139**
4.1	Bones of the Pelvis	140
4.1.1	Os Coxae (Pelvic Bone)	140

4.2	Sacrosciatic Ligament (Broad Sacrotuberous Ligament)	*141*
4.3	Pelvic Peritoneal Pouches *142*	
4.4	Urinary Bladder, Ureters, and Ligaments of the Bladder *142*	
4.5	Male Genitalia *144*	
4.5.1	Penis *144*	
4.5.1.1	Root of the Penis and Cavernous Tissue *145*	
4.5.1.2	Free Part of the Penis and Glans Penis *146*	
4.5.1.3	Retractor Penis Muscle *146*	
4.5.1.4	Apical Ligament *146*	
4.5.1.5	Dorsal Nerve of the Penis *150*	
4.5.2	Male Urethra *150*	
4.5.3	Prepuce *153*	
4.5.4	Superficial Inguinal (Scrotal) Lymph Nodes *153*	
4.5.5	Blood Supply to the Pelvic Viscera and Male Genitalia *153*	
4.5.6	Testes *155*	
4.5.7	Male Accessory Sex Glands *158*	
4.6	Female Reproductive Tract *159*	
4.6.1	Ovaries *159*	
4.6.2	Uterine Tubes *161*	
4.6.3	Uterine Horns *162*	
4.6.4	Uterine Body *162*	
4.6.5	Uterine Cervix *164*	
4.6.6	Vagina *164*	
4.6.7	Female Pudendum *166*	
4.6.7.1	Vestibule *166*	
4.6.7.2	Suburethral Diverticulum *166*	
4.6.7.3	Vulva *167*	
4.6.8	Blood Supply of the Female Genital Tract *167*	
4.6.9	Udder *169*	
4.6.9.1	Suspensory Apparatus and Interior Structures of the Udder *169*	
4.6.9.2	Blood Supply and Venous Drainage of the Udder *170*	
4.6.9.3	Lymphatics of the Udder *172*	
4.6.9.4	Innervation of the Udder *172*	
4.7	Live Cow *172*	
4.8	Lab ID List for the Pelvis and Reproductive Structures *174*	
5	**The Forelimb** *177*	
5.1	Introduction *178*	
5.2	Bones of the Thoracic Limb *178*	
5.2.1	Scapula *178*	
5.2.2	Humerus *180*	
5.2.3	Radius and Ulna *181*	
5.2.4	Carpus (Proximal and Distal Rows) *181*	
5.2.5	Metacarpal Bones (Large Metacarpal or Cannon Bone) *183*	
5.2.6	Digits *184*	
5.3	Muscles and Tendons of the Thoracic Limb *185*	
5.3.1	Extrinsic Muscles of the Forelimb *186*	

5.3.1.1	Trapezius Muscle (Cervical and Thoracic Parts)	*186*
5.3.1.2	Rhomboideus Muscle (Cervical and Thoracic Parts)	*186*
5.3.1.3	Brachiocephalicus Muscle (Cleidocephalicus and Cleidobrachialis)	*187*
5.3.1.4	Omotransversarius Muscle	*188*
5.3.1.5	Latissimus Dorsi Muscle	*188*
5.3.1.6	Superficial Pectoral Muscle (Descending and Transverse Parts)	*188*
5.3.1.7	Deep (Ascending) Pectoral Muscle	*189*
5.3.1.8	Serratus Ventralis Muscle	*189*
5.3.1.9	Subclavius Muscle	*190*
5.3.2	Intrinsic Muscles of the Thoracic Limb	*190*
5.3.2.1	Muscles of the Proximal Limb (Shoulder and Brachium)	*193*
5.3.2.1.1	Supraspinatus Muscle	*193*
5.3.2.1.2	Infraspinatus Muscle	*193*
5.3.2.1.3	Deltoideus Muscle	*194*
5.3.2.1.4	Teres Minor Muscle	*194*
5.3.2.1.5	Teres Major Muscle	*194*
5.3.2.1.6	Subscapularis Muscle	*194*
5.3.2.1.7	Triceps Brachii Muscle (Long, Lateral, Accessory, and Medial Heads)	*194*
5.3.2.1.8	Anconeus Muscle	*195*
5.3.2.1.9	Tensor Fasciae Antebrachii Muscle	*195*
5.3.2.1.10	Coracobrachialis Muscle	*195*
5.3.2.1.11	Biceps Brachii Muscle	*196*
5.3.2.1.12	Brachialis Muscle	*196*
5.3.2.2	Muscles and Tendons of the Distal Limb (Antebrachium and Manus [Carpus, Metacarpus, and Digits])	*196*
5.3.2.2.1	Craniolateral Group (Located on the Cranial and Lateral Forearm)	*196*
5.3.2.2.2	Extensor Carpi Radialis Muscle	*196*
5.3.2.2.3	Common Digital Extensor Muscle (Medial and Lateral Heads and Three Tendons)	*197*
5.3.2.2.4	Lateral Digital Extensor Muscle	*197*
5.3.2.2.5	Ulnaris Lateralis Muscle	*198*
5.3.2.2.6	Extensor Carpi Obliquus Muscle	*199*
5.3.2.3	Caudomedial Muscle Group of the Antebrachium	*199*
5.3.2.3.1	Flexor Carpi Ulnaris Muscle	*199*
5.3.2.3.2	Flexor Carpi Radialis Muscle	*200*
5.3.2.3.3	Pronator Teres Muscle	*201*
5.3.2.3.4	Superficial Digital Flexor with Superficial and Deep Parts: Flexor Manica	*201*
5.3.2.3.5	Deep Digital Flexor Muscle	*201*
5.3.2.3.6	Interosseus Muscle (Suspensory Ligament) with Axial and Abaxial Extensor Branches	*201*
5.4	Retinacula	*203*
5.5	Carpal Canal	*203*
5.6	Ligaments of the Digits	*203*
5.6.1	Proximal Interdigital Ligament	*204*
5.6.2	Distal Interdigital Ligament	*204*
5.6.3	Annular Ligaments (Palmar, Proximal, and Distal Digital Annular Ligaments)	*204*
5.6.4	Digital Annular Ligaments (Proximal and Distal)	*204*
5.7	Hoof (Wall, Sole, Bulb, and White Line)	*205*

5.8	Arteries and Nerves of the Thoracic Limb	205
5.8.1	Nomenclature of Blood Vessels and Nerves in the Distal Limb	206
5.9	Veins of the Forelimb	207
5.10	Lymphatics of the Thoracic Limb	209
5.11	Nerves of the Thoracic Limb	209
5.11.1	Suprascapular Nerve	210
5.11.2	Subscapular Nerve	211
5.11.3	Axillary Nerve	211
5.11.4	Musculocutaneous Nerve	211
5.11.5	Radial Nerve	211
5.11.5.1	Branching of the Radial and Ulnar Nerves in the Distal Limb	212
5.11.6	Median and Ulnar Nerves	212
5.12	Joints of the Forelimbs	212
5.12.1	Shoulder Joint	216
5.12.2	Elbow Joint	217
5.12.3	Carpal Joints	217
5.12.4	Digital Joints	217
6	**The Hind Limb**	**219**
6.1	Bones of the Hind Limb	220
6.1.1	Os Coxae (Hip Bone)	220
6.1.2	Femur (Thighbone)	220
6.1.3	Bones of the Leg (Crus)	223
6.1.4	Tarsal Bones	224
6.1.5	Fused Metatarsals III and IV (Large Metatarsal Bone)	225
6.1.6	Metatarsal Sesamoid Bone	225
6.2	Muscles of the Pelvic Limb	226
6.2.1	Muscles Acting on the Hip Joint	226
6.2.1.1	Gluteal Muscles	226
6.2.1.1.1	Tensor Fasciae Latae Muscle and Fascia Lata	229
6.2.1.1.2	Middle Gluteal Muscle	229
6.2.1.1.3	Deep Gluteal Muscle	230
6.2.1.2	Hamstring Muscles	230
6.2.1.2.1	Gluteobiceps Muscle	230
6.2.1.2.2	Semitendinosus Muscle	230
6.2.1.2.3	Semimembranosus Muscle	230
6.2.1.3	Medial Adductor Thigh Muscles	231
6.2.1.3.1	Sartorius Muscle	231
6.2.1.3.2	Gracilis Muscle	231
6.2.1.3.3	Pectineus Muscle	232
6.2.1.3.4	Adductor Muscle	232
6.2.1.3.5	External Obturator Muscle	232
6.2.2	Muscles Acting on the Stifle Joint	233
6.2.2.1	Quadriceps Femoris Muscle	233
6.2.3	Muscles Acting on the Hock and Digits	234
6.2.3.1	Craniolateral Muscles of the Leg (Crus)	234

6.2.3.1.1	Fibularis (Peroneus) Tertius Muscle	*235*
6.2.3.1.2	Long Digital Extensor Muscle	*235*
6.2.3.1.3	Lateral Digital Extensor Muscle	*236*
6.2.3.1.4	Cranial Tibial Muscle	*237*
6.2.3.1.5	Fibularis (Peroneus) Longus Muscle	*237*
6.2.3.2	Extensor Retinacula	*237*
6.2.3.3	Caudomedial Muscles of the Leg (Crus)	*238*
6.2.3.3.1	Soleus Muscle	*238*
6.2.3.3.2	Gastrocnemius Muscle (Lateral and Medial Heads)	*238*
6.2.3.3.3	Superficial Digital Flexor Muscle	*238*
6.2.3.3.4	Common Calcanean (or Calcaneal) Tendon and Calcanean Bursae	*239*
6.2.3.3.5	Deep Digital Flexor Muscle	*239*
6.2.3.3.6	Popliteus Muscle	*239*
6.2.3.3.7	Interosseus Muscle (Suspensory Ligament)	*239*
6.3	Blood Vessels and Nerves of the Hind Limbs	*239*
6.3.1	Overview of Arterial Blood Supply to the Whole Hind Limb	*240*
6.3.2	Veins of the Hind Limb	*242*
6.3.3	Lymphatic Structures of the Hind Limb	*242*
6.3.4	Nerves of the Hind Limb	*244*
6.3.4.1	Femoral Nerve	*246*
6.3.4.2	Obturator Nerve	*246*
6.3.4.3	Sciatic Nerve	*246*
6.3.4.4	Common Fibular (Peroneal) Nerve	*249*
6.3.4.5	Tibial Nerve	*249*
6.4	Joints of the Hind Limb	*250*
6.4.1	Hip Joint	*250*
6.4.2	Stifle Joint	*250*
6.4.3	Hock (or Tarsus) Joint	*251*
6.5	Live Cow	*251*
6.6	Lab ID List for Forelimb and Hind Limb	*251*
Appendix A	**Dissection Instructions for a Goat Cadaver**	*255*
A.1	Dissection Labs	*255*
A.2	Dissection of Goat Neck and Body Cavities (Labs, 1, 2, and 3)	*255*
A.2.1	Removal of the Thoracic Limb	*255*
A.2.2	Removal of the Pelvic (Hind) Limb	*256*
A.2.3	Skinning of the Neck and Flank on the Side Where the Limbs Are Removed	*256*
A.2.3.1	Neck	*257*
A.2.4	Opening the Thorax and Abdomen for Studying the Topography on the Left and Right Sides	*257*
A.2.5	Thorax	*258*
A.2.5.1	Thoracic Landmarks	*258*
A.2.5.1.1	Basal Border of the Lungs	*258*
A.2.5.1.2	The Diaphragmatic Line of Pleural Reflection	*258*
A.2.5.2	Nerves and Vessels Within the Thorax	*259*

A.2.6	Abdomen (In Situ and on Extirpated Viscera)	*259*
A.2.7	Dissection of Male and Female Pelvis (Lab 4)	*260*
A.3	Head Dissection (Lab 5)	*260*
A.4	Forelimb Dissection (Labs 6 and 7)	*260*
A.5	Hind Limb Dissection (Labs 8 and 9)	*261*
	Videos Captions	*261*

Appendix B Terminology: Common Terminology and Names *263*

Appendix C Further Reading *267*

Index *269*

Contributor

Thomas Passler, DVM, Ph.D., DACVIM
Professor of Food & Fiber Animal Medicine
Department of Clinical Sciences-Auburn University
2026 J. T. Vaughan LATH-Auburn, AL, USA

Preface

The first edition of the *Guide to Ruminant Anatomy: Dissection and Clinical Aspects* was published in 2018. This textbook provides a valuable teaching resource for anatomy instructors and veterinary students worldwide. It covers the anatomy of ruminants based on the bovine and caprine species. We used body regions to organize the book into six chapters that include head and neck, thorax, abdomen, pelvis, forelimb, and hind limb. The first edition was well received by anatomy instructors and veterinary students all over the world.

Each chapter offers learning objectives, detailed explanation, and labeled images based on the dissection of embalmed animals and color illustrations to explain relatively difficult concepts. In addition, a carefully selected list of structures for laboratory identification is available at the end of each chapter. Instructors could modify the lab identification list based on the requirement of their program. Clinical applications are integrated in boxes embedded within the text throughout the book. The objective is to offer clinical perspective on the structures that are emphasized in each chapter.

More notably, the second edition has expanded the companion website with new instructional videos that cover the study material in each chapter. The videos discuss practical concepts and emphasize the important aspects of each body region. They are all narrated by subject matter experts.

We have updated the text and added new photographs in several chapters that include the thorax, abdomen, and pelvis. More noticeably, we have increased the size of the book to 8 × 10 inches to allow for enlargement and better projection of the stellar dissection images depicting goat and cattle anatomy.

Given the emphasis on teaching clinically relevant anatomy, we have focused on updating the clinical applications in each chapter. We hope that students and instructors find the new edition more informative and worthy of their valuable time. The authors welcome any suggestions for future editions.

Mahmoud Mansour, DVM, PhD
Ray Wilhite, PhD
Joe Rowe, DVM
Saly Hafiz, DVM, MS, PhD
Auburn University, AL, USA

Acknowledgments

The authors would like to thank Paul Rumph (Professor Emeritus, Auburn College of Veterinary Medicine) for providing valuable comments and suggestions. We would also like to thank Dr. Eleanor Josephson, Associate Professor of Anatomy, Kevin Delmain, Professor of Veterinary Practice, and Paul Rumph, for their help with the instructional videos associated with this book. Special thanks to Deborah T. Rowe for her excellent line drawings. Her art drawings correlate well with dissection images and help the students understand some difficult concepts.

We would like to thank Professor Robert Judd, Head of the Department of Anatomy, Physiology, and Pharmacology for his support and excellent leadership. Special thanks to Professors Julie Gard and Simon Taylor at the Department of Clinical Sciences for their help with the live animal images. We would also thank Sabrina van Ginkel for her help with the book index. Special thanks to Lauren King and Mary Katherine Fuller (second-year DVM students) for their help with typing the authors' edits in four of the book's chapters.

About the Companion Website

This book is accompanied by a companion website:

www.wiley.com/go/mansour/dissection2

The website consists of:

- Video clips that explain practical aspects of ruminant anatomy.
- Test questions on each section of the book with an answer key.

1

The Head, Neck, and Vertebral Column

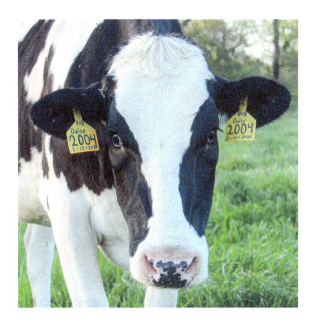

Learning Objectives

- Identify the main bones and some of their palpable features on the bovine skull. Examples of important features include the temporal line, lacrimal bulla, zygomatic arch, facial tuberosity, nasoincisive notch, foramen orbitorotundum, optic canal, supraorbital foramen, infraorbital foramen, mandibular foramen, mental foramen, and body of the mandible.
- Identify the features of the most clinically important frontal and maxillary sinuses. Know the compartments of the frontal sinus (2–3 rostral and 1 caudal). Study the diverticuli of the caudal compartment of the frontal sinus (cornual, nuchal, and postorbital). Note the dividing thin bony septa of the frontal sinus (transverse oblique and median septum). Identify the lacrimal bulla, the most caudal extent of the maxillary sinus. This sinus can be accessed by drilling a hole through the frontal sinus (see Box 1.1). In dehorning operations in goats, you should keep in mind the superficial location and shallow depth of the frontal sinus at the base of the horn.

Guide to Ruminant Anatomy: Dissection and Clinical Aspects, Second Edition. Mahmoud Mansour, Ray Wilhite, Joe Rowe, and Saly Hafiz.
© 2023 John Wiley & Sons, Inc. Published 2023 by John Wiley & Sons, Inc.
Companion website: www.wiley.com/go/mansour/dissection2

- Be able to recall the dental formula and methods for estimating age of cattle and goats using eruption times and changes in the occlusal surface of lower incisor teeth. Know that the incisor and canine teeth in the upper jaw are absent and are replaced by a fibrous structure known as the dental pad.
- Identify clinically important superficial structures on lateral head views (cornual nerve, supraorbital nerve, infraorbital nerve, mental nerve, and dorsal and ventral buccal and auriculopalpebral branches of the facial nerve). Clinically important vessels include the frontal vein, the facial artery (pulse in cattle), and transverse facial artery (pulse in goats). In the neck, identify the external jugular vein, superficial cervical lymph nodes, accessory and great auricular nerves, and parts of the nuchal ligament.
- Identify nerve and blood supply to the horns. You should know the difference in nerve supply of the horn in small and large ruminants, and which nerve or nerves to block in dehorning operations. Note the differences in location and direction of the horn in small and large ruminants. Understand that dehorning is best carried out when the animal is 1–2 weeks of age. Know the meaning of the term epiceras.
- Identify clinically important structures on a median plane of the head (lingual torus and lingual fossa, nasal conchae, medial retropharyngeal lymph node, and other oral, pharyngeal, and laryngeal structures on your laboratory ID list).
- Describe some of the methods and structures associated with enucleation (removal) of the eye that has cancer (i.e., retrobulbar and Peterson's nerve blocks).
- Identify lymph nodes of the head (parotid, mandibular, and lateral and medial retropharyngeal lymph nodes). In the neck, identify the superficial and deep cervical lymph nodes. Know that the lateral retropharyngeal lymph node is the major collection center for lymph from the ruminant head. Understand that the medial and lateral retropharyngeal lymph nodes are incised and examined in meat inspection. You should also know the drainage area for each node.
- Identify major salivary glands of the head (parotid, mandibular, and sublingual).
- Identify neck muscles that form the dorsal and ventral boundaries for the jugular groove (or furrow). Know the difference between jugular groove muscular boundaries in cattle, goats, and sheep. Sheep have a less distinct jugular furrow because of the absence of the sternomandibularis muscle. This muscle forms the ventral boundary in cattle and goats. It is also called the sternozygomaticus muscle in goats.
- Recall the vertebral formula for large and small ruminants. Know vertebral locations for epidural anesthesia in cattle.
- At the end of the head and neck sections watch Videos 1 to 8.

1.1 Skull

Goal: With the help of Figures 1.1–1.9, study the main features of the bovine and caprine skulls on dorsal, lateral, caudal, and ventral views. You should place emphasis on the main paranasal sinuses and bony landmarks for blocking clinically important nerves of the head (e.g., temporal line [cornual nerve], zygomatic arch [auriculopalpebral nerve], infraorbital and mental foramina [infraorbital and mental nerves, respectively], and foramen orbitorotundum [oculomotor, trochlear, ophthalmic, and abducent nerves]). Consult Boxes 1.2–1.5 for clinical application related to features of the skull.

Before you start your dissection of the head, study the bovine skull. Make comparisons with goat and sheep skulls whenever indicated.

The skull is part of the axial skeleton. In addition to the skull, the **axial skeleton** includes bones of the **vertebral column, ribs,** and the **sternum.**

The functions of the skull include protection of the brain, sensory organs, and the upper gastrointestinal and respiratory tracts.

The mandibles and the hyoid apparatus articulate with the skull but are technically not part of the skull. However, they will be studied with the bones of the skull.

The most striking features of the adult bovine skull are the flattened dorsum (frontal bone), the presence of the **cornual process** (the bony part of the horn),

facial tuberosity (a bony prominence on the lateral surface of the maxilla), and the lack of upper incisor teeth and their replacement with the **dental pad** in the live animal.

The dorsum of the skull in goats and sheep is slightly dome-shaped compared with the flat frontal bone in adult cattle. However, in young calves, the skull is dome-shaped, like the skull in small ruminants.

Look at the dorsal view of the bovine skull and, with the help of Figures 1.1 and 1.2, study the following bones and features: **frontal bone, cornual process** of the frontal bone (if present in your specimen),

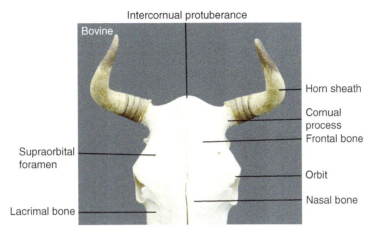

Figure 1.1 Bovine skull: caudodorsal view. The epidermal part of the horn (horn sheath or capsule) and the bony part (cornual process) form the horn. Akin to the hoof, the horn sheath and the cornual process are glued together by dermal tissue that contains blood vessels and nerve endings of the cornual nerve and artery. The cornual process and the horn capsule are removed in dehorning operations.

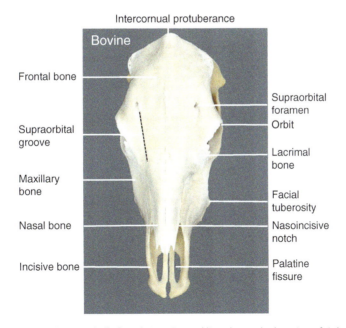

Figure 1.2 A polled (no horns present) bovine skull: dorsal view. Dotted line shows the location of right supraorbital groove. In the live animal, the supraorbital groove houses the supraorbital vein (called the frontal vein after passing through the supraorbital foramen). The bovid may have multiple supraorbital foramina (single in small ruminants).

lacrimal bone, nasal bone, incisive bone, nasoincisive notch, intercornual protuberance, supraorbital groove, and **supraorbital foramen.**

Study the nerves passing through some of the foramina listed on your laboratory ID list (Table 1.1).

Note that the **cornual process** in cattle lies several centimeters caudal to the eye or bony orbit. It extends in lateral and dorsal directions (Figure 1.1). In goats, it lies relatively close to the caudal border of the eye and extends in a caudal rather than lateral direction (Figure 1.3).

The cornual process grows from the frontal bone. Much like the hoof structures, the horn has a bony part (cornual process), dermal and epidermal (horn sheath) parts layered on the cornual process.

The epidermal **horn sheath** and the cornual process form the horn. If the horn sheath is not separated from the cornual process, you should be able to identify both the cornual process and horn sheath on the skull as shown in Figure 1.1.

Turn the skull so that the lateral surface is facing you. With the help of Figures 1.3 and 1.4, identify the **facial tuberosity, maxilla, body of the mandible, infraorbital foramen, temporal line,** and **the bony rim of the orbit.** Identify the **zygomatic arch** and note that it is formed by two bones, the **zygomatic bone rostrally,** and the **zygomatic process of the temporal bone caudally** (Figure 1.4). The caudal part of the zygomatic bone is called the **temporal process of the zygomatic bone**.

On the lateral facial surface of the skull, ruminants have a circumscribed **facial tuberosity** (Figure 1.4) compared with a longitudinal long bony ridge known as the facial crest in the horse.

> **Box 1.1**
>
> Drilling a circular hole in the skull or other bones is known as trephination. This hole is generally made to drain inflammatory exudate and flush sinuses in the skull with antiseptic solution. Diseases of the frontal sinus result from microbial infections mostly from dehorning operations in cattle. Consult Figure 1.9d.

> **Box 1.2**
>
> In the bovine, the supraorbital groove is palpable. It houses the supraorbital or **frontal vein**. In rostral frontal sinus surgery (i.e., trephination), the frontal vein must be avoided.

Table 1.1 Major foramina of the bovine skull and nerves passing through them. Understand that there are vessels that accompany these nerves (not listed). CN V1, ophthalmic subdivision of CN V; CN V2, maxillary subdivision of CN V.

Foramen/canal	Nerve
Supraorbital foramen	Supraorbital nerve (continuation of frontal nerve, a branch of the ophthalmic division of the trigeminal nerve)
Maxillary foramen–infraorbital canal–infraorbital foramen	Maxillary nerve (subdivision of the trigeminal nerve continued by the infraorbital nerve through the infraorbital foramen)
Mandibular foramen–mandibular canal–mental foramen	Inferior alveolar nerve, mental nerve (continuation of the inferior alveolar), branches of the mandibular subdivision of the trigeminal nerve
Foramen orbitorotundum	Oculomotor nerve (CN III), trochlear nerve (CN IV), ophthalmic (CN V-1) subdivision of the trigeminal nerve, maxillary (CN V-2) nerve subdivision of the trigeminal nerve, and abducent nerve (CN VI)
Optic canal	Optic nerve (CN II)
Caudal palatine foramen–major palatine foramen	Major palatine nerve, a branch of the maxillary nerve subdivision of the trigeminal nerve
Sphenopalatine foramen–nasal cavity	Caudal nasal nerve, branch of the maxillary nerve, a subdivision of the trigeminal nerve

> **Box 1.3**
>
> In dehorning operations in cattle, the **temporal line** is used as a palpable landmark to block the **cornual nerve** that innervates the horn in cattle. The cornual nerve emerges from the orbit and courses toward the base of the horn along the temporal line. The **cornual artery**, which supplies the horn, must also be ligated or its branches cauterized (for more details of the nerves that supply the horn; see Box 1.18).
>
> In adult goats, three nerves must be blocked if regional anesthesia is selected. These nerves are:
>
> 1) The **cornual nerve:** block is between the lateral canthus of the eye and the lateral part of the base of the horn.
> 2) The cornual branches of the **infratrochlear nerve:** block is more medial than that of the cornual nerve between the medial canthus of the eye and medial edge of the base of the horn.
> 3) Cornual branches of the **great auricular nerve:** at the back of the ear.
>
> Additionally, a ring nerve block is sometimes performed by depositing a local anesthetic around the base of the horn to achieve maximal pain suppression.
>
> In goats, general anesthesia is sometimes used as a better alternative than local anesthesia.
>
> The horn can then be sawed off using a hacksaw or obstetrical wire.
>
> **Horn buds** (called horn buttons) are typically eliminated in young animals to prevent horn growth. Several procedures, including chemical or heat cautery, are used to prevent the growth of the horn buds. Several dehorner devices such as tube or spoon dehorners, lever-type dehorners, and surgical saws are used to remove horns when they are very small.
>
> In dehorning of adult goats, care must be taken not to expose the brain cavity because of the proximity of the cornual process and parietal bone.

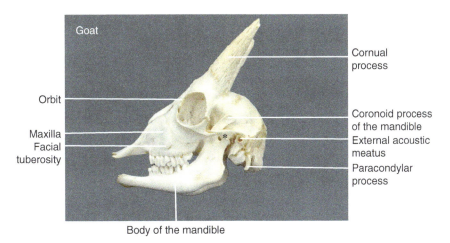

Figure 1.3 Goat skull: lateral view. The horn sheath (epidermal part) is removed. * Temporomandibular joint (TMJ). Note the proximity of the cornual process to the parietal bone. In dehorning of mature goats, the cut must not be made too far caudally to avoid exposure of the brain.

Identify the **infraorbital foramen** on the lateral surface of the maxilla (Figure 1.4). The infraorbital nerve (terminal branch of the maxillary nerve) emerges on the face through this foramen.

Note that the bony orbit is complete in ruminants by fusion of the **zygomatic process of the frontal bone** (ZF) and the **frontal process of the zygomatic bone** (FZ) (Figures 1.4 and 1.5). This is also true for the horse skull.

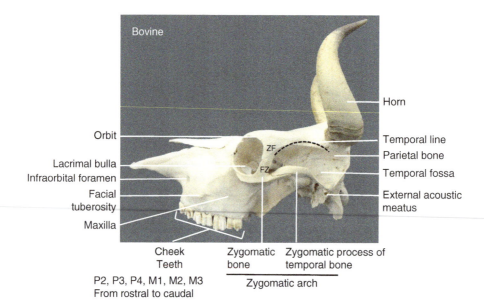

Figure 1.4 Bovine skull: lateral view. The bony orbit is complete where the frontal process of the zygomatic bone (FZ) and the zygomatic process of the frontal bone (ZF) meet. The zygomatic arch is palpable in the live animal and is formed by two bones: the zygomatic bone and the temporal process of the zygomatic bone (TZ) rostrally and the zygomatic process of the temporal bone caudally. **Temporal line** (dotted) is used as a landmark for blocking the cornual nerve in dehorning operations in adult cattle. M, molar; P, premolar. P1 is not present in the upper or lower jaws.

Box 1.4
The infraorbital nerve passes out of the skull through the infraorbital foramen. The infraorbital nerve block is sometimes used in cattle to repair nasal laceration and/or to place nasal rings in bulls. Alternatively, a local anesthetic drug, such as lidocaine, can be injected directly at the site of the surgical procedure (local nerve block). Consult Box 1.18.

In the dog, the orbit is incomplete, and the gap on the orbital rim is bridged by a rigid fibrous structure known as the orbital ligament.

Note the prominent but very thin **lacrimal bulla** within the rostral confinement of the orbit (Figure 1.4). The maxillary sinus extends caudally into the lacrimal bulla.

The angle between the temporal process of the zygomatic bone and the frontal process of the zygomatic bone (FZ) is used as landmark for needle insertion when anesthetizing nerves emerging from the **foramen orbitorotundum** that course to the eye (Figure 1.5).

In ruminants, the foramen orbitorotundum represents the combination of the orbital fissure and round foramen present in other species (e.g., dog). The ophthalmic, maxillary, oculomotor, trochlear, and abducent nerves pass from the brainstem to the orbital space through the foramen orbitorotundum to supply various structures of the eye.

Box 1.5
The lacrimal bulla is vulnerable to puncture in enucleation (removal) of the eye by the retrobulbar technique. Read more about the retrobulbar technique in the nerve block section (Box 1.6).

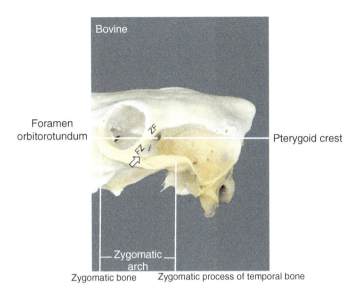

Figure 1.5 The bovine skull showing the bony landmarks for Peterson's nerve block: caudolateral view. The white arrow points to the angle where the needle is inserted to deposit an anesthetic close to the foramen orbitorotundum. This angle is formed by the bifurcation of the zygomatic bone caudally into the frontal process of the zygomatic bone (FZ) and the temporal process of the zygomatic bone (TZ). The pterygoid crest and coronoid process of the mandible are encountered and avoided as a long-curved needle is advanced toward the foramen.

> **Box 1.6**
>
> Anesthesia for enucleation of the eye can be performed by two standardized techniques known as retrobulbar (or modified retrobulbar) technique or by Peterson's nerve block.
>
> In Peterson's nerve block, the angle between the frontal and the temporal process of the zygomatic bone is used for needle insertion where an anesthetic is deposited close to the foramen orbitorotundum to block several nerves coursing to the eye. The coronoid process of the mandible and the pterygoid crest should be avoided.
>
> Because Peterson's nerve block requires advanced technical skill, the retrobulbar technique is considered as an easier alternative. The medial and lateral canthi of the eye and upper (superior) and lower (inferior) eyelids are used as landmarks for anesthetic injection at four points. In this procedure, care should be taken to avoid damaging the thin lacrimal bulla, a caudal extension of the maxillary sinus within the orbital region (Figure 1.4).

Look at the caudal aspect of the skull and, with the help of Figure 1.6, identify the **occipital condyles** and the large **foramen magnum** between the occipital condyles. The spinal cord exits the cranium through foramen magnum. The **paracondylar processes** (also called jugular processes) run parallel to the occipital condyles. The digastricus muscle that opens the jaw originates from the paracondylar process. Identify the **external occipital protuberance** on the caudal aspect of the skull ventral to the **intercornual protuberance**. The funicular part of the nuchal ligament attaches to the external occipital protuberance. The intercornual protuberance, located between the horns, forms the highest point of the bovine skull.

In small ruminants, the nuchal crest (or poll) forms the highest point. The nuchal crest is not present in cattle, but they instead have a nuchal line (Figure 1.6).

On the ventral aspect of the skull and with the help of Figure 1.7, identify the basilar part of the occipital bone (basioccipital or basilar part), palatine fissure, tympanic bulla, and the choana (plural choanae), a funnel-shaped caudal opening of the nasal cavities

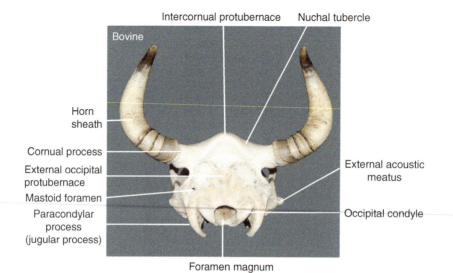

Figure 1.6 Bovine skull showing features of the occipital bone: caudal view. The foramen magnum is the exit pathway for the spinal cord. The external occipital protuberance is the attachment site for the funicular part of the nuchal ligament. In small ruminants, the nuchal crest (poll) forms the highest point of the skull. The nuchal crest is not present in cattle.

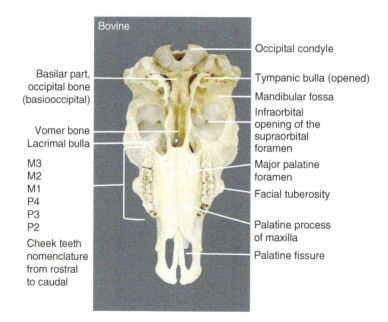

Figure 1.7 The bovine skull: ventral view. * Choanal region, caudal opening of the nasal cavity into the nasopharynx in the live animal. M, molar; P, premolar. The premolar teeth start with P2 in both the upper and lower jaws (the upper P2 are removed to show the shallow alveolar sinuses [teeth sockets in lay terms]). The upper and lower P1 are considered absent in ruminants (see lower P2 in Figure 1.8a). The roots of the cheek teeth in ruminants are shallow compared with horses and it is possible to remove upper cheek teeth without entering the maxillary sinus.

into the nasopharynx. Because of time constrains and lack of clinical relevance, most of the structures on the ventral aspect of the skull may not be part of your identification list. Ask your instructor for advice.

1.2 Mandible

Goal: Identify the regions of the mandible, and vessels and nerves passing through the mandibular and mental foramen.

The mandible has horizontal (**body**) and vertical (**ramus**) parts (Figure 1.8). The junction of the ramus and body forms the **angle** of the mandible.

On the proximal aspect of the ramus, identify the caudally pointing **coronoid process**. The **condylar process** extends caudally from the ramus where it articulates with the mandibular fossa of the skull to form the **temporomandibular joint** (TMJ). A **mandibular notch** separates the coronoid and condylar processes.

The coronoid process in the horse is vertically oriented. The angular process present in dogs is lacking in ruminant and equine mandibles.

On the medial side of the ramus, identify the **mandibular foramen** (Figure 1.8b), the point of entry to the mandibular canal within the body of the mandible. The inferior alveolar nerve enters the mandibular foramen and traverses the mandibular canal giving alveolar branches to the mandibular teeth (Table 1.1). It emerges on the lateral surface as the mental nerve through the mental foramen.

On the rostrolateral surface of the body, identify the **mental foramen**. The mental nerve (sensory) passes out of the mandibular canal as a continuation of the inferior alveolar nerve. It conveys sensation from the skin and mucosa of the lower lips.

Find the mandibular symphysis on the medial side of the mandible (Figure 1.8b). This is a fibrous joint that connects the left and right mandibles. The mandibular symphysis in cattle is weaker than that of the horse and ossifies late in life. Fracture of the mandible is rare in cattle but can occur in young calves following manipulation of the head with a snare. Now you are ready to see Video 1 that demonstrates the features of the bovine skull (Chapter 1, Video 1).

1.3 Paranasal Sinuses

Goal: Identify the maxillary sinus, the rostral and caudal frontal sinuses, and the diverticuli associated with the caudal frontal sinus on the bovine skull (Figure 1.9). Other paranasal sinuses (Figure 1.10) are minor spaces with less clinical significance. Compare and contrast the cavities of the frontal and maxillary sinuses in the bovid with those of small ruminants. At the end of this section, watch **Videos 1 part 1 and 2 that summarizes the features of the bovine skull and paranasal sinuses.**

Adult ruminants possess a complex set of paranasal sinuses (empty spaces between the external and internal plates of the bones of the cranium and bones of the face). Not all of them are of clinical interest. In young calves, the paranasal sinuses are poorly developed.

Sinus infections with mucoid or purulent discharge or blockage of normal drainage through the nasal cavity represent important clinical issues in bovine medicine.

Small ruminants have the same set of sinuses present in cattle, but they are relatively shallow and lack some of the communications present in cattle.

The following is a complete list of all the sinuses that are present in the adult bovine.

1) **Frontal sinus,** divided into:
   - Rostral compartment: forms a minor part of the frontal sinus and has 2–3 small chambers (lateral, intermediate, and medial compartments)
   - Caudal compartment: forms a major part of the frontal sinus.

   The caudal compartment of the frontal sinus has three diverticuli **cornual, nuchal,** and **postorbital diverticuli.**
2) Sphenoid sinus: lies in the rostral part of the floor of the cranium and extends into the orbital wing of the sphenoid bone. It communicates with the middle nasal meatus via ethmoidal meatuses.

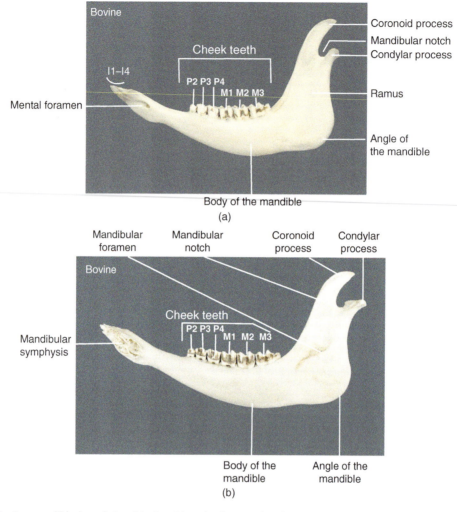

Figure 1.8 (a) Bovine mandible: lateral view. I, incisor; M, molar; P, premolar. The coronoid process in the horse is vertically oriented compared with caudally inclined coronoid processes in ruminants. (b) Bovine mandible: medial view. Ruminants lack the angular process, a feature present in the mandible of dogs and cats.

3) Ethmoid sinus: multiple spaces within the turbinates of the ethmoid bone.
4) Conchal sinuses: dorsal, middle, and ventral conchal sinuses. In the horse, the dorsal conchal sinus communicates with the frontal sinus forming the frontochoncal sinus.
5) **Maxillary sinus:** the cavity medial to the maxilla and dorsal to the upper cheek teeth. It extends into the lacrimal sinus and lacrimal bulla.
6) Palatine sinus: the cavity within the hard palate. It is present in ruminants and pigs.
7) Lacrimal sinus: excavation of the lacrimal bone. It is present in ruminants and pigs.

The **maxillary sinus** is a large space predominately medial to the maxilla and above the upper cheek teeth (Figure 1.9c). It extends into the lacrimal bulla within the bony orbit and communicates with the lacrimal sinus dorsally, and the palatine sinus medially. Unlike the horse, the maxillary sinus in cattle is not divided by a septum into caudal and rostral compartments.

The maxillary, palatine, ventral conchal, and lacrimal sinuses drain into the **middle nasal meatus**. The frontal, sphenoid, ethmoid, and middle conchal sinuses have individual openings into the **ethmoid meatuses** at the most caudal part of the nasal cavity (Figure 1.10).

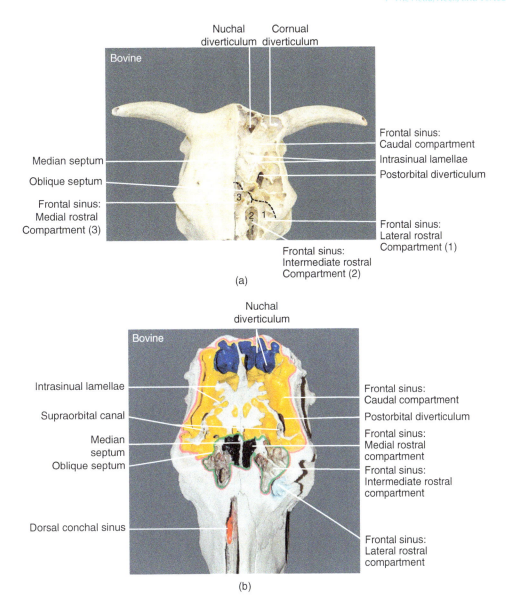

Figure 1.9 (a) Bovine skull with sculptured frontal sinus: dorsal view. An oblique transverse septum (dotted line) divides the frontal sinus into rostral and caudal compartments. The line extends obliquely from the mid-dorsal border of the orbit to the median septum. The median septum separates the left and right frontal sinuses. The caudal compartment of the frontal sinus has three diverticuli: the cornual (within the cornual process), nuchal (rostral to the nuchal tubercle), and postorbital (caudal to the orbit) diverticuli. The bony supraorbital canal, which houses the supraorbital vein, passes through the caudal compartment of the frontal sinus. (b) Compartments of the bovine left and right frontal sinuses. Bovine skull showing caudal (yellow and blue) and rostral (multiple colors) compartments and diverticuli of the frontal sinus: dorsal view. The caudal compartment of the frontal sinus is larger than the rostral compartment and has three diverticuli (postorbital, nuchal, and cornual). The cornual diverticulum is absent in this skull (no horns present; Figure 1.9a). The rostral compartment of the frontal sinus is divided into three smaller spaces (lateral, intermediate, and medial parts). The rostral and caudal compartments of the frontal sinus communicate with ethmoidal meatuses (not visible). Another major paranasal sinus in cattle is the maxillary sinus (Figure 1.9c). Minor sinuses of less clinical significance include the lacrimal, palatine, sphenoid, and conchal sinuses (Figure 1.10).

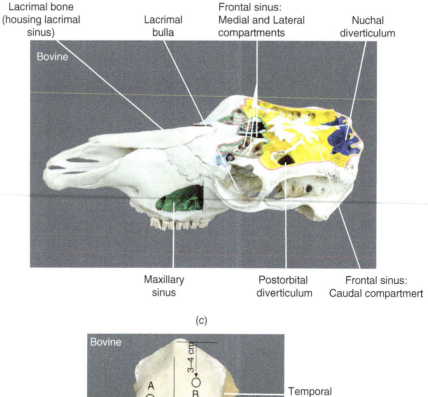

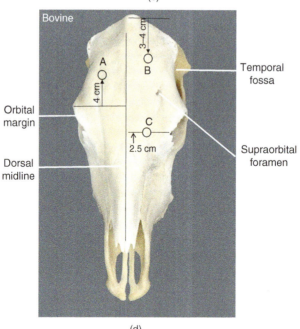

Figure 1.9 (*Continued*) (c) Bovine skull showing the maxillary and frontal sinuses: dorsolateral view. The lacrimal bulla is a very thin and excavated bony structure. It represents the caudal extent of the maxillary sinus. The maxillary sinus communicates with the lacrimal sinus (at the junction of frontal and lacrimal bone) and with the nasal cavity through the middle nasal meatus. * Frontal sinus (lateral compartment). (d) Selected trephination sites of the frontal sinus (small circles). Site A: postorbital diverticulum, located about 4 cm caudal to the caudal edge of the orbit and above the temporal fossa. Site B: caudal part of frontal sinus (major part of frontal sinus), drilled 4 cm rostral from topmost of the head and midway between the base of the horn and the dorsal midline. Site C: rostral frontal sinus, drilled 2.5 cm laterally from the dorsal midline on a perpendicular midline passing through the center of the orbit.

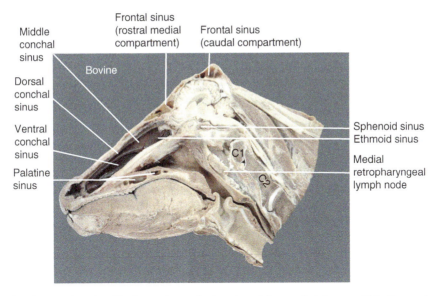

Figure 1.10 Bovine head: sagittal section. The figure shows the location of the conchal sinuses within the nasal conchae. The frontal, sphenoid, ethmoid, and middle conchal sinuses open into the ethmoid meatuses at the caudal aspect of the nasal cavity. The palatine sinus is the space within the caudal part of the hard palate. C1, atlas; C2, axis.

The palatine sinus is not present in carnivores (dogs and cats). In the horse, the palatine and sphenoid sinuses merge forming the sphenopalatine sinus.

The **frontal sinus** has multiple compartments (Figure 1.9a–c). Using a bovine skull with the sinuses exposed, study the maxillary sinus and the caudal and rostral compartments of the frontal sinus (Figures 1.9a–c and 1.10). Consult Box 1.7 and Figure 1.9d for tephination sites.

In cattle, the frontal sinus is more elaborate compared with the shallow frontal sinus in goats (Figures 1.9a–c and 1.11). On the bovine skull where the dorsal plate of the frontal bone is removed, note that the frontal sinus is divided by an **oblique transverse septum** into two or three relatively small **rostral compartments** and one large **caudal compartment** (Figure 1.9a–c). The frontal sinus extends within a cavity involving the frontal, parietal, occipital, and temporal bones.

A **median septum** separates the left and right frontal sinuses (Figure 1.9a,b). The 2–3 compartments of the rostral frontal sinus vary with age but include lateral, intermediate, and medial parts. The caudal

---

Box 1.7

Trephination of the frontal sinus (Figure 1.9d) is the most commonly performed surgery. This surgery is usually performed in a standing animal restrained in a squeeze chute. Light sedation and local anesthesia are used at predetermined sites.

The main trephination sites for draining the diverticuli of the frontal sinus are shown in Figure 1.9d:

1) Main part of the caudal frontal sinus (at a point 3–4 cm rostral from the topmost of the head and midway between the base of the horn and the dorsal midline.
2) The postorbital diverticulum (at a point 4 cm caudal to the caudal edge of the orbit above the temporal fossa).
3) The rostral part of the frontal sinus (at a point 2.5 cm laterally off the dorsal midline on a perpendicular line passing through the center of the orbit).

Extension of caudal frontal sinus into the horn (cornual diverticulum) may carry the risk of sinus infection when adult cattle or goats are dehorned.

compartment of the frontal sinus represents the major component of the frontal sinus and is well developed in older animals.

Note that the interior of the frontal sinus is variably divided by very shallow and irregular spongy bony partitions (**intrasinual lamellae**) that can be seen forming incomplete septa in the dry skull (Figure 1.9a–c). One of these septa forms the bony wall for the **supraorbital canal** in the rostral part of the caudal compartment of the frontal sinus (Figure 1.9b). The canal carries the frontal vein, which should be kept in mind in trephination procedures.

The **caudal compartment of the frontal sinus** covers most of the brain area and extends laterally into the horn and squamous part of the temporal bone and caudally into the occipital bone, forming three distinct diverticuli (extensions) for this compartment. These diverticuli include the **cornual diverticulum** extending into the cornual process of the horn; the **nuchal diverticulum** extending caudally into the area close to the interparietal bone and rostral to the nuchal tubercle; and the **postorbital diverticulum** located caudal to the orbit spanning a space within the parietal bone and squamous part of the temporal bone (Figure 1.9a,b). In dehorning operations, opening of the cornual diverticulum exposes the frontal sinus to microbial infections.

In goats, the lateral part of the rostral frontal sinus communicates with the horn and not the caudal compartment.

On lateral view of opened bovine skull (Figure 1.9c), identify the **maxillary sinus** located predominantly deep to the body of the maxilla and dorsal to the upper cheek teeth. Note that it communicates with lacrimal sinus dorsocaudally, and with the palatine sinus over the infraorbital canal along the caudal surface of the hard palate. It also extends caudally into the lacrimal bulla within the bony orbit. Rostrally, it may extend to the level of the facial tuberosity. The maxillary sinus drains into the nasal cavity through the nasomaxillary opening into the **middle nasal meatus**.

Note that the roots of the last 3–4 cheek teeth may project into the maxillary sinus. But, unlike in the horse, the roots of the cheek teeth are shallower in ruminants, and it is possible to remove these teeth without entering the maxillary sinus.

Identify the palatine sinus on the sagittal section of the bovine head (Figure 1.10).

Small ruminants have the same sets of paranasal sinuses present in the bovid but differ in some of the compartments and their communications. For example, the frontal sinus is composed only of lateral and medial compartments that open into the middle nasal meatus of the nasal cavity. The lateral compartment is similar to the caudal compartment of the frontal sinus in cattle (Figure 1.11). Additionally, the maxillary sinus is divided by the infraorbital canal into medial and lateral compartments. The lateral compartment communicates with the lacrimal bulla while the medial compartment communicates with the palatine sinus.

In summary, the maxillary sinus drains into the middle nasal meatus of the nasal cavity. It communicates with the lacrimal bulla caudally and the lacrimal sinus dorsocaudally.

Details of other sinuses (palatine, sphenoid, and conchal) are less important and are not discussed here.

1.4 Vertebral Column

Goal: Know regional differences in the shape of the vertebrae, the vertebral formula in small and large ruminants, and the sites for epidural anesthesia and collection of cerebrospinal fluid (CSF). Understand that degenerative changes in vertebral articulations may lead to retiring of bulls from breeding services. Consult Box 1.8 for clinical applications related to the vertebral column.

The vertebral formula for cattle and small ruminants is similar in the cervical (C) and thoracic (T) regions but differs slightly in the lumbar (L), sacral (S), and caudal (Cd) regions.

The vertebral formula is C7, T13, L6, S5, Cd 18–20 in **cattle**; C7, T13, L6 (7), S5, Cd 16–18 in **goats**; and C7, T13, L6 (7), S4, Cd 16–18 in **sheep**.

The anatomy of the vertebrae (see Figures 2.1, 2.2, and 3.1) and joint articulations is similar among cattle, goats, and sheep. In the articulated skeleton, the summation of the vertebral foramina forms the vertebral canal. The vertebral canal contains the spinal cord and its coverings and the clinically important internal vertebral venous plexus. Review some of the clinical aspects associated with the vertebral column in Box 1.8.

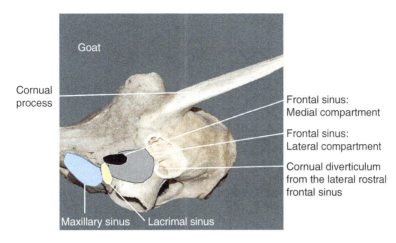

Figure 1.11 Goat skull excavated to show part of the frontal sinus: dorsal view. The left horn is removed to show cornual diverticulum from the lateral frontal sinus. In small ruminants, the frontal sinus is composed of lateral (relatively large) and medial (small) frontal sinus located mostly below the frontal bone. The lateral frontal sinus is equivalent to the caudal frontal sinus in the ox. Note that the compartments of the frontal sinus are shallower compared with cattle. Shaded areas show the extent of the frontal, lacrimal, and maxillary sinuses.

Box 1.8

1) In addition to the external jugular vein in the neck region, the **median caudal or "tail" vein** is one of the common locations where blood can be collected from cattle. When the tail is raised, the median caudal vein can be accessed in proximal ventral third of the tail between two adjacent tail vertebrae. In this location, the caudal vertebrae have hemal arches that should be avoided.
2) Site for collection of the CSF is similar to other species and can be performed at the atlantooccipital (AO) joint; however, this procedure requires general anesthesia. A more convenient sampling site is the lumbosacral space, which allows collection of CSF samples in standing or sternally recumbent animals using no or light sedation.
3) Degenerative changes could occur in the articulation between L6 and S1 region in bulls. This could lead to failure of the bull to serve.
4) Access to the epidural space for induction of epidural anesthesia can be performed at three interarcuate sites depending on the area of interest: (i) L1–L2; (ii) L6 (7)–S1; and (iii) Cd1–Cd2. Epidural punctures should be carried out cautiously as they carry the risk of hemorrhage if the internal vertebral venous plexus is punctured.
5) In situations where the caudal vena cava is blocked by an enlarged rumen (gas tympany) or liver displacement, venous blood could alternatively pass through intervertebral veins that join the internal vertebral venous plexus within the vertebral canal.

1.5 Teeth and Age Estimation of Cattle and Small Ruminants (Goats and Sheep)

Goal: Understand basic ruminant dental anatomy and be able to approximate the age of cattle and small ruminants. Be familiar with the nomenclature of the teeth surfaces (outer vestibular, inner lingual [lower mandibular arcade] or inner palatine [upper maxillary arcade], contact [mesial and distal], and occlusal or masticating). Consult Boxes 1.9 and 1.10 for some of the features of the teeth in ruminants.

Ruminants have brachydont (incisors) and hypsodont (cheek) teeth. In general, brachydont incisors have a typical tooth construction like those in humans, dogs, and cats with a crown above the gum line (covered in enamel), a neck at the gum line, and one or more roots below the gum line (covered in cementum). In contrast, hypsodont teeth (cheek premolar and molar teeth) have a crown and root but no neck. An important difference from brachydont is that the crown of a hypsodont tooth is divided into coronal (above gum line) and reserve portion (below the gum line) both covered in enamel. As such, a hypsodont tooth continues to grow throughout the animal's life via exposure of the embedded reserve portion of the crown. Horses have mostly hypsodont teeth except for the brachydont canines and first premolars (wolf teeth), but unlike ruminants, the lower and upper incisors are hypsodont.

Estimating age of beef, breeding, or dairy cattle adds value to producers and ranchers when selling their stock. Age determination is also important for buyers of cattle (e.g., when buying animals in cattle shows or exhibitions).

You should understand that documenting birth records (e.g., by year branding or ear tags) is a reliable way of determining age. In the absence of that, a veterinarian may be asked to estimate the age of a cow by the looking at teeth on the lower jaw (especially the lower incisor teeth). As we will see shortly, ruminants do not have upper incisors or upper canines.

Age estimation depends on determining eruption times for the type of teeth present (deciduous or permanent) and on identifying the degree of wear on the lingual surface of the lower incisors (by a process called leveling, which will be discussed shortly).

Before you can practice estimating age, we suggest that you read all the following sections on teeth and watch **Videos 2 and 3 (part 1 and 2 each)**. A thorough understanding of type of incisor teeth present (deciduous and/or permanent) and the degree of wear on their lingual surfaces is essential.

1) Teeth can be grouped according to form, function, and whether they have been developmentally preceded by deciduous teeth. The four groups are **incisors (I), canines (C), premolars (P)**, and **molars (M)**. The premolars and molars collectively are called the **cheek teeth**. The cheek teeth are in the caudal part of the mouth and are present in both the upper and lower jaws. They are called upper (or maxillary) and lower (or mandibular) cheek teeth (Figures 1.4, 1.7, and 1.8).

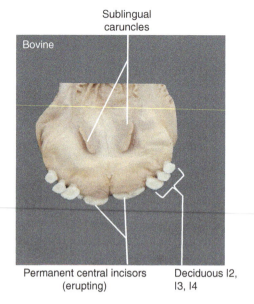

Figure 1.12 Bovine lower jaw showing the permanent central incisors (I1) just erupting while the rest of the incisor teeth (2–4) are still deciduous. This suggests an 18-month-old cow.

2) In calves, there are 20 **deciduous** teeth (also called **temporary, milk,** or **baby teeth**), 8 of which are incisors and 12 are premolars. There are no deciduous molars. Adult ruminants have 32 **permanent** teeth. Of these, 8 are incisors, 12 are premolars, and 12 are molars. Incisors are located only on the lower mandibular jaw (4 on the left side and 4 on the right side). See Figures 1.12 and 1.13. Cheek teeth are located on both the lower and upper jaws (6 on left and right sides of each jaw). See Figures 1.7 and 1.8.

3) The deciduous teeth will be lost as an animal matures and will be replaced sequentially by permanent teeth starting with the central incisors erupting at approximately 18 months of age in cattle (Figure 1.12). Followed outward by the first intermediate incisors at approximately 27 months, the second intermediate incisors at approximately 36 months, and the corner incisors (canines) at approximately 45 months.

4) A dental formula is an abbreviated statement of the number and types of teeth. Generally, placental mammals typically have up to four upper and four lower premolar teeth (in both deciduous and permanent formulas). When a species has fewer

premolars, the reduction occurs in the more rostral members of the group. Because the first premolar (**P1**) is absent in both the upper and lower jaws, the first rostral cheek tooth is designated as premolar two (**P2**) in young and adult ruminants (Figures 1.4, 1.7, and 1.8).

5) The most striking feature of dentition in ruminants is the lack of incisors and canines in the upper jaw. Their place is occupied by a cornified elastic fibrous structure known as the **dental pad** (Figure 1.13).

6) The canines of the lower jaw have the appearance of incisors and are assimilated with the true incisors to form a continuous arched arcade of four pairs of lower incisors (three true incisors plus one functional incisor [or adapted canine] on each half of the jaw). The four pairs of incisors are named as **I1** (**central or pincher**), **I2** (**first intermediate**), **I3** (**second intermediate**), **I4** (**corner**) incisors from rostral (front) to caudal (back), respectively (Figure 1.13a).

7) The incisors have a spatula or shovel-like appearance (Figures 1.14 and 1.15a). As in other species, each tooth has a **crown, neck**, and **root**. The crown and the relatively narrow neck are visible above the gum and are both encased in enamel (Figure 1.13b). The peg-like neck (especially in very young or old cattle) joins the root that is invisible below the gum. The crown is composed of a thin, white, outer **enamel** and an inner core of **dentin**. The root contains blood vessels and nerves within a pulp cavity and is encased by an outer layer of **cementum**. Grossly, permanent incisors are relatively larger than deciduous incisors. They are also yellowish in color and lack a distinct neck. In contrast, deciduous teeth are whiter in color with a distinct neck and a triangular shape (see Figure 1.14).

8) In ruminants, the anchoring of incisor teeth within their alveoli is not as rigid as is found in other species and there may normally be slight movement of these teeth.

9) Because the canine teeth are similar in shape to incisor teeth, authors differ when representing them in the dental formula. Some identify them as canines while others include them with the incisors. Therefore any of the following formats for the dental formula is acceptable:

- **Permanent teeth dental formula:**

$$2 \times \left(I\,0/3,\, C\,0/1,\, P\,3/3,\, M\,3/3 \right) = 32$$

or

$$2 \times \left(I\,0/4,\, P\,3/3,\, M\,3/3 \right) = 32$$

- **Temporary (deciduous, milk, or baby) teeth dental formula:**

$$2 \times \left(DI\,0/3,\, DC\,0/1,\, DP\,3/3 \right) = 20$$

or

$$2 \times \left(DI\,0/4,\, DP\,3/3 \right) = 20.$$

Abbreviations: I = incisors, C = canines, P = premolars, D = deciduous, DI = deciduous incisors, DC = deciduous canines, DP = deciduous premolars

10) Teeth have several surfaces including the **labial surface** (toward the lips; Figure 1.13), the **lingual surface** (toward the tongue; Figure 1.15a), the **occlusal surface** (contact surface between an upper and lower tooth), the **mesial surface** (nearer the center line of the dental arch; Figure 1.15b), and the **distal surface** (further away from the center line of the dental arch; Figure 1.15b). The labial surface is mostly convex, and the lingual surface is concave (Figure 1.16). The outer surface of the lower and upper cheek teeth is described as the **vestibular** or **buccal** surface.

11) The space that separates the incisors from the cheek teeth is called the **diastema.** However, understand that this term can be applied for any space between two adjacent teeth.

12) The anatomy of ruminant cheek teeth is similar to that found in horses. Both premolars and molars have a complex, infolded arrangement of enamel and cementum. In addition, they have one or two infundibula. This composition results in an occlusal surface that can withstand the intense grinding of plant material to which they will be subjected. To account for the inevitable wear, the cheek teeth are hypsodont in that they continue to grow in length after eruption. This growth does not last as long in cattle as in horses, but after growth stops, the cheek teeth are somewhat pushed from their alveoli. The upper premolar teeth have a single infundibulum

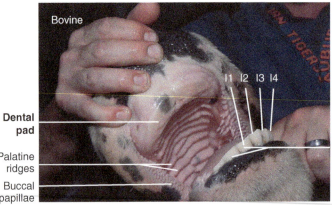

(a)

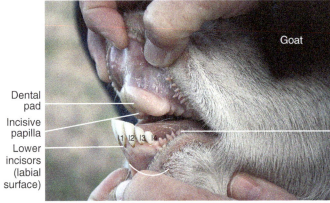

(b)

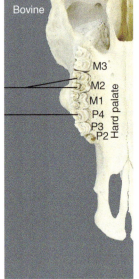

(c)

Figure 1.13 (a) Bovine mouth showing internal structures that include the **dental pad** on the upper jaw and **lower incisor teeth**. The dental pad replaces the upper incisors and canine teeth in ruminants. I1 (central or pincher), I2 (first intermediate), I3 (second intermediate), and I4 (corner incisor) on the left side of the mandible. (b) Opened mouth of small ruminant showing the dental pad (replaces upper incisors and canines) and deciduous lower incisors (I1–I4): left lateral view. The incisive papilla is a small projection located caudal to the dental pad where the incisive ducts open on either side of the papilla. The incisive ducts connect dorsally with paired vomeronasal organs located above the hard plate on the floor of the nasal cavity. The vomeronasal organs are olfactory tubular structures that transmit sexual stimuli (pheromones) to the brain. They are associated with what is known as the Flehmen response. Source: Helena Bowen and Richard Bowen / Wikimedia. (c) Occlusal surface of upper premolar and molar teeth. Note that the upper premolar teeth have a single infundibulum while the molar teeth each have two.

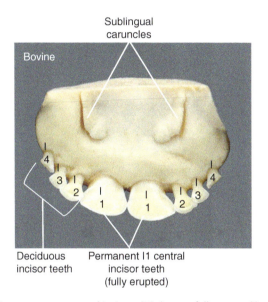

Figure 1.14 Lower bovine jaw showing *permanent* central incisors (I1) that are fully erupted but not in wear. The remaining set of incisors (first intermediate [I2], second intermediate [I3], and corner [I4] incisors) are deciduous. Estimated age of this cow is 24 months (2 years). Note the **small size** and **triangular, peg-shaped** appearance of deciduous I2–I4 compared with the **broad-shaped** appearance of the fully erupted permanent central incisors (I1).

Box 1.9

The cheek teeth arcade of the upper jaw is wider than that of the lower jaw (this is called anisognathia). Engagement of the occlusal surfaces of the upper and lower cheek teeth during feed grinding creates sharp edges over time. The sharp edges will be located on the lingual surface of lower teeth and on the labial surface of the upper teeth. Floating (leveling) of teeth sharp edges is performed in equine practice and may be necessary in older cattle and small ruminants that are observed to have trouble eating (dropping of feed) or are missing premolar or molar teeth.

---

and the molar teeth each have two. Only the lower molars have infundibula with each molar having two. As with horses, there is extensive cementum found above the gum. These features result in the occlusal surface having cementum, enamel, and dentine arranged in intricate patterns. The occlusal surface, when viewed laterally, appears to have an interlocking serrated pattern.

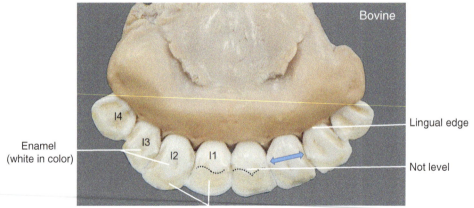

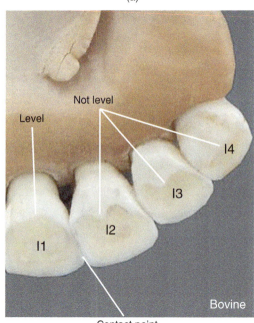

Figure 1.15 (a) Bovine lower mandible showing permanent lower incisors that are all fully erupted and in **wear** but **not level** yet. Note the shovel-like appearance of teeth characteristic of ruminant incisors. The enamel–dentin junction line on the lingual surface of incisors is serrated or **wavy** (i.e., not level; see dotted wavy line on I1). Estimated age of this cow is 5 years. The corner incisors (I4) mandibular canines have fully developed, and their shapes is similar to the other true incisors. Blue arrow denotes the lingual surface. (b) Permanent incisors in the left half of a lower bovine jaw. All permanent incisors in this mouth are in wear with I1 level. Note the round lingual surface of the central incisor (I1) that indicates leveling. I2–I4 are not level and have wavy or serrated lingual surfaces. The approximate age of this cow is 6 years.

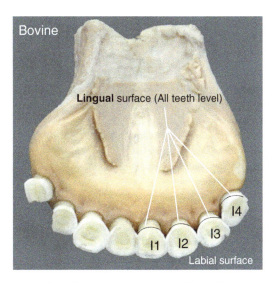

Figure 1.16 Lower bovine jaw showing all eight incisors are **permanent** and **level.** Note the round and smooth arc lines at the enamel–dentin junctions of the lingual surfaces. Estimated age of this cow is above nine years of age.

Box 1.10

The **diastema** between the corner incisor and second premolar offers a space to make it easy to pry open the mouth, grasp the tongue, and pull it sideways for clinical examination of the teeth or for drenching an animal with drugs. (Figure 1.13a). The eruption of the permanent central incisors (I1) is used as a guide to determine eligibility for brucellosis vaccinations in heifers. According to the USDA APHIS, heifer calves should be vaccinated for brucellosis between 4 and 12 months of age. The presence of permanent central incisors will disqualify a heifer for this vaccination.

1.5.1 Definitions and Criteria for Estimating the Age of Ruminants

The general criterion for age estimation in ruminants depends on knowing the approximate eruption times of deciduous and permanent incisor teeth, and on recognition of wear changes on the occlusal surfaces of the lower permanent incisors (i.e., level and not level incisor teeth).

The determination of age is not an exact science. The criteria used for age estimation depends on expected dates for eruption (typically, a range for each pair of incisors), and on the state of **wear** (level or not level) of the lower incisors. The types of fodder (soft or harsh diet), breed (genetics), rate of maturation, and geographic location where an animal is raised could individually or collectively influence eruption dates and types of changes on the occlusal surfaces of incisors.

Before you can successfully estimate cattle age, you need to understand the meaning of the terms **eruption, wear,** and **level** as applied to dentition of ruminants.

Eruption means that a tooth has pierced the gum and is visible above the gum line. For example, the central permanent incisors (I1) are typically erupted at 18 months of age (Figure 1.12).

Wear means that the encasing thin enamel wears out over time causing visible exposure of the underlying dentin on the occlusal surface. Initially, the enamel–dentin junction of the occlusal surface creates a wavy outline on the caudal (lingual) surface of an incisor tooth (Figure 1.15a). A permanent tooth with a wavy appearance on the lingual surface is described as **not level** (Figure 1.15a).

An incisor pair is described as **level** when the enamel–dentin junction of the **lingual surface** has turned from jagged (**serrated** or **wavy**) appearance to a smooth, round, or arc appearance (Figures 1.15b and 1.16).

The meaning of the term **level** in dentition of ruminants is different from that used in equine dentition. In equine dentition, the term level means that the enamel of the infundibulum (cup) and the outer surface enamel are separated by dentin.

Except for variations in the eruption time of permanent incisors (Table 1.5), the dentition of small ruminants generally resembles that of cattle. The teeth of sheep are often exposed to very rough wear.

Several "lay" terms are used to describe old cattle in which teeth were lost or wear significantly down toward the direction of the gum line. For example, a cow that has lost some incisors is described as "**broken mouth**." An animal with significant teeth wear in which the incisor teeth became shorter and smoother than when fully erupted is described as "**short mouth**." The wear of the teeth in a short mouth animal does not yet reach the gum line. Additionally, an animal with all the incisors missing or completely worn down smooth to the gum line is described as "**smooth mouth**." The term "**gummer**" is sometimes used for a cow with a smooth mouth. Usually by 15 years some teeth may have fallen out and the rest may stand out as thin **rods** or **pegs.**

An animal that lacks noticeable teeth problems, with no broken or missing teeth is described as "**solid mouth**."

1.5.2 Steps for Estimating the Age of Cattle

Read the following section and study features of the teeth on Figures 1.12, 1.14, 1.15, and 1.16. Use the information in Tables 1.2, 1.3, 1.4, and 1.5 to practice the art of aging in ruminants.

1) First, decide if the incisor teeth present are all deciduous, all permanent, or a combination of permanent and deciduous. **Deciduous incisors** are generally smaller, whiter, narrower, and more triangular than permanent incisors (Figure 1.12). **Permanent incisors** are larger, less triangular, and darker in color, with varying shades of yellow (stained) than deciduous teeth (Figure 1.14).
2) When only deciduous incisors are present, the eruption of deciduous incisor teeth generally varies. According to the US Food Safety and Inspection

Table 1.2 Eruption times and wear of **permanent teeth in cattle**. Use eruption times, wear, and leveling of incisors for age estimation. *I1–I4 are said to be "level" at 6, 7, 8, and 9 years, respectively (Table 1.3). The lower range in eruption times represents the earliest period for eruption to happen while the upper range represents the latest time for eruption to occur. Table 1.5 shows a schema on how to remember eruption times of permanent incisors.

Teeth	Eruption times (age)	Wear (but not level*) times
Permanent incisors-all present	42–48 months (3½–4 years)	
I1 (central)	18–24 months (1½–2 years)	24–30 months (2–2½ years)
I2 (first intermediate)	24–30 months (2–2½ years)	30–36 months (2½–3 years)
I3 (second intermediate)	36–42 months (3–3½ years)	42 months (3½ years)
I4 (corner incisor or canine)	42–48 months (3½–4 years)	60 months (5 years)
Permanent premolars		Not applicable
P2 (premolar 2)	24–30 months (2–2½ years)	
P3 (premolar 3)	18–30 months (1½–2½ years)	
P4 (premolar 4)	30–36 months (2½–3 years)	
Permanent molars		
M1 (molar 1)	6 months	
M2 (molar 2)	12–18 months (1–1½ years)	
M3 (molar 3)	24–30 months (2–2½ years)	

Table 1.3 Leveling times of permanent incisors in cattle starts from central (I1) out to the corner (I4) incisors, respectively.

Incisor pair that are level	Leveling in years
I1 (central)	6
I2 (first intermediate)	7
I3 (second intermediate)	8
I4 (C) (corner incisor or canine)	9

Service, about 75% of well-bred calves have all deciduous incisors erupted at birth. On average, deciduous incisors erupt between **birth** to **2 weeks** of age (Figure 1.12). Replacement of deciduous incisors with permanent teeth typically begins at about **18 months** of age when the central permanent incisors (I1) erupt. Cattle having only erupted and fully developed deciduous teeth are estimated to be **less** than 18 months of age.

Table 1.4 Eruption of **permanent** and **deciduous teeth** in **goats** and **sheep**. Generally, estimation of eruption times of permanent incisors in small ruminants is derived by subtraction of 6 months from the eruption times of permanent incisors in cattle except for I1 (Tables 1.2 and 1.5). The eruption time for I1 is similar in cattle and small ruminants (i.e., 18 months).

Teeth	Eruption times of permanent teeth	Eruption times of deciduous teeth
Permanent incisors		
I1 (central)	12–18 months (1–1½ years)	At birth
I2 (first intermediate)	18–24 months (1½–2 years)	At birth
I3 (second intermediate)	30–36 months (2½–3 years)	At birth
I4 (corner incisor or canine)	36–48 months (3–4 years)	Birth or (1–3 weeks)
Permanent premolars		
P2 (premolar 2)	18–24 months (1½–2 years)	Birth–4 weeks (3 weeks)
P3 (premolar 3)	18–24 months (1½–2 years)	Birth–4 weeks (3 weeks)
P 4 (premolar 4)	18–24 months (1½–2 years)	Birth–4 weeks (3 weeks)
Permanent molars		
M1 (molar 1)	3 (3–4) months	Not present
M2 (molar 2)	9 (8–10) months	Not present
M3 (molar 3)	18 (18–24) months (1½–2 years)	Not present

Table 1.5 Schema for remembering eruption times of permanent incisors in cattle and small ruminants in months. List incisors (I1–I4) in column A. Next, write the numbers 1 to 4 (from top to bottom) in the left half of column B. In the right half of column B, write the numbers 5 to 8 (from bottom to top). The two-digit numbers created across the rows in column B translate into eruption times for I1, I2, I3, and I4 in cattle, respectively. For estimation of age in small ruminants, subtract 6 months from cattle numbers except for I1. The eruption time for I1 is similar in cattle and small ruminants (i.e., 18 months). C, canine; I, incisor.

A. Incisor number and name	B. Bovine: eruption times of permanent incisors (months)		C. Goat and sheep: eruption times of permanent incisors (months)
I1 (central)	↓1	8	18
I2 (first intermediate)	2	7	27 – 6 = 21
I3 (second intermediate)	3	6	36 – 6 = 30
I4 (C) (corner incisor or canine)	4	↑5	45 – 6 = 39

3) Cattle with **permanent** incisors. As an animal ages, permanent incisors erupt sequentially from rostral to caudal replacing their corresponding deciduous incisors (I1–I4, centrals out to the corners; see eruption times in Table 1.2). The latest eruption time for eruption of permanent I4 (corner incisors) is 48 months (~4 years). It may take an additional 12 months for cattle to have fully erupted, fully developed, permanent incisors that have some type of wear but not level (Figure 1.15a). Therefore, an animal with all fully erupted permanent but non-level incisors (i.e., adult teeth) should be estimated at around five years of age (Figure 1.15a). Beyond five years of age, the degree of wear on the occlusal surface of incisors (leveling) can be used as guidance for age estimation. Leveling is bound to occur at mostly predictable times for I1, I2, I3, and I4, respectively (Table 1.3).
4) At four years of age, all permanent teeth (incisors, premolars, and molars) are erupted. When these teeth are fully erupted and fully developed, the animal is referred to as having a "**full mouth**."
5) Estimation of age in cattle beyond five years of age depends on **leveling** criteria, as defined earlier. In a scenario where you have decided that the animal's age is over five years (fully erupted permanent incisors with visible wear on all the occlusal surfaces), then you should determine if any of the permanent incisors are **level.**
6) I1, I2, I3, and I4 are said to be level at **approximately six, seven, eight,** and **nine years**, respectively (Figure 1.16 and Table 1.3). As defined earlier, leveling means that an incisor pair is worn down so that the enamel–dentin junction line on the lingual surface is smoothly curved.
7) Estimation of age in cattle beyond leveling (i.e., over nine years) is guesswork. The following information can be used as a rough guide, but it is less reliable.
   I1, I2, I3 are "pegs" and I4 is level: 10–12 years ("**short mouth**")
   All incisors are small and rounded pegs: 15 years
   Mixture of missing and small rounded pegs: more than 15 years
8) Age estimation of goats and sheep with permanent incisors. Generally, eruption of permanent incisors in goats is six months earlier than the eruption dates for cattle (Table 1.4).
9) Suggestion of how to remember eruption times of permanent incisors. A relatively easy way to remember approximate eruption dates in "months" is presented in **Table 1.5**.

1.6 Joints of the Head

Goal: Identify the bony components for each joint using an articulated skeleton. You do not need to dissect the joints of the head on your specimen.

The joints of the head include the TMJ (Figure 1.3), the atlanto-occipital (AO) and mandibular symphysis (Figure 1.8b). The TMJ and AO are condylar synovial joints. The mandibular symphysis is fibrous. Review the features of these joints on the skeleton.

1.6.1 Temporomandibular Joint

The TMJ is a synovial articulation between the obliquely oriented **condylar process** of the mandible and the **mandibular fossa** of the squamous temporal bone (Figure 1.3). The joint has a fibrocartilaginous disc that compensates for the irregularities of articular surfaces. The **articular disc** divides the joint cavity into dorsal and ventral compartments. The general location of the joint in the live animal can be estimated as a mid-way point on an imaginary line between the base of ear and the ipsilateral lateral canthus of the eye.

1.6.2 Atlantooccipital Joint

The atlantooccipital (AO) is a synovial joint between the cranial articular foveae of the **atlas** (C1 vertebra) and the **occipital condyles** on the skull. Consult Box 1.11 for clinical application.

1.6.3 Mandibular Symphysis

The mandibular symphysis is a fibrous joint between the rostral ends of the contralateral mandibles (Figure 1.8b). In cattle, this joint ossifies later in life and is much weaker than that of the horse.

> **Box 1.11**
>
> The atlantooccipital (AO) joint capsule is a site for the collection of CSF. With the animal under general anesthesia, the joint is punctured between the dorsal arch of the atlas and the dorsal aspect of foramen magnum using a long spinal needle.

1.6.4 Vertebral Joints

For most vertebral articulations caudal to the axis (C2), there are two types of joints: (i) **fibrocartilaginous joint** between two successive vertebral bodies, and (ii) **plane (flat) synovial joint** between cranial and caudal articular processes of two successive vertebrae.

An intervertebral disc bridges the gaps between vertebral bodies. The intervertebral disc is composed of two parts: an outer **annulus** (or anulus) **fibrosus** and a central **nucleus pulpous**. Consult Box 1.12 for clinical application.

> **Box 1.12**
>
> The term spinal (vertebral) spondylopathy is defined as any vertebral disease, such as osteomyelitis, spinal abscessation, and ankyloses (spondylosis). Trauma in young calves could cause intervertebral disease in the thoracolumbar region.

1.7 Muscles of the Head

Goal: Identify major muscle groups based on their function (e.g., muscles of facial expression or muscles of mastication). Know the innervation of each muscle group and the clinical signs associated with motor nerve damage to any of the specific muscle groups.

Understand that the muscles of the head receive more attention in the dog and horse than in ruminants. It may be sufficient to identify the superficial muscles of the head in ruminants and understand the major groups and their innervation.

Based on your prior knowledge, your instructor will decide which head muscles you would need to dissect. In our program at Auburn College of Veterinary Medicine, we require that students identify only two head muscles. The first is the **sternomandibularis muscle** in cattle, which is also known as **sternozygomaticus** in goats. This is a neck muscle that originates from the manubrium of the sternum and attaches on the mandible (bovine) or the zygomatic arch (goat) (Figures 1.17 and 1.18). The sternomandibularis is absent in sheep (consult Box 1.13).

The second muscle is the **masseter**, a muscle of mastication (Figure 1.17).

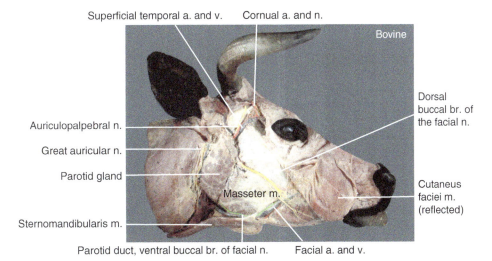

Figure 1.17 Dissection of superficial structures of the bovine head: lateral view. Note that the **cutaneous faciei** muscle is reflected rostrally and dorsally to uncover facial vessels (artery and vein), nerves, and the parotid duct.

Box 1.13

The sternomandibularis muscle in cattle (sternozygomaticus in goats) forms the ventral boundaries of the jugular groove for the external jugular vein. This muscle is absent in sheep, making the ovine jugular groove less distinct. The external jugular vein is used as the prime site for venipuncture and for the placement of indwelling catheters in ruminants. Unlike in cats and dogs, venous catheters can also be placed in the ear veins of ruminants.

To study the muscles of the head, understand that these muscles are broadly similar in goats and cattle and any variation does not merit attention. With the help of Figures 1.17 and 1.18, identify the muscles listed on your lab ID list.

After removal of the skin and the **cutaneous faciei muscle**, many superficial muscles of the head will be identified on the lateral view. Few muscles will be identified on the medial (sagittal) view.

Like those of the horse, the muscles of the head in ruminants can be broadly divided into eight groups:

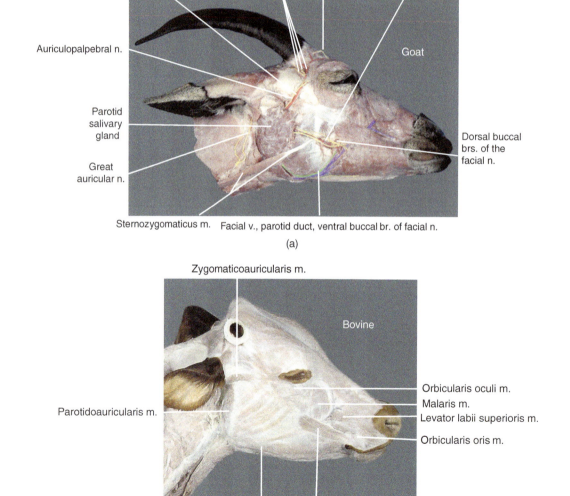

Figure 1.18 (a) Superficial structures of goat head: lateral view. Note the distinct tendon of the sternozygomaticus muscle inserting on the zygomatic arch. (b,c) Selected superficial muscles of the bovine (b) and caprine (c) heads.

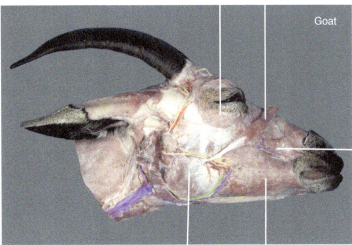

Figure 1.18 *(Continued)*

1) **Cutaneous muscles**
2) **Muscles of facial expression**
3) **Muscles of mastication**
4) **Pharyngeal muscles**
5) **Laryngeal muscles**
6) **Hyoid muscles**
7) **Lingual muscles**
8) **Extraocular muscles.**

To save time and focus on clinically important muscle groups, we suggest identifying the muscles listed on your lab ID list. If you studied the horse or dog head muscles, you should be familiar with the nomenclature and muscle groups in ruminants. There follows a brief discussion of the head muscle groups. Most of these muscles will not be dissected but you should understand the innervation and action of muscles of facial expression, muscles of mastication, and laryngeal and pharyngeal muscles.

1.7.1 Cutaneous Muscles

Goal: Identify the cutaneous faciei in cattle and platysma in goats.

The major cutaneous muscles of the head are the **cutaneous faciei** in cattle (Figures 1.17 and 1.18b), and the **platysma** muscle in goats and sheep (Figure 1.18c).

The cutaneous faciei muscle in cattle twitches the skin around the face. It is present in the horse and is equivalent to the facial part of the platysma in dog and small ruminants.

The cutaneous faciei originates from the fascia around the lateral mandible and blends with the orbicularis oris muscle (the orbicularis oris is a muscle of facial expression around the mouth).

Remove the cutaneous muscles of the head and superficial fascia to trace the more important superficial structures of the head (e.g., salivary glands, lymph nodes, nerves, and blood vessels).

1.7.2 Muscles of Facial Expression

Goal: Know innervation for the muscles of facial expression. Identify the orbicularis oculi only.

The muscles of facial expression are also known as mimetic muscles. They are responsible for closing of the eyelids and mouth and for movements of the lips, nose, and ears. Motor branches from the **facial nerve (CN VII)** innervate them.

There are several muscles in this category (Figure 1.18b,c). However, the most important superficial mimetic muscles include **orbicularis oculi** (closes the eyelids), **frontalis** (elevates the upper eye lid), **malaris** (depresses the lower eyelid and helps in widening the palpebral fissure), **buccinator** (forms the foundation of the cheek), **orbicularis oris** (surrounds the mouth), **levator nasolabialis** and **levator labii superioris muscles** (elevate the nose and upper lip), and **depressor labii inferioris** (depresses the lower lip). There is no need to identify these muscles.

1.7.3 Muscles of Mastication

Goal: Know innervation for the muscles of mastication. Identify the masseter muscle only. If need be, the rest of the mastication muscles could be studied in prosected specimens.

The muscles of mastication (or masticatory muscles) assist with chewing food (opening and closing the jaws). They include **masseter, temporal, digastricus, medial**, and **lateral pterygoid** muscles.

The muscles of mastication in the horse are like those of the bovine with minor differences in shape and size (e.g., digastricus has three parts in the horse but two parts in cattle).

Muscular motor branches of the **mandibular nerve** (subdivision of the trigeminal nerve, CN V) innervate muscles of mastication.

The digastricus muscle opens the jaw, and the rest of the mastication muscles (temporalis, masseter, medial, and lateral pterygoids) close the jaw.

Use a cow skull and mandible to identify the general location of the muscles of mastication. Identify the masseter muscle on your specimen.

The **masseter muscle** covers the ramus and caudal body of the mandible. It originates from the zygomatic arch and facial tuberosity and inserts on the ramus of the mandible (Figure 1.17).

The **temporal muscle** (or temporalis) is indistinct in ruminants when compared with that of the horse and dog. It is deeply located in the laterally located temporal fossa of the skull (Figure 1.4). Thin rostral auricular muscles cover the temporal muscle. The rostral auricular muscles are thin and belong to the muscles of facial expression.

The **digastricus muscle** has caudal and rostral bellies in the dog. In the horse, it has an occipitomandibular part in addition to the rostral and caudal bellies. In ruminants, the digastricus is considered to have one part because the tendinous separation between the rostral and caudal bellies is indistinct. Additionally, the left and right muscles are connected across the intermandibular fossa. The **digastricus muscle** originates from the paracondylar process of the occipital bone (Figure 1.6) and inserts on the caudomedial surface of the mandible. There is no need to dissect it.

The **medial** and **lateral pterygoid muscles** occupy the pterygopalatine fossa deep to the zygomatic arch. There is no need for dissection of the pterygoid muscles.

1.7.4 Pharyngeal Muscles

Goal: Know the nomenclature and function of pharyngeal muscles. Pharyngeal muscles are studied in detail in small animals (dogs and cats). They will not be covered in detail or dissected here. There follows a brief synopsis of their nomenclature and innervation. There is no need to identify them.

1.7.4.1 Nomenclature of Pharyngeal Muscles

The prefix in the name of a pharyngeal muscle indicates its origin, which could either be a laryngeal cartilage or bone of the hyoid apparatus (**crico-, thyro-, hyo-, or stylo-**). The suffix is always the word -**pharyngeus** for all the pharyngeal muscles.

The pharyngeal muscles of interest include **cricopharyngeus, thyropharyngeus, hyopharyngeus**, and **stylopharyngeus**. These muscles can be identified as one group on the dorsolateral surface of the esophagus.

The pharyngeal muscles originate from the laryngeal cartilages and from the hyoid apparatus. They assist with food swallowing (deglutition). The left and right muscles insert on the median dorsal wall of the esophagus. Collectively, they act as an upper esophageal sphincter to propel the food down the esophagus. The pharyngeal muscles contract en masse.

Branches from cranial nerves IX (**glossopharyngeal**) and X (**vagus**) supply the pharyngeal muscles.

1.7.5 Laryngeal Muscles

Goal: Know the function and innervation of the cricoarytenoideus dorsalis muscle only. There is no need to dissect the laryngeal muscles.

The muscles of the larynx are divided into (i) **intrinsic laryngeal muscles** that connect various cartilages of the larynx; and (ii) **extrinsic laryngeal muscles** that connect the thyroid cartilage with the sternum or the thyroid cartilage with the hyoid apparatus. These muscles are studied more extensively in the horse and dog. They will not be dissected.

The first (intrinsic) group includes the **cricoarytenoideus dorsalis**, **cricothyroideus**, and **thyroarytenoideus** muscles. The **thyroarytenoideus muscle** is located deep to the lamina of the thyroid cartilage. Therefore, the lamina of the thyroid cartilage should be reflected or fenestrated to uncover the thyroarytenoideus muscle. The thyroarytenoideus has two parts: the vocalis muscle rostrally, and the ventricularis muscle caudally.

The **cricoarytenoideus dorsalis** is the only intrinsic laryngeal muscle that dilates the glottis; the rest of the intrinsic laryngeal muscles close the glottis.

The second (extrinsic) group includes a long thin **sternothyroideus** muscle that spans the distance between the sternum (manubrium) and thyroid cartilage, and the short **thyrohyoideus** muscles between the lateral surface of the thyroid cartilage and thyrohyoid bone of the hyoid apparatus.

The caudal (recurrent) laryngeal nerve innervates all the laryngeal muscles except the cricothyroideus muscle. The cranial laryngeal nerve, a branch of the vagus nerve (CN X), innervates the latter.

1.7.6 Hyoid Muscles

> **Goal:** There is no need to dissect the hyoid muscles. Your instructor may prepare a prosected specimen for identification of the superficial hyoid muscles.

The hyoid muscles are attached to the bones of the hyoid apparatus. There are several muscles in this group. All the hyoid muscles are of minor significance and will not be dissected.

Identify the most superficial hyoid muscles, including the **mylohyoideus, geniohyoideus,** and **thyrohyoideus muscles**.

The long hyoid muscles, the **omohyoideus** and **sternohyoideus**, have their origin from the shoulder and sternum, respectively. They are located below the trachea.

1.7.7 Lingual Muscles

> **Goal:** Know the function and innervation of the lingual muscles. There is no need to dissect them.

The lingual muscles are divided into **intrinsic lingual muscles** (form the substance of the tongue) and **extrinsic lingual muscles** (move the tongue).

The lingual muscles receive more attention in the study of the dog anatomy. They are innervated by the **hypoglossal nerve (CN XII).**

1.7.8 Extraocular Muscles

> **Goal:** Identify the action and innervation of the extraocular muscles, but there is no need for their dissection. If needed, your instructor will prepare a prosected specimen. In our program, the extraocular muscles are typically dissected in the dog and/or the horse.

The extraocular muscles move the eyeball. They are similar among domestic animals. There are seven extraocular muscles. Four **rectus muscles (dorsal, ventral, lateral,** and **medial), two oblique muscles (ventral** and **dorsal oblique**), and one retractor muscle (**retractor bulbi**). The action of the extraocular muscles is synonymous with their names. They are innervated by several cranial nerves.

A thin **levator palpebrae superioris** is located on the dorsal surface of the dorsal rectus muscle. It is not part of the extraocular muscles because it inserts on the superior eyelid. The action of the levator palpebrae superioris muscle is synonymous with its name, in that it elevates the upper eyelid.

The **oculomotor nerve (CN III)** innervates five muscles. They include all rectus muscles except the lateral rectus muscle. In addition, it innervates the ventral oblique muscle and levator palpebrae superioris.

The **abducent nerve (CN VI)** innervates two muscles: the lateral rectus and retractor bulbi muscles.

The **trochlear nerve (CN IV)** innervates one muscle: the dorsal oblique muscle.

A thin connective tissue sheet known as the **periorbita** envelops the extraocular muscles.

The action and innervation of the extraocular muscles are more clinically important in dogs and horses, especially when conducting cranial nerve examination.

The anatomy of the eye muscles is like that of the horse. (For a more detailed description of eye muscles, see *Equine Anatomy Guide: The Head and Neck* by Mansour et al., 2016.)

Dissection of the extraocular muscles is time-consuming because of their deep location within the orbit and deep to the zygomatic arch. In general, the extraocular muscles are not clinically important in ruminants; we recommend that students become familiar with their innervation and general area of location. If needed, a prosected specimen can be used to demonstrate their location.

1.8 Blood Vessels, Lymph Nodes, and Nerves of the Head

1.8.1 Blood Vessels (Arteries and Veins)

Goal: Identify some of the major branches of the common carotid artery including the facial artery in cattle, the transverse facial artery in goat, and the superficial temporal and cornual arteries in both cattle and goats. Unlike in other domestic animals, the internal carotid artery is much modified in ruminants. Of the veins of the head, identify the external jugular, maxillary, linguofacial, facial, and frontal veins. Note that the facial artery is absent in small ruminants where the lingual artery is the direct branch off the external carotid artery (no linguofacial trunk). A pulse can be evaluated from the facial artery in cattle and the transverse facial artery in goats. At the end of this unit, watch **Videos 5, 6, and 7**.

1.8.1.1 Arteries of the Head

Only clinically important arteries of the head and neck are discussed here.

Study arteries of the head on a bovine head cut off the neck. The head can be split into equal halves along the midline. Use one side for blood vessels and nerves. With help of Figure 1.19(a), skin the head and carefully reflect the cutaneous muscles of the head.

Branches of the **common carotid artery** supply the head and neck. Identify bilaterally located common carotid arteries located within the **carotid sheath**.

The **carotid sheath** is found close to the esophagus in the visceral space of the neck.

Branches of the common carotid artery in ruminants are like other domestic animals. The regression of the internal carotid artery in ruminants after birth is one exception. The internal carotid artery supplies the brain in other species. In ruminants, the brain is supplied by branches from the maxillary and occipital arteries forming a complex network of fine arteries known as the *rete mirabile*. The rete mirabile will not be dissected.

In the bovine head, follow the **external carotid artery** that serves as the major cranial continuation branch of the common carotid artery beyond the occipital artery. It gives off several branches that include the **linguofacial trunk** (gives the **lingual** and **facial arteries**), **caudal auricular,** and **superficial temporal arteries**. It continues as **maxillary artery** to supply the deep structures of the head. The maxillary artery gives several deep branches that are of no clinical value and should not be dissected.

The most clinically important arteries in ruminants that you should identify are the **cornual artery** (Figure 1.19b) that supplies the horns in the ox, buck, and ram; the **facial artery** (Figure 1.19b) in cattle (absent in small ruminants); and the **transverse facial artery** in goats (Figure 1.20). Identify the facial artery running along the ventral border of the masseter muscle accompanied by the ventral buccal branch of the facial nerve, facial vein, and parotid duct (Figure 1.19a).

The cornual artery is a branch of the **superficial temporal artery** (Figures 1.17, 1.18, and 1.19a,b). Note the clinical significance of the cornual artery (Box 1.14).

Identify the **superficial temporal, cornual, facial,** and **transverse facial arteries** on lateral views of a goat and cow heads (Figures 1.18a and 1.19a,b).

In goats and bovine, the **transverse facial artery** courses with the dorsal buccal branch of the facial nerve. Identify the **dorsal buccal nerve** and transverse facial artery as they cross the lateral surface of the masseter muscle in goats (Figure 1.18c).

The transverse facial artery is present in both small ruminants and in cattle. It is a branch of the superficial temporal artery.

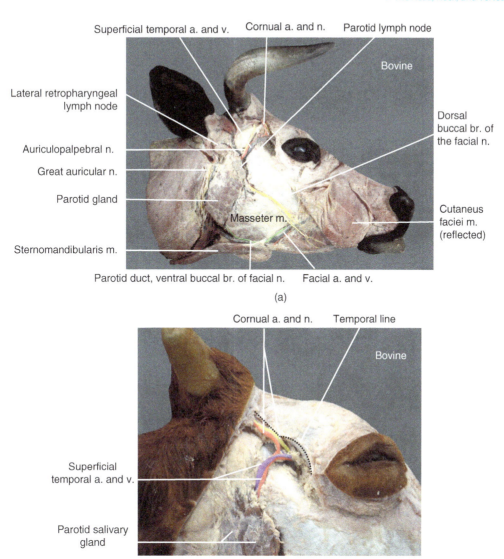

Figure 1.19 (a) Bovine head: lateral view. The cutaneous faciei muscle is reflected cranially to uncover the superficial vessels and nerves of the bovine head. The parotidoauricularis muscle that covers the parotid salivary gland is removed. (b) Bovine head: lateral view. Close-up view of the superficial temporal artery and vein, and cornual artery and nerve. In dehorning operations, the cornual nerve is blocked along the bony temporal line. The cornual artery is a branch of the superficial temporal artery.

Box 1.14

Ligation of the **cornual artery** is suggested in the dehorning operation of adult cattle. While that sure would be helpful, understand that the cornual artery cannot be clamped at the origin during dehorning procedures. Rather, hemostasis is provided by ligation or cauterization following horn removal.

> **Box 1.15**
>
> The facial artery is used for pulse evaluation in cattle. The artery crosses the ventral border of the mandible in front of the masseter muscle accompanied by the facial vein, ventral buccal branch of the facial nerve, and parotid duct (Figure 1.19a). The facial artery is absent in goats and instead the transverse facial artery serves the role of the facial artery for pulse evaluation in goats.
>
> In horses, the facial, masseteric, and transverse facial arteries are sites for pulse evaluation.

Note that the facial artery and transverse facial arteries are used for pulse evaluation in cattle and goats, respectively (Box 1.15). The rostral branches of the facial artery supply blood to lips and muzzle region. They will not be discussed.

Named branches from the facial artery (inferior and superior labial arteries) are variously distributed in the rostral head below and above the lips to supply the muzzle region (they will not be dissected). A similar pattern exits for branches of the **facial vein**, which is satellite to the facial artery (Figure 1.20).

1.8.1.2 Veins of the Head

Goal: Identify the external jugular, maxillary, linguofacial, facial, dorsal nasal, angularis oculi, and frontal veins. Know the clinical significance of the external jugular and frontal veins.

The superficial veins of the head drain into the **external jugular vein**, which carries venous blood from the head and neck back toward the right side of the heart. The external jugular vein joins other veins at the thoracic inlet to form the cranial vena cava. It is a major site for venipuncture.

As in other species, the external jugular vein is formed by confluence of the **maxillary** and **linguofacial** veins (Figure 1.22).

The **frontal vein**, a large vein, runs in the supraorbital groove medial to the eye (Figures 1.2 and 1.20). It is clinically important in cattle and must be avoided when surgically entering the rostral frontal sinus.

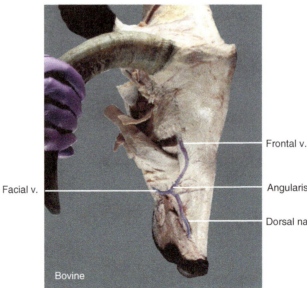

Figure 1.20 Bovine head: dorsal view. The facial vein travels dorsally across the face and gives rise to the lateral and dorsal nasal veins. The **facial vein** is continued dorsally by the angularis oculi vein (courses to medial canthus of the eye) and the **frontal vein** (courses more dorsally in the supraorbital groove toward the supraorbital foramen). At the supraorbital foramen, the frontal vein becomes the supraorbital vein. The supraorbital vein drains into the ophthalmic plexus within the bony orbit.

The frontal vein is continued rostrally by the angularis vein (passes to the medial canthus of the eye) and caudally by the supraorbital vein (passes through the supraorbital foramen to join the ophthalmic plexuses within the orbit of the eye).

Identify the facial vein and its continuation by the frontal vein over the orbit (Figure 1.20).

1.8.2 Lymph Nodes of the Head and Neck

Goal: Identify the major lymph nodes or lymphocenters of the head and know which is important in meat inspection (Figures 1.19a, 1.21, 1.22, and 1.23). Abnormal appearance of lymph nodes suggests pathology in the area drained by those nodes. Watch Videos 5 and 6.

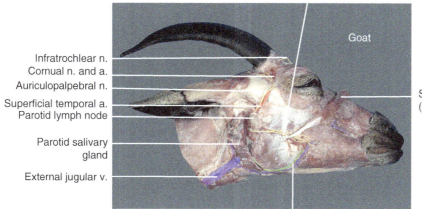

Figure 1.21 Caprine head: lateral view. Parotid gland, parotid lymph node, vessels, and nerves of the goat head.

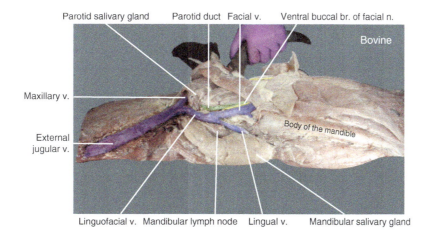

Figure 1.22 Right bovine sagittal head and neck section: ventrolateral view. Note that the external jugular vein is formed by the confluence of the maxillary and linguofacial veins.

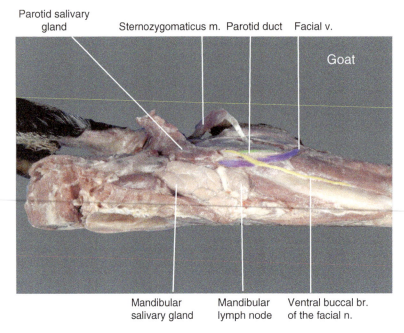

Figure 1.23 Caprine right half head and neck: ventrolateral view. Note that the mandibular salivary gland is located caudal and medial to the mandibular lymph node.

The major lymph nodes or lymphocenters of the head and neck are like those of other domestic animals. They include **(i) parotid, (ii) mandibular, (iii) retropharyngeal (medial** and **lateral retropharyngeal)**, and **(iv) deep cervical** (cranial, middle, and caudal groups) (Figure 1.24).

Other lymphoid structures include five tonsils: pharyngeal, palatine, tubal, lingual, and tonsils of the soft palate.

Identify the **medial retropharyngeal lymph nodes** on midsagittal section of the bovine head. The **parotid, lateral retropharyngeal**, and **mandibular lymph nodes** should be identified on lateral and ventral views of the head with the help of Figures 1.19a, 1.21, 1.22, and the following description:

- **Parotid lymph node:** located in the rostral border of the of parotid salivary gland.
- **Lateral retropharyngeal lymph node:** ventral to the wing of the atlas and medial to the caudal aspect of the mandibular salivary gland.
- **Mandibular lymph nodes:** 1–3 lymph nodes that are located rostral and lateral to the mandibular salivary glands close to the caudal angle of the mandible. They are oval in shape.

Lymph is channeled from distinct areas of the body to a target lymph node (inflow) by the way of **afferent** lymphatic vessels. Lymph vessels leaving lymph nodes (out flow) to join the next lymph node or vein are known as **efferent** lymphatic vessels.

A single or group of lymph nodes form a single unit known as a **lymphocenter.** For example, the **lateral retropharyngeal lymphocenter** contains one large lymph node. It is the main collection center for lymph fluid from the entire head in ruminants. Identify the lateral retropharyngeal lymph node located on the lateral head below the wing of the atlas (Figure 1.24).

From the lateral retropharyngeal lymphocenter, the lymph outflow is to the tracheal lymphatic duct of the neck. The pathway of the lymph from the tracheal duct is variable and lymph could be channeled either to the large veins at the thoracic inlet or directly to the thoracic duct (the duct will be identified later with the thorax). Consult Box 1.16 for clinical applications related to lymph centers of the head.

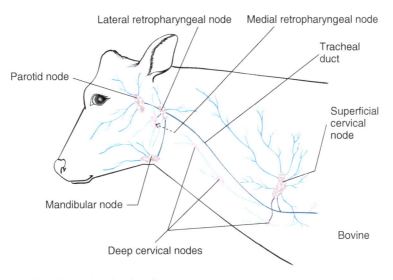

Figure 1.24 Lymphocenters of the bovine head and neck.

Box 1.16

The parotid lymph node is located along the rostral edge of the parotid salivary gland. It drains the region of the eye. In cattle, this node is usually inspected in slaughterhouses to determine cancer of the eye. In goats, the parotid lymph node is the lymph node most frequently affected by caseous lymphadenitis (CL), a common disease caused by *Corynebacterium paratuberculosis*. The main lymph collection in the center of the head, the lateral retropharyngeal, is also inspected to rule out general head infections.

The medial retropharyngeal lymph node may become inflamed and could interfere with swallowing and breathing by causing compression in the region of the larynx and/or oropharynx. Identify the medial retropharyngeal lymph node on a medial (sagittal) section of the head.

1.8.3 Nerves of the Head

Goal: Know the nomenclature of cranial nerves and their broad functions, especially if you are learning these nerves for the first time. Identify the **cornual nerve** (branch of the maxillary subdivision of the trigeminal nerve that supplies the horn in the bovid (Figure 1.19b); the **dorsal and ventral buccal** and **the auriculopalpebral nerve branches of the facial nerve** (CN VII). Know the function and clinical significance of the cornual nerve (blocked in dehorning operations), dorsal buccal nerve of CN VII (subject to injury on lateral recumbency), and auriculopalpebral nerve (blocked to prevent blinking of eye during eye examination). Review foramina for CNN branches on the bovine skull (Table 1.1).

Twelve (12) pairs of **cranial nerves** (CNN) supply the structures of the head. Names and roman numerals designate these nerves. The numerals reflect the rostral to caudal sequence of origin from the brainstem. **Parasympathetic fibers** are present in **cranial nerves III, VII, IX, and X**.

1.8.3.1 Summary of Cranial Nerves and Their Functions

Below is a brief overview of CNN names and functions. The formina by which they pass from the brainstem to outside of the skull or enter the skull (for sensory CNN) are discussed. The courses of CNN in the brain are discussed in a neuroscience course. Some of the branches that you need to know are disused with the head or eye.

Olfactory nerve (CN I). The olfactory nerve conveys the sense of smell. Its fibers pass from the olfactory mucosa on the ethmoid concha to the olfactory bulb of the brain through the **cribriform plate**. There is no need to identify this nerve.

Optic nerve (CN II). The optic nerve conveys the special sense of vision. Its fibers pass through the **optic canal**. Identify the optic nerve on the eyeball or section (see Section 1.13). On the axial section of the eye, the optic nerve is identified as the optic disc (see Section 1.13).

Oculomotor nerve (CN III). The oculomotor controls eye movement by innervating four extraocular muscles. The parasympathetic fibers in CN III cause constriction of the pupil and control the shape of the lens (accommodation). The oculomotor nerve passes out of the skull through the **foramen orbitorotundum**. Identify this foramen on the skull but there is no need to identify this nerve.

Trochlear nerve (CN IV). This controls eye movement by supplying one extraocular muscle (dorsal oblique muscle). It passes out through the **foramen orbitorotundum**. There is no need to identify this nerve.

Trigeminal nerve (CN V). The trigeminal nerve has three branches that include two sensory divisions (**maxillary** [V1] and **ophthalmic** [V2] **nerves**), and one mixed division that has both sensory and motor fibers (**mandibular** nerve [V3]). Overall, the trigeminal subdivisions convey the sense of touch, pain, and temperature (hot and cold). The mandibular subdivision of the trigeminal nerve innervates muscles of mastication.

All the trigeminal nerve divisions, except the mandibular division, pass out through the **foramen orbitorotundum**. Several branches of the trigeminal nerve convey general sensation (pain, touch, and temperature) from the head. Others such as the lingual branch of the mandibular nerve convey general sensation (pain, touch, and temperature) from the tongue. Identify the location of the **supraorbital, infraorbital,** and **mental nerves** and know their functions.

Abducent nerve (CN VI). The abducent nerve controls eye movement by innervating two extraocular muscles (lateral rectus and retractor bulbi muscles).

> **Box 1.17**
>
> Cranial nerve damage can be manifested in different clinical presentations depending on the functions of the cranial nerve involved.
>
> The dorsal buccal branch of the facial nerve (CN VII), for example, is vulnerable to damage in lateral recumbency during general anesthesia when the head is not properly padded.

It passes through the **foramen orbitorotundum**. No need to identify this nerve.

Facial nerve (CN VII). The facial nerve supplies motor innervation to the muscles of facial expression. It has parasympathetic components that regulate tear and saliva production. It supplies salivary glands, lacrimal glands, and secretion in the nasal cavity. It also conveys taste sensations from the rostral two-thirds of the tongue. Consult Box 1.17 for clinical application.

Individual branches of the facial nerve that are of clinical interest include the **dorsal** and **ventral buccal branches** that supply most muscles of facial expression, the **auriculopalpebral nerve** that controls movement of the ear (auricular muscles) and closing and opening of the palpebral fissure (orbicularis oculi muscle). The facial nerve exits the skull through the **stylomastoid foramen**. Identify the **buccal branches** and **auriculopalpebral nerve** (Figures 1.19a and 1.21).

Vestibulocochlear nerve (CN VIII). The vestibulocochlear nerve conveys the special sense of hearing and balance. There is no need to identify this nerve.

Glossopharyngeal nerve (CN IX). The glossopharyngeal nerve, as its name suggests, is related to the tongue and the pharynx. It innervates the pharyngeal muscles and pharyngeal mucosa. The parasympathetic component in the CN IX carries the special sense of taste from the caudal third of the tongue. It also regulates saliva production along with the facial nerve.

The glossopharyngeal nerve exists its origin in the brainstem through the **jugular foramen**. There is no need to identify this nerve.

Vagus nerve (CN X). The vagus nerve is the longest of the cranial nerves and is known as the "wanderer" nerve because it supplies vast areas of the body from the head to caudal abdomen. It has a mixture of motor parasympathetic, visceral sensory, and motor somatic fibers. It regulates movement (peristalsis) and general sensation of the viscera in the thorax and abdomen.

In the cranial region of the body, it innervates some of the pharyngeal muscles and pharyngeal mucosa along with the glossopharyngeal nerve. The vagus nerve stimulation slows the heart rhythm in contrast to the opposite effect of the sympathetic system. In the neck, the vagus nerve is intimately associated with the sympathetic trunk. It is known as the **vagosympathetic trunk**. Identify the vagosympathetic trunk in the neck region (see Section 1.15.2). The branches of the vagus will be discussed with the thoracic cavity.

Motor branches of the vagus, the **recurrent laryngeal (caudal laryngeal)** and **cranial laryngeal nerves**, supply the laryngeal muscles.

The vagus nerve passes through the **jugular foramen**.

Accessory nerve (CN XI). The accessory nerve innervates some muscles of the neck, including the **trapezius muscle** located over the dorsal border of the scapula (see Section 1.15.1). The accessory nerve controls movement of the head and shoulder. It has **dorsal** and **ventral branches**.

Identify the **dorsal branch** of the accessory nerve passing to the deep (medial) surface of the trapezius muscle (see Section 1.15.2).

The accessory nerve passes through the **jugular foramen**.

Hypoglossal nerve (CN XII). The hypoglossal nerve controls the movement of the tongue. Its somatic motor fibers innervate the intrinsic and extrinsic muscles of the tongue. The hypoglossal nerve exits the skull through the **hypoglossal canal**.

Examination of specific cranial nerves is more important in small animals (dogs and cats) and in horses. It does not often have practical application in ruminants. However, regional nerve blocks on the head have important clinical utility in cattle (anesthesia in dehorning operations, eye removal, eye examination, and suturing of lacerations on the muzzle region).

The most important superficial nerves of the head include branches of the facial nerve (CN VII), and the trigeminal nerve (CN V). Identify the **auriculopalpebral, dorsal,** and **ventral buccal branches of the facial nerve**, **cornual nerve** (branch of maxillary subdivision (V1) of the trigeminal), the **infraorbital nerve** (continuation of the maxillary division of the trigeminal nerve), and **mental nerve** (continuation of inferior alveolar nerve). The inferior alveolar nerve itself is a branch of the mandibular division of the trigeminal nerve (V2). Consult Box 1.18 on information on regional anesthesia in ruminant head.

Note the course of the ventral buccal nerve along the ventral edge of the masseter muscle and body of the mandible (Figures 1.19a and 1.21). Compare this location with the location of the dorsal buccal branch. The ventral buccal branch is reasonably more protected by the medial edge of the body of the mandible, and the ventral and rostral edges of the masseter muscle.

The course of the ventral buccal branch of the facial nerve in ruminants is different from that in the horse and dog. In the latter species, the dorsal and ventral buccal branches of the facial nerve cross the lateral

---

Box 1.18

Regional anesthesia in ruminant head

In cattle, physical restraint and local anesthesia are used as a safe alternative to general anesthesia when performing surgical procedures on the head. Examples of these procedures include dehorning and eye removal because of cancer (ocular squamous cell carcinoma).

In dehorning operations, the following nerves are blocked in cattle and goats.

In cattle

- The **cornual nerve** (arises from the zygomaticotemporal nerve, a branch of the maxillary division of the trigeminal nerve [CN V]) is blocked midway along the temporal line between the lateral canthus of the eye and the lateral base of the horn (Figure 1.19b).
- The **great auricular nerve** (branch of the second cervical nerve [C2]) is blocked between the horn and the base of the ear or by a ring block around the base of the horn.

In goats

- In addition to the **cornual** and **great auricular nerves**, the **infratrochlear nerve** (branch of the ophthalmic division of the trigeminal nerve) is blocked midway between the medial canthus of the eye and medial base of the horn (medial to the cornual nerve block).

Box 1.18 (Continued)

- Because it is difficult to block all the branches of the above three nerves in small ruminants, general anesthesia is the preferred option when performing dehorning in adult goats.
- Dehorning in both cattle and goats is best performed on young animals (1–2 weeks of age) by removal of the epiceras (germinal epithelium located at the border of the tiny cornual process). Cauterization can be used to remove both the **epiceras** and **scent glands** in male goats. These glands are located between the horns. They are activated by testosterone, the male steroid hormone. During the breeding season they produce a strong odor (considered offensive by owners) that attracts female goats.

Other nerve blocks include:

- Infraorbital nerve block for nasal laceration or placing of a nose ring in bulls.
- Auriculopalpebral nerve block for eye examination. The auriculopalpebral nerve is the branch of the facial nerve (CN VII) that crosses the zygomatic arch to supply the orbicularis oculi muscle (from the palpebral branch of the auriculopalpebral nerve). The auriculopalpebral nerve block is performed by the injection of an anesthetic agent under the skin midway between the lateral canthus of the eye and the base of the ear at the level of the zygomatic arch.
- Enucleation (removal) of the eye due to cancer is performed by either retrobulbar or Peterson's nerve block. Peterson's nerve block is more difficult to perform than the retrobulbar nerve block. It requires familiarity with the bony prominences at the site of injection. The landmarks for needle placement are the angle made by the frontal process of the zygomatic bone and the zygomatic process of the squamous temporal bone or for simplicity at the angle formed by the caudal bifurcation of the zygomatic bone into frontal and temporal process (Figure 1.25). The coronoid process and pterygoid crest could hinder needle placement (review these bony landmarks in Figure 1.25). More details on how to perform retrobulbar nerve blocks are discussed in Box 1.19.

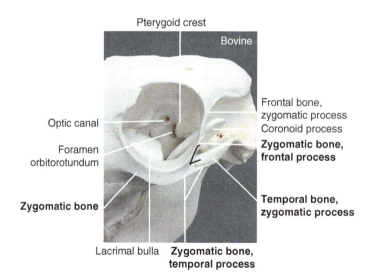

Figure 1.25 Bovine skull and articulated mandible: caudolateral view. Figure shows the landmarks for Peterson's nerve block for enucleation of the eye. The angle formed by the frontal process of the zygomatic bone and the zygomatic process of the temporal bone is used for anesthetic injection. This angle could also be described as the caudal bifurcation of the zygomatic bone into frontal and temporal process (bolded). The ramus of the mandible (coronoid process) and the pterygoid crest are in the needle pathway and should be avoided.

> **Box 1.19**
>
> **Four-point retrobulbar nerve block**
>
> The retrobulbar nerve block is used as an easier alternative to the more challenging Peterson's nerve block for (i) enucleation of the eye, or (ii) surgery of the cornea. The aim is to anesthetize the nerves (cranial nerves III, IV, V [V1], and VI) coursing through foramen orbitorotundum to supply the eye.
>
> The needle placement for retrobulbar technique is performed by injecting a local anesthetic at four sites behind the globe of eye. The sites include injections at the medial and lateral canthi of the eye, and above the superior and inferior eyelids. Care should be taken to avoid puncturing the eyeball or damaging the lacrimal bulla. Fingers could be used to deflect the globe of the eye away from the tip of the syringe when advancing the needle.

surface of the masseter muscle, making the dorsal and ventral buccal branches of the facial nerve equally vulnerable to compression forces (e.g., in lateral recumbency during general anesthesia). In ruminants, only the dorsal buccal branch is vulnerable to damage from prolonged lateral recumbency.

In Peterson's eye block in the ox, the local anesthetic is deposited to anesthetize nerves coursing through **foramen orbitorotundum**. Identify this foramen on the skull. Nerves passing through foramen orbitorotundum in cow, sheep, and pig include:

- CN III (oculomotor nerve)
- CN IV (trochlear nerve)
- CN V (ophthalmic [V-1] and maxillary [V-2] divisions of trigeminal nerve)
- CN VI (abducent nerve).

1.9 Salivary Glands

Goal: Identify the major salivary glands (parotid, mandibular, and sublingual) and the course of their ducts. Secretion of saliva from salivary glands is an important source of electrolytes (bicarbonates), mucus, and digestive enzymes. Copious production of saliva in ruminants is essential for food fermentation in the forestomach (rumen and reticulum).

The major salivary glands of ruminants are generally like other domestic animals and include (i) **parotid**, (ii) **mandibular**, and (iii) **sublingual** (**monostomatic** and **polystomatic divisions**).

Other salivary glands of minor importance include *dorsal*, *middle*, and *ventral buccal salivary glands*. There is no need to identify the buccal salivary glands.

With the help of Figures 1.17, 1.18, 1.22, and 1.23 and the following description, identify the **parotid, mandibular,** and **monostomatic sublingual glands.** *Reflect the parotidoauricularis muscle to expose the parotid salivary gland. Be careful to preserve the maxillary vein (located in the gland substance) and facial nerve deep to the gland.*

The **parotid salivary gland** is located medial to the thin parotidoauricularis muscle between the ventral border of the mandible and the wing of the atlas. It is rectangular in shape. The **parotid duct** arises from the rostral border of the gland in small ruminants and ventrolateral aspect in cattle. It opens in the upper vestibule of the mouth close to the upper molar 2 (M2) cheek tooth. The duct courses along the ventral border of the masseter muscle and the body of the mandible before it turns dorsally on the lateral side of the head.

Identify the **parotid duct** in the ox coursing along the ventral and rostral edges of the masseter muscle accompanied by the **facial vein, facial artery,** and **ventral buccal branch** of the facial nerve. The parotid gland is relatively smaller than that of the horse (Figures 1.17 and 1.18). In goats, the parotid duct has a similar course but the facial artery is missing.

The **mandibular salivary gland** lies in the caudal border of the mandible and curves rostrally into the intermandibular area. The gland has a crescent shape and is relatively larger than the parotid salivary gland. Identify the ventral part of the mandibular salivary gland in the intermandibular region (Figure 1.23). Be sure to differentiate between the mandibular salivary gland and mandibular lymph node. The dorsal part of the mandibular salivary gland lies deep to the parotid salivary gland and wing of the atlas.

The **mandibular** and monostomatic sublingual ducts open at the **sublingual caruncle**. Identify the sublingual caruncle on the floor of the lower jaw of your specimen or on a plastinated specimen (Figure 1.15).

1.10 The Pharynx

Goal: Identify the major parts of the pharynx on a median sagittal section of the head (Figure 1.26).

The pharynx is defined by some anatomists as the crossing place for food and air. It has three parts: (i) **oropharynx,** (ii) **nasopharynx**, and (iii) **laryngopharynx**. Identify the three parts on mid-sagittal section of the head (Figure 1.26).

1.10.1 Oropharynx

The oropharynx is the space below the soft palate that extends from the root of the tongue to the rostral surface of the epiglottic cartilage (Figure 1.26). It contains the **palatine tonsil.** It is relatively narrow.

1.10.2 Nasopharynx

The nasopharynx is located dorsal to the soft palate (Figure 1.26). It extends from the choanae to the end of the soft palate. It contains the opening of the auditory tube. In ruminants, the nasopharynx is incompletely divided by a pharyngeal septum. It contains the pharyngeal tonsils and the tubal tonsils in its caudal region.

1.10.3 Laryngopharynx

The laryngopharynx is located dorsal to the larynx and joins the esophagus caudally (Figure 1.26). The lumen of the laryngopharynx is closed by what is clinically known as the upper esophageal sphincter.

The **soft palate** continues from the hard palate coursing caudally. It separates the nasopharynx dorsally from the oropharynx ventrally. The free margins of the soft palate form two mucosal arches:

1) **Palatoglossal arch:** extends from the lateral margins of the soft palate to the root of the tongue. Using the sagittal section, pull the tongue toward you to demonstrate the palatoglossal arch coursing from the soft palate to the root of the tongue.
2) **Palatopharyngeal arch:** extends from the caudal part of the soft palate to fan over the entrance of the esophagus.

1.11 Tongue

Goal: Identify the **torus linguae** and **lingual fossa** on the bovine tongue and know their clinical

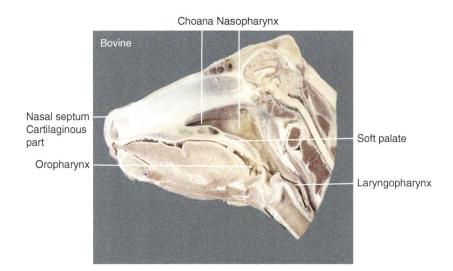

Figure 1.26 Bovine median sagittal section of the head passing through the nasal septum. Study the major regions of the pharynx that include the oropharynx, nasopharynx, and laryngopharynx. The nasal septum has a small caudal bony part, and a large cartilaginous rostral part that does not project distal to the choana.

significance. Know that the hypoglossal nerve (CN XII) innervates the intrinsic and extrinsic muscles of the tongue. Other cranial nerves of the tongue convey general sense of pain, touch, and temperature (trigeminal, CN V and CN IX) and special sense of taste (facial and glossopharyngeal nerves, CN VII and CN IX).

The tongue is the principal organ of prehension in cattle. Small ruminants use their lips for prehension.

The tongue is subject to trauma and laceration associated with sharp objects or infectious processes. The extrinsic and intrinsic muscles of the tongue are innervated by the hypoglossal nerve (CN XII).

The tongue of ruminants has two unique features of clinical interest. Using Figures 1.27 and 1.28, identify the raised caudal part of the tongue known as the **lingual torus** (or **torus linguae**). Additionally, a distinct transverse depression can be seen in the middle of the tongue in front of the lingual torus. This depression is known as lingual **fossa** (or **fossa linguae**).

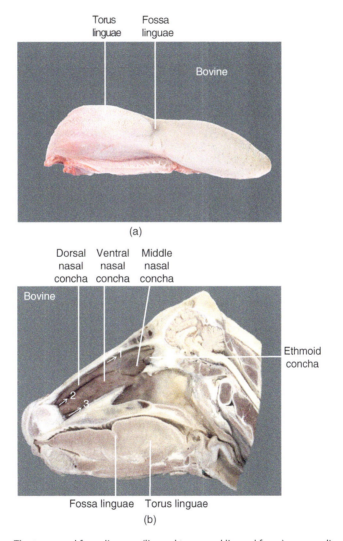

Figure 1.27 (a) Bovine tongue. The torus and fossa linguae (lingual torus and lingual fossa) are peculiar features on the bovine tongue. Note their clinical significance in Box 1.20. (b) Bovine median sagittal section of the head. The nasal septum has been removed to demonstrate the nasal and ethmoid conchae. The paper-thin spaces between the nasal conchae (arrows) are the dorsal nasal meatus (1), middle nasal meatus (2), and ventral nasal meatus (3). A common nasal meatus is the space that communicates with 1–3 meatuses and is located immediately lateral to the nasal septum and medial to the nasal and ethmoid conchae.

> **Box 1.20**
>
> Food tends to collect in the **lingual fossa.** The fossa is considered a potential site for harboring microbes. It has a delicate mucosa that can easily be pierced by sharp contaminated objects.
>
> A bacterial tongue infection known commonly as **wooden tongue** or Actinobacillosis is caused by a bacterium from the genus *Actinobacillus*. It causes a hard swollen tongue, a retropharyngeal abscess and could spread to the respiratory system causing pleuropneumonia. It primarily affects cattle but can be seen in sheep.
>
> The **torus linguae,** the concave elevation at the root of the tongue, can present an obstacle to the passage of a balling gun or cattle mouth Frick speculum. The gun must be carefully passed over the torus linguae before dispensing the bolus, otherwise the ball will be chewed and spilled out.

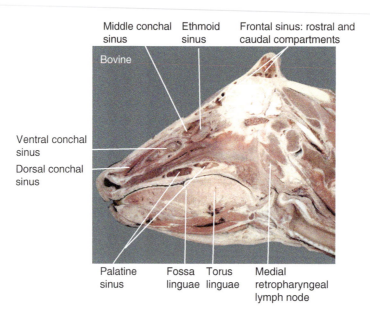

Figure 1.28 Median sagittal section of the bovine head. Conchae are opened to show the sinusal space within each.

1.12 The Larynx and Hyoid Apparatus

Goal: Identify bones and cartilages of the larynx and hyoid apparatus and some of the associated muscles (cricoarytenoideus dorsalis) on a sagittal section of the head or prosected specimen. Compare clinical significance with the horse and dog.

1.12.1 Larynx

The laryngeal cartilages include the **cricoid, thyroid, arytenoid,** and **epiglottis** from caudal to cranial, respectively (Figure 1.29). They are generally similar to other species with slight variations that merit some attention. Consult Box 1.21 for clinical relevance of the larynx.

A feature of the ruminant thyroid cartilage relevant in palpation of the larynx is the prominence at its caudoventral aspect. This feature is located more cranially in the equine larynx.

Use a hemi-dissected ox larynx and compare it with that of the horse.

In ruminants, the cuneiform processes of the arytenoid cartilages are absent but the corniculate processes are very prominent when inspected by laryngoscope. Additionally, the aryepiglottic fold curves sharply as it connects the base of the epiglottis to the arytenoid cartilage.

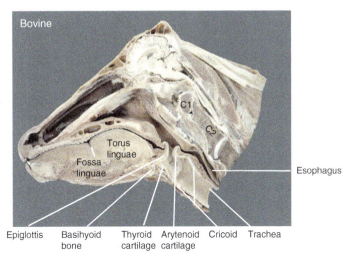

Figure 1.29 Bovine median sagittal section of the head. Identify laryngeal cartilages from caudal to rostral.

Box 1.21
Anatomy of the larynx is clinically more important in horses because of a condition known as laryngeal hemiplegia. Laryngeal hemiplegia (also called roaring) is mostly caused by damage to the left recurrent laryngeal nerve, a branch of the left vagus nerves. The condition is produced by a partial paralysis of the intrinsic laryngeal muscles, especially the cricoarytenoideus dorsalis muscle.

On a sagittal section of the larynx, identify the **vocal fold** and laryngeal cartilages (Figure 1.29).

Neither the vestibular folds nor the laryngeal ventricles are present in ruminants.

Be familiar with the term glottis. The **glottis** is defined as the valvar region that controls the entrance to the trachea. The vocal processes of the arytenoid cartilages, the vocal folds, and the opening cleft (**rima glottidis**) form the glottis. In laryngoscopy, the size of the rima glottidis varies with the stage of respiration and abduction of the vocal folds.

1.12.2 Hyoid Apparatus

The bones of the hyoid apparatus are broadly like those of the horse except for a short lingual process and relatively distinct epihyoid bone (Figure 1.30).

With the help of Figure 1.30, identify the **stylohyoid, epihyoid, ceratohyoid, basihyoid, lingual process of the basihyoid,** and **thyrohyoid bones.** All the hyoid bones are paired except for the basihyoid and lingual process.

The thyrohyoid bone articulates with the rostral cornu of the thyroid cartilage of the larynx.

1.13 The Eye

Goal: Identify the major structures and layers of the eyeball. Keep in mind the importance of the parotid lymph node in diagnosing cancers of the eye in cattle. If you have studied the anatomy of the eye before, your instructor may opt for omitting the eye from your syllabus. The anatomy of the eye is best studied on prosected specimens using a fresh and/or fixed cow eyeball.

Understand that the anatomy of the eye is clinically more important in small animals and in equine practice. Bovine ocular squamous cell carcinoma "cancer of the eye" is the common disease of the eye in cattle and is generally treated by enucleation (surgical removal) of the eye (see Box 1.22).

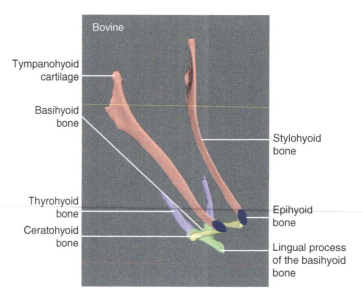

Figure 1.30 Bones of the bovine hyoid apparatus.

> **Box 1.22**
>
> - In cattle, the eye is surgically removed when cancer of the eye is diagnosed. You need to review the landmarks for needle placement for enucleation of the eye. These are discussed in Figure 1.25.
> - The parotid lymph node is inspected for diagnosis of eye cancer in slaughterhouses.
> - The most common cancer of the eye in cattle is squamous cell carcinoma.
> - Infectious bovine keratoconjunctivitis, or pink eye, is the most common ocular bacterial disease of cattle. It is spread between herds by the face fly *Musca autumnalis* and causes ulceration of the cornea.
> - Diseases of eye in animals include glaucoma (increased intraocular pressure) and cataract (increased opacity of the lens with aging). Glaucoma can be caused by inadequate drainage of the aqueous humor which is continuously produced by the ciliary body.

The eye in ruminants is located within a complete bony orbit. This is similar to the horse but different from the dog where the orbit rim is incomplete. A dense collagenous orbital ligament bridges the gap.

Ocular disorders are common in cattle and can be a result of nutritional, congenital, infectious, traumatic, or neoplastic factors.

Because the dissection of the eye is typically covered in equine anatomy and anatomy of small animals, the structures of the eye are not included in your lab ID of the head. Nevertheless, we have included the most salient information here. Identify the structures of the eye in bold typeface in this section with the help of Figures 1.31, 1.32, 1.33, 1.34, 1.35, and 1.36.

The eyeballs of horses and cattle are recessed in the bony orbit with a large **fat pad** behind the eye. The fat pad serves as a protection cushion against physical trauma.

1.13.1 Superficial Features of the Eye

Identify the superficial features of the eye including the superior and inferior **palpebrae** (upper and lower eyelids).

The thin translucent mucosal layer covering the interior of the eyelids is the **palpebral conjunctiva**. The palpebral conjunctiva reflects on the white of the eye (sclera) as **bulbar conjunctiva**. Inflammation of the conjunctiva is known as conjunctivitis (See Box 1.23).

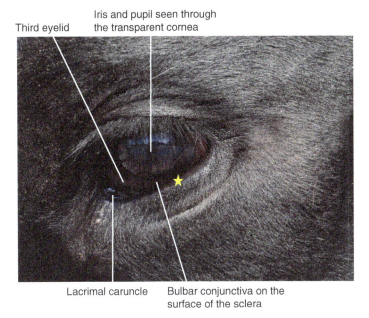

Figure 1.31 External features of the bovine eye. Note that the bovine iris is wide horizontally. Yellow star denotes the location of the palpebral conjunctiva on the lower eyelid. The bulbar conjunctiva covers the surface of the sclera (white of the eye).

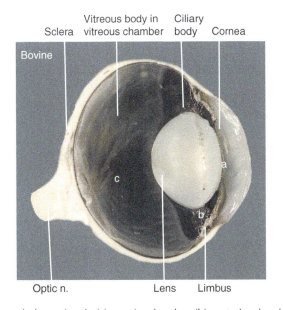

Figure 1.32 Bovine eye: section through the optic axis. (a) anterior chamber; (b) posterior chamber; (c) vitreous chamber.

The angle between the palpebral and bulbar conjunctiva is the **fornix**. The space formed by the angle of reflection or fornix is the **conjunctival sac**. Dorsal and ventral conjunctival sacs are thus recognized.

Superior and inferior **puncta** (singular form is punctum) can be located near the **medial canthus** (or commissure) of the eye on the superior and inferior lids, respectively. This is where tears collect to pass from the puncta through lacrimal canaliculi to the **lacrimal sac**.

From the lacrimal sac, the tears pass through a single duct, the **nasolacrimal duct**, to empty in the

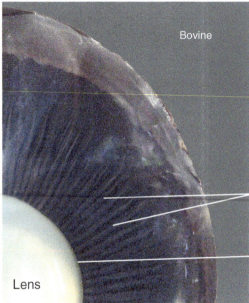

Figure 1.33 Posterior view of the eye, equatorial section of the bovine eye. Note the topographic relationship of the ciliary processes of the ciliary body, zonules (less visible), and lens.

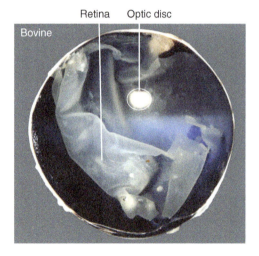

Figure 1.34 Vitreous chamber of a bovine eye (the vitreous body was removed): posterior view. Note that the retina appears as a thin transparent membrane peeled off from the dark outer choroid layer. The retina is more firmly attached at the optic disc.

rostral part of the nasal cavity and out through the nose.

The **lacrimal gland, conjunctiva,** and the **gland of the third eyelid** are the main producers of tears.

Box 1.23

Staining from increased tearing (epiphora) and congestion of the conjunctival blood vessels is visible grossly especially with conjunctivitis (inflammation of the conjunctiva of the eye).

Inflammation of the conjunctiva of the eye in cattle can be caused by a disease known as pinkeye (infectious bovine kerato-conjunctivitis, or IBK)) caused by the bacterium *Moraxella bovis*.

1.13.2 Layers of the Eye

The eyeball has three concentric layers known as eye tunics. From exterior to interior, the eye tunics are (i) outer **fibrous tunic**; (ii) middle **uvea** (or vascular tunic); and (iii) inner **nervous** tunic. Use Figures 1.32–1.36 to study the eye parts and tunics.

The outer fibrous tunic is composed of the **sclera** (white of the eye) and **cornea** (transparent and avascular). The relatively dark junction between the sclera and cornea is known as the **limbus**.

The middle vascular tunic is pigmented and is composed of the **iris** and **ciliary body** anteriorly, and **choroid** posteriorly.

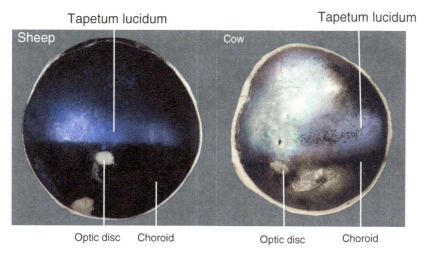

Figure 1.35 Fundus of the eye (view of the interior posterior surface of eye that includes the area of the optic disc). Sheep (left) and bovine (right) eye axial sections showing tapetum lucidum and optic disc. The vitreous bodies and retinae have been removed.

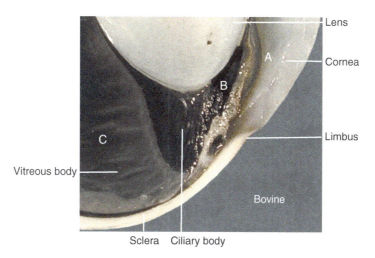

Figure 1.36 Bovine eye: axial section. Magnified anterior portion of the eye. Note the anterior chamber between the cornea and iris (a); the posterior chamber between the iris and ciliary body (b); and the vitreous chamber with vitreous body between the ciliary body and choroid (c).

The choroid has outer pigmented and inner vascularized parts. Blood vessels that supply the eye are located in the uvea.

The **iris** can be viewed through the transparent cornea. The bovine iris is wide horizontally and has **iridic granules** (**corpora nigra**) that are more prominent on the upper edge of the iris.

The size of the pupil is regulated by two smooth muscles: **constrictor** and **dilator pupillae**.

The constrictor pupillae muscle constricts the pupil in response to increased light intensity. It is innervated by parasympathetic fibers from the oculomotor nerve (CN III). The parasympathetic fibers of the oculomotor also supply the **ciliary muscle** (smooth muscle at the base of the ciliary body). The ciliary muscle regulates accommodation of the lens (changes in lens shape from default oval shape to round shape). Rounding of the lens assists with near vision.

The dilator muscle increases the size of the pupil opening in response to fear and darkness. It is innervated by the sympathetic system that originates in cranial thoracic segments of the spinal cord.

Sympathetic fibers to the eye travel from the thoracic region through the vagosympathetic trunk in the neck to synapse in the cranial cervical ganglion at the base of the skull.

Postganglionic axons leave the cranial cervical ganglion to supply the structures of the head, including the dilator pupillae of the eye.

The **ciliary body** is composed of radially oriented **ciliary processes** (Figure 1.33). Projecting from the tips of the ciliary processes to circumference of the lens are the **zonular fibers**.

The ciliary muscle regulates tension on the zonules. When the ciliary muscle contracts, the zonules relax and the shape of the lens then changes from oval to round, allowing the eye to focus on close objects.

The **innermost** nervous layer is the **retina** (Figure 1.34). The retina consists of a posterior (visual or sensitive) area that covers the choroid, and anterior nonvisual (or non-sensitive or non-nervous) area that covers the back of the ciliary body and iris. Histologically, the retina has several layers.

The posterior view of the eye is called the **fundus**. Identify the white circular **optic disc** in the fundus (Figure 1.35). The optic disc is an area where the axons of the optic nerve exit the eye to convey visual impulses to the brain.

Identify the choroid in the posterior chamber of the eye. The area of choroid that has metallic blue and green colors is called the **tapetum lucidum** (Figure 1.35). The tapetum lucidum reflects light at night to increase visualization. The nature of the structure of the tapetum lucidum is different among domestic animals. It is fibrous in herbivores (cattle and horse) and cellular in carnivores (dogs and cats).

1.13.3 Sectioning of the Eyeball

Using a sharp scalpel, section the eye either in a horizontal or vertical plane. Identify the chambers of the eye. Be gentle when you cut through the eyeball. Fluid (aqueous humor and vitreous body) will ooze out.

1.13.3.1 Chambers of the Eye

With the help of Figures 1.32 and 1.36, use the tip of your probe to identify the following eye chambers.

- **Anterior chamber:** the space between the cornea and iris.
- **Posterior chamber:** a narrow space between the iris and lens. The anterior and posterior chambers contain aqueous humor. The aqueous humor is a clear watery fluid continuously produced by the ciliary body.
- **Vitreous chamber:** the large space behind the ciliary body. In the live animal, the vitreous chamber is filled with a jelly-like substance known as the **vitreous body**. The vitreous body gives the round shape of the eye and helps keep the retina tucked to the interior of the choroid.

1.13.4 Drainage Pathway of the Aqueous Humor

The aqueous humor is continuously produced by the ciliary body and circulates from the posterior chamber, through the pupillary opening, to the anterior chamber. From the anterior chamber, it passes to the angle between the iris and cornea (known as the **iridocorneal angle**) to where it passes through the trabecular meshwork before emptying into the scleral venous plexus to join the venous circulation.

1.14 Neck Skeleton

Goal: Study the features of the cervical vertebrae, and the articulations of the skull with the atlas (atlantooccipital joint) and the atlas with the axis (atlantoaxial joint).

With the help of a bovine articulated skeleton and Figure 1.37, spend a moment to study the osteology of the neck. Like other mammals, ruminants have seven cervical vertebrae (**C1–C7**). The first (C1) and second vertebrae (C2) are the **atlas** and **axis**, respectively.

Note that the atlas and axis have modified shapes and peculiar features compared with the rest of the cervical vertebrae. The atlas differs from a typical cervical vertebra as it lacks a body and instead has dorsal and ventral arches. The ventral arch is large and replaces the "body" found in other vertebrae.

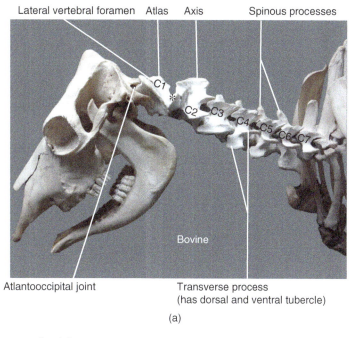

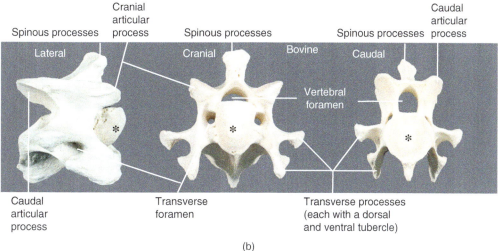

Figure 1.37 (a) Bovine cervical vertebrae. Note the large wings of the atlas (palpable in the live animal). The atlas has lateral vertebral foramen (on the dorsal arch) and alar foramen (in the wings, not visible here). Transverse foramina are present on the wings of the atlas in horses and dogs but are absent in ruminants. Note the dorsal and ventral tubercles of transverse processes of C2–C7 (two-pronged transverse processes; see (b). *Atlantoaxial joint. C7 has a large spinous process. (b) Three close-up views (lateral, cranial, and caudal) of a bovine cervical vertebra. In the articulated skeleton, the summation of the vertebral foramina forms the vertebral canal. 1, cranial vertebral notch; 2, caudal vertebral notch. The articular surfaces of the cranial articular processes are directed dorsomedially. The articular surfaces of the caudal articular processes are directed ventrolaterally.

Note the lateral vertebral foramen on the dorsal arch. Additionally, the atlas has large transverse processes commonly called the **wings of the atlas.** The wings of the atlas differ from the two-pronged transverse processes of C2–C7 vertebrae. Being large and superficial, the wings of the atlas are palpable in the live animal.

The atlas has lateral vertebral and alar foramina but lacks the transverse foramina that pierce the transverse processes of C2–C6 vertebrae. The vertebral artery and nerve pass cranially through the transverse foramina of C6–C2 vertebrae and the lateral vertebral foramen of the atlas to supply the brain.

In the atlas, the first cervical spinal nerve exits the vertebral canal through the lateral vertebral foramen. The nerve divides into dorsal and ventral branches after it exits the lateral vertebral foramen. The ventral branches of the first cervical spinal nerve pass through the alar foramen.

Locate the lateral vertebral foramen on the dorsal craniolateral surface of the dorsal arch of the atlas.

In contrast to ruminants, which lack a transverse foramen, the atlas in horses and dogs has a transverse foramen.

Oxen and horses have cranially located **alar foramina**. This foramen is incomplete in the dog and is called the alar notch. This foramen conveys the ventral branch of C1 cervical spinal nerve.

Note the modified articulations between the atlas and skull (**atlantooccipital joint**) and atlas and axis (**atlantoaxial joint**) (Figure 1.37a, b).

The axis also differs from the rest of the cervical vertebrae. It has an elongated spine and modified cranial articular process known as the **dens**, or **odontoid process**. Note these features on the skeleton.

1.15 Neck Muscles, Nerves, and Vessels

Goal: Identify the esophagus, external jugular vein, nuchal ligament, and the muscles that form the dorsal and ventral boundaries for the jugular groove or jugular furrow. Understand that the location of the esophagus on the left side of the neck and its relation to the trachea are important when passing a stomach tube. Compare the muscular boundaries for the external jugular groove (or furrow) in goats, sheep, and cattle. Identify the major structures within the carotid sheath (common carotid artery and vagosympathetic trunk) and major lymph nodes in the neck (superficial cervical lymph nodes). Do not attempt to identify the deep cervical lymph nodes. Identify the dorsal branch of the accessory nerve (CN XI) coursing to the trapezius muscle. **At the end of the neck section, watch Videos 7 and 8.**

1.15.1 Neck Muscles

Goal: Identify the dorsal and ventral muscular boundaries of the jugular groove.

The neck muscles can be divided into superficial and deep groups. There is little merit in studying the deep neck muscles.

With the help of Figures 1.38, 1.39, and 1.40, identify the superficial muscles of the neck including the clinically relevant muscles that form the boundaries for the **jugular groove** (or **jugular furrow**) (Figures 1.38 and 1.39).

The muscles that form the dorsal and ventral boundaries of the jugular furrow include the brachiocephalicus muscle dorsally (cleidomastoideus plus cleidooccipitalis muscles), and the sternomandibularis muscle ventrally. In goats, the sternomandibularis muscle is known as the sternozygomaticus muscle. The sternozygomaticus muscle is absent in sheep (Box 1.24).

1.15.1.1 Superficial Neck Muscles

Study the superficial muscles of the neck in detail on the dorsolateral and ventral aspects of the neck (Figures 1.40 and 1.41). We omitted the middle and deep muscles from our discussion, but you need to transect all of them en masse to uncover the nuchal ligament.

1.15.1.1.1 Brachiocephalicus Muscle

The **brachiocephalicus muscle** is a broad compound muscle that forms the dorsal boundary for the jugular furrow. The brachiocephalicus is located on the dorsolateral surface of the neck and runs obliquely along the area between the brachium and dorsolateral surface of the skull. It comprises three fused muscles. The **clavicular intersection** (remnant of the clavicle at the shoulder) is technically considered the origin for the three parts of the brachiocephalicus muscle. The clavicular intersection divides the brachiocephalicus muscle into cranial and caudal parts (Figure 1.39).

The cranial portion of the brachiocephalicus has two parts, **cleidooccipitalis** dorsally, and **cleidomastoideus** ventrally. The cleidomastoideus lies directly

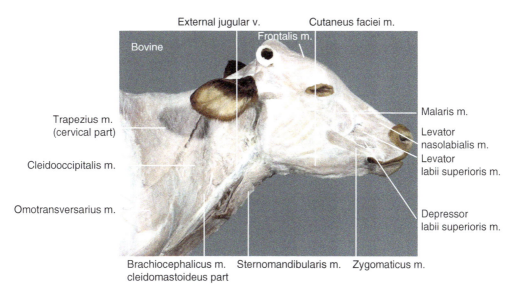

Figure 1.38 Bovine superficial neck and head muscles. Identify the **dorsal** and **ventral** boundaries of the jugular groove formed by the cleidomastoideus muscle (ventral part of the brachiocephalicus muscle) and sternomandibularis muscle (superficial part of the sternocephalicus muscle), respectively. The deep part of the sternocephalicus muscle is formed by the sternomastoideus muscle.

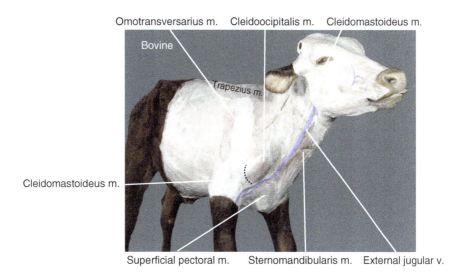

Figure 1.39 Bovine superficial muscles of the neck. Clavicular intersection shown by the dotted line. Trapezius muscle has cervical and thoracic parts.

> **Box 1.24**
>
> Note that the sternozygomaticus muscle is absent in sheep, making the jugular groove less distinct in this species when compared with the ox and goat.

dorsal to the external jugular vein (Figure 1.40a). These parts can also be named as separate muscles: the **cleidooccipitalis** and **cleidomastoideus muscles** (Figure 1.40a). The cleidooccipitalis muscle is absent in the horse but present in the dog.

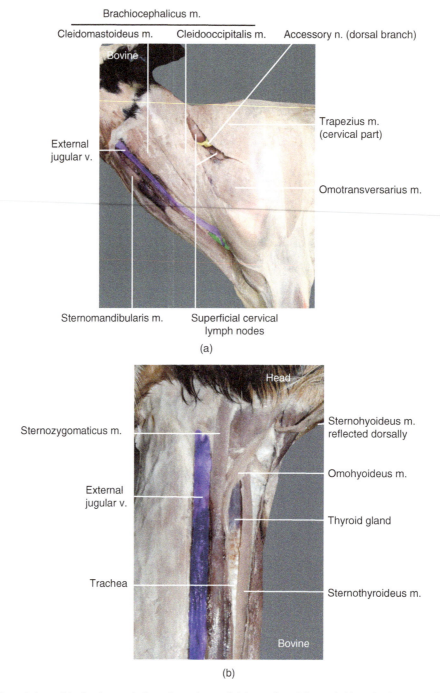

Figure 1.40 (a) Left lateral view of the bovine neck. Dorsolateral superficial muscles of the neck. Note the location of the large superficial cervical lymph nodes between the cervical part of the trapezius, omotransversarius, and cleidooccipitalis muscles. (b) Ventral neck muscles (goat). The thin sternohyoideus and sternothyroideus muscle are separated and the sternohyoideus is reflected cranially. The two muscles are fused at their origin from the manubrium (called sternothyrohyoideus muscle when fused). The sternohyoideus inserts on the basihyoid at the midline. The sternothyroideus muscle inserts laterally on the lamina of the thyroid cartilage. The two muscles help with swallowing by drawing the larynx and hyoid apparatus caudally.

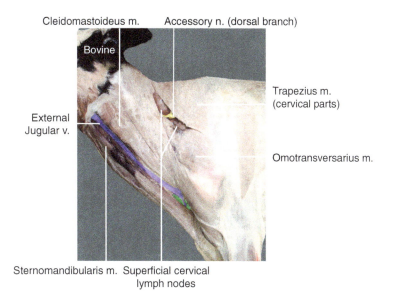

Figure 1.41 Dorsal branch of the accessory nerve (yellow in figure) coursing deep to the cervical part of the trapezius muscle.

The caudal part of the brachiocephalicus extends from the shoulder (clavicular intersection) to the brachium. It is known as the **cleidobrachialis muscle** (Figure 1.39).

1.15.1.1.2 Omotransversarius Muscle

The omotransversarius muscle extends from the scapula in the shoulder region to the wing of the atlas (transverse process of C1) (Figure 1.40a).

Note that the dorsal branch of the **accessory nerve (CN XI)** courses caudally along the dorsal surface of the omotransversarius muscle. This nerve supplies several neck muscles including the omotransversarius, brachiocephalicus, and trapezius muscle, a shoulder girdle muscle (Figure 1.40a).

Find the **superficial cervical lymph nodes** at the cranial border of the scapula and in the space between the omotransversarius and cervical part of the trapezius muscle. Use Figure 1.40(a) to locate the **omotransversarius muscle** and the **superficial cervical lymph nodes**.

1.15.1.1.3 Trapezius Muscle

The trapezius muscle has cervical and thoracic parts. Identify the cervical and thoracic trapezius parts of the trapezius muscle (Figure 1.40a). This is a triangular, fan-shaped muscle that originates on the dorsal border of the neck (cervical part) and withers (thoracic part) and inserts distally on the spine of the scapula. The dorsal branch of accessory nerve (CN XI) innervates both parts (Figure 1.40a).

1.15.1.1.4 Sternocephalicus Muscle

The sternocephalicus muscle is a large V-shaped ventral neck muscle that originates from the sternum (manubrium) and first costal cartilage and inserts on the head. It has two parts: the **sternomandibularis** (**sternozygomaticus** in goats) and **sternomastoideus** muscles. The names of these parts are descriptive of their origin and insertion points. These parts are sometimes called the mandibular and mastoid parts of the sternocephalicus muscle.

The sternomandibularis inserts on the mandible in cattle (Figure 1.17), and on the zygomatic arch in goats (Figure 1.18c). The sternozygomaticus is absent in sheep.

The sternocephalicus (specifically, the sternomandibularis part) and brachiocephalicus (specifically, the cleidomastoideus part) muscles form the ventral and dorsal parts of the muscular boundaries for the jugular furrow, respectively.

1.15.1.1.5 Sternothyroideus and Sternohyoideus Muscles
The left and right **sternothyroideus** and **sternohyoideus** muscles are relatively thin, flat muscles located in between the left and right sternocephalicus muscle on the ventral neck (Figure 1.40b). They cover the ventral surface of the trachea. They extend from the sternum (manubrium) to the thyroid cartilage (sternothyroideus muscle) and basihyoid bone of the basihyoid apparatus (sternohyoideus muscle). These muscles are fused in the caudal neck and at their origin from the manubrium of the sternum but are separated at their insertion points on the lateral lamina of the thyroid cartilage (sternothyroideus muscle) and basihyoid bone (sternohyoideus muscle).

Trace the sternothyrohyoideus muscles from their origin at the sternum to their insertion on the lateral surface of the thyroid lamina and on the ventral surface of the basihyoid bone (Figure 1.40b).

1.15.1.2 Deep Neck Muscles

As mentioned earlier, the deep neck muscles will not be dissected. Those who are interested in the dissection of these muscles should read the following summary and consult other textbooks (see Appendix B) for more details and figures. The deep cervical muscles, depending on their location, either extend or flex the neck or move the neck sideways. Here is a summary of their nomenclature and location.

Neck muscles located deep to the superficial layer on the dorsolateral aspect of the neck can be classified into middle and deep layers. These muscles are generally located dorsal to the cervical vertebrae. They are also considered as extensors of the neck. Reflection of the trapezius cervicis and brachiocephalicus muscles will expose a middle layer composed largely of the serratus ventralis cervicis ventrally, rhomboideus cervices muscle dorsally, and the omotransversarius muscle in between them. The omotransversarius is a strap muscle that inserts to the wing of the atlas. The large muscle deep to the rhomboideus cervicis is the splenius muscle.

The rhomboideus in ruminants has cervical and thoracic parts but lacks the capitis part found in dogs. The **hump** in zebu cattle such as Brahman cattle (*Bos indicus*) is produced by the enlargement of the rhomboideus muscle. European breeds (*Bos taurus*) lack a hump.

Reflect the serratus ventralis cervicis to expose the longissimus group of muscles running longitudinally parallel with the cervical vertebrae. These muscles represent the cranial extension of an intermediate portion of the epaxial musculature (muscles of the trunk lying dorsal to the transverse processes of the vertebrae in the abdominal, thoracic, and cervical vertebrae). The epaxial muscles in the neck region include longissimus cervicis, longissimus atlantis, and longissimus capitis.

The muscle located deep to the splenius is the semispinalis capitis that has two parts: the complexus and biventer. Reflect semispinalis capitis muscle to expose the nuchal ligament (see Section 1.16).

Muscles lying along and ventral to the transverse processes of cervical vertebrae (hypaxial muscles) include the intertransversarius muscle, dorsal and ventral scalenus, longus capitis, and multifidus cervicis. The muscle that covers the ventral surfaces of the vertebral bodies is the longus colli muscle. Collectively, these muscles flex the neck.

Short neck muscles in the occipital region lying just behind the skull are classified into obliquus capitis caudalis and obliquus capitis cranialis lying cranial and caudal to the wing of the atlas, respectively.

Dorsal to obliquus muscles are rectus capitis dorsalis major and rectus capitis dorsalis minor. The rectus capitis dorsalis (major part) originates from the spine of C2 (axis) and inserts on the nuchal region near the external occipital protuberance. Major part of the muscle is further divided into superficial and deep parts. The minor portion of the rectus capitis dorsalis originates from the dorsal surface of the atlas and inserts on the caudal surface of the skull. There is no need to spend time dissecting the deep muscles of the neck.

1.15.2 Nerves of the Neck

Goal: Identify the bilateral nerves of the neck that include the **accessory nerve, recurrent laryngeal nerve,** and the **vagosympathetic trunk** (Figures 1.41 and 1.42).

Branches of eight cervical spinal nerves supply structures of the neck. Identify only **C2** and its **great auricular** branch that conveys sensation from the caudal surface of the horn (Figure 1.18a).

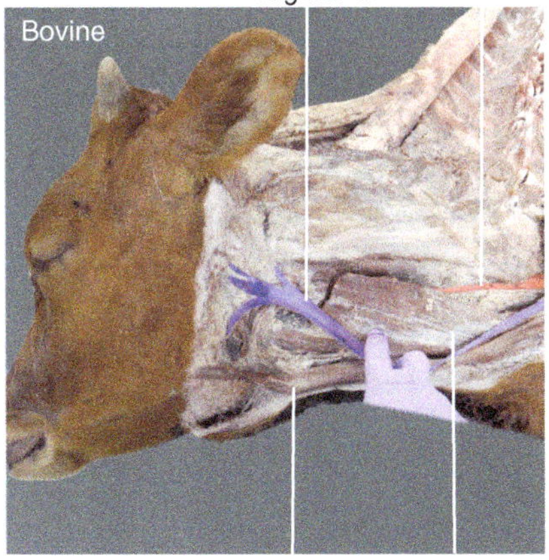

Figure 1.42 Goat neck: ventral view. Dissection of common carotid artery and vagosympathetic trunk by spreading the ventral neck muscles apart using a Gelpi self-retaining retractor. The common carotid artery and the vagosympathetic trunk are partially separated. Spreading of the mid-ventral neck muscles (combined sternothyrohyoideus muscles) is also used for exposure of the trachea.

The **accessory nerve** (CN XI) courses from the skull to the neck under the wing of the atlas. Here it divides into dorsal and ventral branches.

Dorsal branch: passes dorsal to the second cervical nerve (C2). It supplies the cleidooccipitalis and trapezius muscles. Follow the dorsal branch of the accessory nerve across the dorsal surface of the **omotransversarius** muscle to supply the omotransversarius and trapezius muscles (Figure 1.41).

Ventral branch: passes ventral to C2. It supplies the sternomandibularis (sternozygomaticus in small ruminants), sternomastoideus, and cleidomastoideus muscles.

The **vagosympathetic trunk** is located dorsal to the **common carotid artery** in the carotid sheath (Figure 1.42a).

Find the **recurrent laryngeal nerve** lateral to the trachea. As the nerve approaches the larynx, the name of the nerve is changed to the **caudal laryngeal nerve**. Find the caudal laryngeal nerve in the proximity of the **thyroid gland**.

The caudal laryngeal nerve supplies all the laryngeal muscles except the cricothyroideus muscle, which is supplied by the **cranial laryngeal nerve**. The cranial laryngeal nerve originates from the vagus nerve (CN X) soon after it emerges from the skull. The caudal laryngeal nerve originates from the vagus in the thoracic region.

1.15.3 Blood Vessels of the Neck

Goal: Identify the **external jugular vein** in the jugular furrow (Figures 1.41 and 1.43). The branches of the external jugular vein were previously discussed with the vessels of the head (Figure 1.22). Open the carotid sheath and identify the **common carotid artery** along with other contents that include the vagosympathetic trunk, internal jugular vein in the ox (absent in small ruminants), and tracheal trunk. Branches of the common carotid artery were also discussed with the vessels of the head.

The muscular boundaries of the **jugular groove** that houses the **external jugular vein** are discussed earlier with the neck muscles. It is bounded ventrally by the **sternomandibularis** and dorsally by the **brachiocephalicus** muscles (Figures 1.38, 1.39, and 1.41). The brachiocephalicus muscle in ruminants is a multipart muscle with three divisions: cleidobrachialis, cleidomastoideus, and cleidooccipitalis muscles. The sternocephalicus muscle is also a compound muscle with mandibular and mastoid parts: sternomandibularis and sternomastoideus muscles, respectively.

Transect the sternomastoideus muscle (mastoid portion of the sternocephalicus) that covers the common carotid artery in the caudal part of the neck. This muscle forms the medial boundary of the external jugular vein (Figure 1.43).

Dissect the fascia from the carotid sheath to uncover the **common carotid artery**, **internal jugular vein**, and the **vagosympathetic trunk**. The trunk is located on the dorsal surface of the common carotid artery (Figure 1.42). The branches of the common carotid artery were discussed with the vessels of the head.

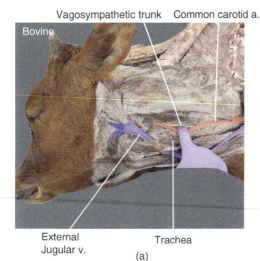

The **nuchal ligament** in cattle is substantial and is like that in the horse but is different in size and shape from that of the dog. It is elastic in nature and has both **funicular** and **laminar (or lamellar) parts** (Figure 1.44). The nuchal ligament is located deep to the dorsal muscles of the neck above the cervical spines.

The nuchal ligament in goats consists of two parts as in cattle.

The nuchal ligament supports the heavy weight of the head as well as head movement.

With the help of Figure 1.44 and the following description, study the two parts of the nuchal ligament and their insertion on a cow skeleton.

Funicular part: consists of paired cord-like structures. It runs from the skull (external occipital protuberance) caudally to the summits of the highest spines of the withers. It is round cranially, and flat caudally. The funicular part continues caudally as the supraspinous ligament. A **supraspinous bursa** is located between the ligament and the summit of T1 thoracic vertebral spine.

Figure 1.43 Dissection of the external jugular vein and common carotid artery (bovine of the neck: left lateral view). The brachiocephalicus muscle (dorsal boundary of the external jugular vein) is removed to uncover the common carotid artery. The external jugular vein is pulled down to demonstrate the sternomastoideus muscle that forms the medial border of the jugular furrow. It is transected in the cranial neck.

1.16 Nuchal Ligament

Goal: Identify the funicular and laminar parts of the nuchal ligament and their attachments. Understand the function and clinical significance of the nuchal ligament.

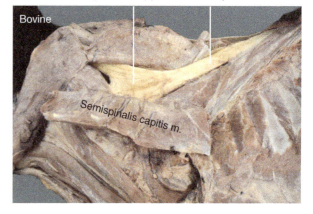

Figure 1.44 Bovine nuchal ligament: left lateral view of deep neck muscles. The semispinalis is freed from the nuchal ligament and reflected ventrally. The funicular part of the nuchal ligament courses between the first few thoracic vertebrae to the external occipital protuberance. The laminar part spans the distance from C2 to C7 and merges with the funicular part. It has cranial (paired) and caudal (unpaired) parts.

Laminar or lamellar part: the laminar part is located ventral to the funicular part. It consists of a pair of flat sheets cranially, and an unpaired sheet caudally. The cranial pair sheets extend between C2 and C4. The caudal unpaired sheet extends from C6/7 to T1.

In bullfights, the picador gouges and damages this ligament, making it difficult for the bull to hold the head high. For clinical relevance of the nuchal ligament, see Box 1.25.

Box 1.25

The nuchal ligament acts as a barrier to the spread of cervical abscesses between the left and right sides of the neck. It also helps direct inflammatory exudate fluid ventrally in the direction of gravity away from the chest. When administering medications to cattle via subcutaneous or intramuscular injection, a triangular area of the neck is used. This area is outlined by the nuchal ligament dorsally, jugular furrow ventrally, and shoulder caudally. Injections given at other sites could cause damage to more valuable cuts of meat and should be avoided.

1.17 Surface Topography (Head and Neck)

Goal: This section is intended to provide some information on palpable structures on the head and neck of live cattle. It is provided to help students carry out palpation exercises and give applied context to gross anatomy (Figures 1.45, 1.46, 1.47, 1.48, 1.49, and 1.50).

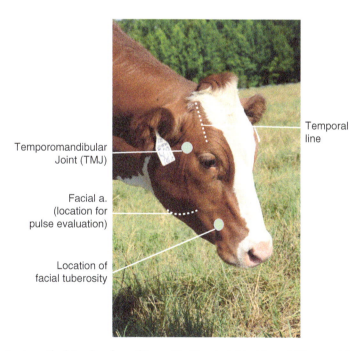

Figure 1.45 Palpable structures on the lateral surface of live cattle. The straight white solid line caudal to the eye depicts the temporal line, a landmark for localization of the cornual nerve and cornual artery. The curved white dotted line depicts the course of the facial artery, facial vein, and parotid duct. The filled circles depict approximate locations of temporomandibular joint and the facial tuberosity.

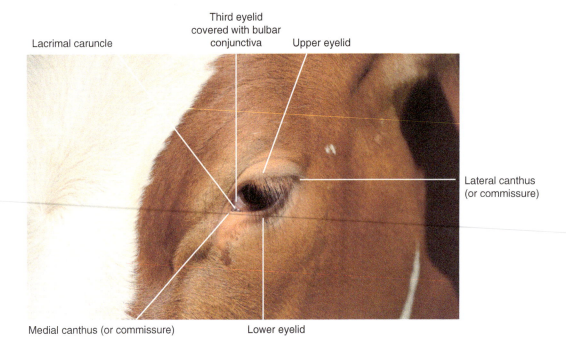

Figure 1.46 External features of the eye. The inner surface of the upper (superior) and lower (inferior) eyelids is lined with palpebral conjunctiva. The third eyelid is covered by bulbar conjunctiva of the third eyelid.

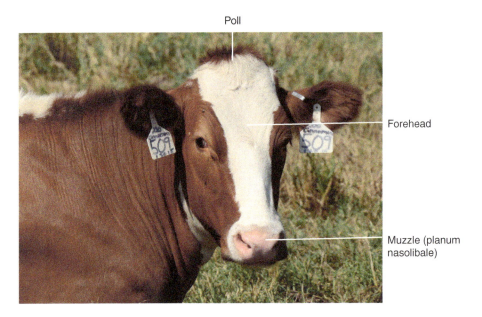

Figure 1.47 Common terms for areas on the bovine head. The poll (intercornual protuberance) is the highest point on the bovine skull.

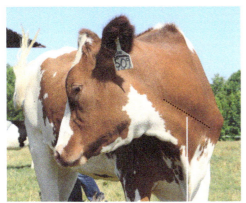

Jugular groove
(or furrow)

Figure 1.48 Jugular groove or furrow containing the external jugular vein, a major site for venipuncture in domestic animals including cattle. The muscular boundaries for the jugular groove include the brachiocephalicus muscle dorsally (specifically the cleidomastoideus part), and sternomandibularis muscle ventrally (superficial part of the sternocephalicus). Pulling the head up and to the opposite side is helpful in visualization of the jugular groove.

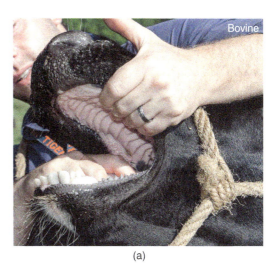

(a)

Figure 1.49a Technique for opening the mouth and holding it open for teeth inspection or medication. Pry the mouth open by placing several fingers at the corner of the mouth inside the space behind the incisor teeth (diastema). Note that the tongue is grabbed and pulled to one side to hold the mouth open.

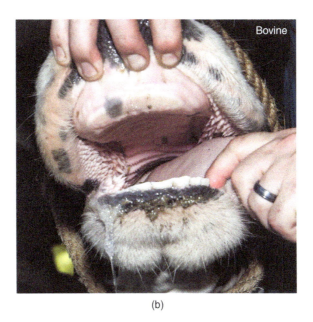

(b)

Figure 1.49b Another technique for mouth opening. A rope or custom cattle halter is helpful in restraining the animal by an assistant. The mouth is opened, and tongue pulled to one side through the diastema.

Box 1.26

The **median caudal vein** (Figure 1.50) in cattle is located under the ventral midline of the tail in association with a satellite artery, the **median caudal artery**. The vein can be used for the withdrawal of a small quantity of blood from the tail. Because of the proximity to the artery, venous blood collected from this site may become mixed with arterial blood. The artery can also be used for pulse evaluation. The vein should be accessed between two successive caudal vertebrae as both the vein and artery are protected with hemal arches in their course under vertebral bodies. You should avoid fecal contamination when collecting blood from the median caudal vein.

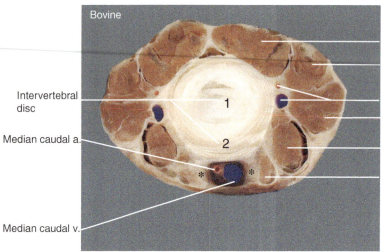

Figure 1.50 Cross-section of a cow tail showing location of the **median caudal vein** (tail vein) and **median caudal artery** on the midline of the ventral surface of the proximal third of the tail. *Hemal arch. 1, nucleus pulposus; 2, anulus fibrosus of the intervertebral disc. See Box 1.26 for clinical application related to the tail vein.

1.18 Lab ID List for the Head and Neck

There is no need to identify items in *italics*.

A. **Skeletal features of the bovine skull (bones, foramina, paranasal sinuses, mandibles, and teeth).**
   Identify the structures that pass through listed foramina.
   1. Optic canal
   2. Foramen orbitorotundum
   3. Supraorbital foramen
   4. Infraorbital foramen
   5. Mental foramen
   6. Facial tuberosity
   7. Temporal line
   8. Temporal fossa
   9. Supraorbital groove
   10. Horn (horn sheath, cornual process)
   11. Intercornual protuberance
   12. External occipital protuberance
   13. Zygomatic arch (zygomatic bone and zygomatic process of the temporal bone)
   14. Incisor teeth (1–4)–lower jaw (central–first intermediate–second intermediate–corner)
   15. *Crown (spatula-shaped incisor tooth)*
   16. *Neck (peg-shaped in old cow or goat)*
   17. *Root (embedded in gum)*
   18. *Incisor tooth surfaces: labial, lingual, and occlusal surfaces*
   19. Cheek teeth (P2–P3–P4; M1–M2–M3)
   20. Diastema
   21. Frontal bone (cornual process)
   22. Zygomatic process of the frontal bone
   23. Frontal process of the zygomatic bone

24. Temporal process of the zygomatic bone
25. Zygomatic process of the temporal bone
26. Pterygoid crest
27. Frontal sinus
    a. Rostral compartment
    b. Caudal compartment
        i. Cornual diverticulum
        ii. Nuchal diverticulum
        iii. Postorbital diverticulum
    c. Oblique septum
    d. Median septum separating left and right frontal sinuses
28. Maxillary sinus
29. Palatine sinus
30. Lacrimal bone
31. Lacrimal bulla
32. Nasal bone
33. Incisive bone
34. Nasoincisive notch
35. Maxilla
36. Rim of the orbit

B. Mandible

37. Coronoid process
38. Condylar process
39. Ramus
40. Mental foramen
41. Mandibular foramen (identify structures passing through this foramen)
42. Mandibular symphysis

C. Dental formula

43. Permanent teeth: 2 × (I 0/4, P 3/3, M 3/3) = 32 total
44. *Temporary teeth*: 2 × (DI 0/4, DP 3/3) = 20 total

D. Muscles (some will be identified on the neck, see section J).

45. Cleidomastoideus m. (ID on the head or neck)
46. Masseter m.
47. Sternocephalicus m. (ID on head or neck)
    a. Sternomandibularis m. on cow head (absent in sheep)
    b. Sternozygomaticus m. (goat)
    c. Sternomastoideus m.

E. Nerves and vessels supplying structures on the head

Nerves

48. Auriculopalpebral n. (know where the nerve is blocked and clinical significance)
49. Cornual n. (know where the nerve is blocked and clinical significance)
50. *Great auricular n.* (C2) (know function)
51. *Infratrochlear n.* (goat) (know function)
52. Facial n.
    a. Dorsal buccal branch of VII
    b. Ventral buccal branch of VII

Arteries

53. Facial a. in bovine (pulse, absent in goats)
54. Transverse fascial a. (pulse in goat. Present in bovine)
55. Superficial temporal a.
56. Cornual a.

Veins

57. Facial v. (bovine)
58. *Transverse facial v.* (goat)
59. Frontal v. (cow)
60. Linguofacial v.
61. Maxillary v.
62. Angularis oculi v.

F. Salivary glands

63. Parotid salivary gland
64. Mandibular salivary gland
65. Monostomatic sublingual
66. Parotid duct

G. Lymph nodes of the head

67. Parotid lymph node
68. Mandibular lymph node
69. Medial retropharyngeal lymph node (medial view)
70. Lateral retropharyngeal lymph node (bovine)

H. External features

71. *Scent glands in goats* (know general location only)
72. *Epiceras* (know function)
73. Nasolabial plate
74. *Opening of the nasolacrimal duct* (know location)

I. **Oral/pharyngeal structures (on paramedian section)**
   75. Dental pad
   76. Incisive papilla
   77. *Nasopharynx*
   78. *Oropharynx*
   79. *Laryngopharynx*
   80. Soft palate
   81. Dorsal, ventral, and middle concha
   82. Dorsal, middle, and ventral nasal meatuses
   83. Laryngeal cartilages (cricoid–thyroid–arytenoid–epiglottis)
   84. Basihyoid
   85. Tongue
       a. Torus linguae (lingual torus)
       b. Fossa linguae (lingual fossa)

J. **Neck**
   86. Nuchal ligament (funicular and laminar parts)
   87. Vertebral formula:
       Cattle: C7–T13–L6–**S5**–Cd variable (Cd 18–20)
       Goat: C7–T13–L6 (7)–**S5**–Cd variable (Cd 16–18)
       Sheep: C7–T13–L6 (7)–**S4**–variable (Cd 16–18)

Muscles of the neck
   88. Sternocephalicus m. in ox and goat (two parts: sternomandibularis + *sternomastoideus*)
       a. Sternomandibularis m. (ID on cow's head, absent in sheep)
       b. Sternozygomaticus m. (in goat, same as sternomandibularis in cow)
   89. Brachiocephalicus m. (three parts: cleidobrachialis + cleidooccipitalis + *cleidomastoideus, may be absent*)
   90. Trapezius m. (cervical part)
   91. Omotransversarius m. (in sheep, it fuses to cleido-occipitalis m.)
   92. Rhomboideus m. (two parts: cervical + thoracic)
   93. *Sternohyoideus m.*
   94. *Sternothyroideus m.*
   95. *Pharyngeal muscles (cricopharyngeus and thyropharyngeus muscles same as other species)*

Lymph nodes of the neck
   96. Superficial cervical lymph nodes (also known as pre-scapular lymph nodes)

Nerves of the neck
   97. Accessory nerve (dorsal and ventral branch)
   98. Recurrent laryngeal n. (ID left nerve in the thorax and its continuation in neck as Cd laryngeal n.)
   99. Vagosympathetic trunk
   100. *Great auricular n.*

Other structures in the neck region
   101. Common carotid a.
   102. Trachea
   103. Esophagus (cervical part)
   104. External jugular v. (ID dorsal and ventral boundaries for the jugular groove)
   105. Thyroid gland
   106. Cervical thymus (in young animals)

2
The Thorax

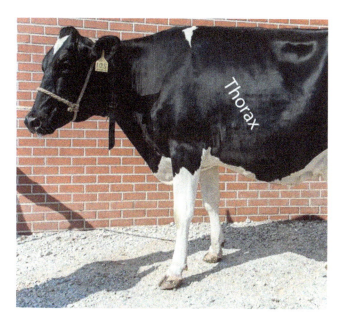

Learning Objectives

- List the anatomic boundaries for the auscultation areas of the lungs and heart.
- Identify lung lobes and the thoracic part of the thymus (large in young calves and may extend into the neck).
- Identify the tracheal bronchus (special bronchus for ventilation of the cranial lobe of the right lung) and know its clinical significance.
- Know the term mediastinum and the contents of the cranial, middle, and caudal mediastinum.
- Identify mediastinal (cranial, middle, and caudal) and tracheobronchial lymph nodes. Know the clinical significance of the caudal mediastinal lymph nodes.
- Know the term pluck (tongue, trachea, esophagus, heart, and lungs) used in meat inspection in a slaughterhouse setting.

Guide to Ruminant Anatomy: Dissection and Clinical Aspects, Second Edition. Mahmoud Mansour, Ray Wilhite, Joe Rowe, and Saly Hafiz.
© 2023 John Wiley & Sons, Inc. Published 2023 by John Wiley & Sons, Inc.
Companion website: www.wiley.com/go/mansour/dissection2

- Identify major thoracic nerves and autonomic ganglia (similar to other species).
- Identify left and right azygos veins. Compare the presence of these veins in other species (horse and dog).
- Identify the brachiocephalic and pulmonary trunks, and thoracic lymphatic duct on the left side of the thorax.
- Study the topography of the heart (atrial versus auricular surfaces) and the internal structures within the atria and ventricles. List the layers comprising the pericardium.
- At the end of the thorax section, watch Videos 9, 10, and 11.

2.1 Introduction

The thoracic cage is formed by the **thoracic vertebrae** dorsally, **ribs** laterally, and **sternum** ventrally. The thorax of ruminants differs from that of the equine thorax in the number of ribs and vertebrae (typically, 18 ribs in the horse and 13 ribs in ruminants). In cattle, the ribs are flat and wide with relatively narrower intercostal spaces compared with round ribs with relatively wider intercostal spaces in horses.

It is of clinical interest to be able to identify the areas suitable for lung auscultation and auscultation of heart sounds (valves) as part of a complete physical examination. You should be able to identify the ribs that make the surface landmarks for the **basal border of the lungs, the points of maximum intensity of the heart valves (puncta maxima)**, the triangular area for lung auscultation, and the **diaphragmatic line of pleural reflection**.

Understand that the point of the elbow (olecranon tuber) approximates the sixth rib and the most cranial extent of the diaphragm.

In the interior of the chest, study the lung lobes and note the differences between the equine and ruminant lungs. Bovine lungs are somewhat asymmetrical and are distinguished by their pronounced lobation and very evident lobulation when compared with that of the horse.

Study the contents of the mediastinum (composed of the mediastinal pleurae and all of the contents between them) that separates the pleural cavity into left and right cavities) and the lymphatic structures including thymus in young animals.

2.2 Bones of the Thorax

Goal: Identify various parts of the ribs and thoracic vertebrae and know the number of ribs and thoracic vertebrae. Understand the surface landmarks for the thoracic inlet, basal border of the lung, and diaphragmatic line of pleural reflection. Consult Boxes 2.1–2.3 for review of some clinical applications.

Box 2.1

Note the flat structure of ribs with narrower intercostal spaces in ruminants when compared with the round ribs of the horse. Rib fractures, although rare, may occur in young calves during difficult calving (dystocia).

Box 2.2

In performing lung auscultation in a live animal, you should place your stethoscope in front of the basal border of the lung and caudal to the caudal border of the triceps brachii muscle.

Identify the diaphragmatic line of pleural reflection on the live animal. A needle inserted cranial to the diaphragmatic line of pleural reflection will typically end up in the pleural cavity. In contrast, a needle inserted caudal to the diaphragmatic line of pleural reflection will typically be in the peritoneal cavity of the abdomen.

Box 2.3
Surgical incision into the thorax through the intercostal muscles should be made midway through the intercostal space between the ribs. This is necessary to avoid damaging the intercostal vessels and nerves running at the caudal border of each rib.

The thorax of ruminants typically includes 13 thoracic vertebrae and 13 pairs of ribs (Figure 2.1). The floor of the thorax is formed by the sternum.

The sternum is composed of seven sternebrae that connect with costal cartilages of 8 out of the 13 ribs. The ribs that are attached to the sternum are known as the sternal ribs. The remaining five pairs of ribs are connected indirectly to the sternum by their costal cartilages and are designated as asternal ribs.

With the help of Figure 2.2 (lateral, cranial, and caudal views of vertebrae), study the structures that form a typical thoracic vertebra. Study the **head, neck, tubercle,** and **body** of a rib using Figure 2.1 for guidance.

Typically, a rib is composed of a dorsal osseous part and a ventral **costal cartilage**. The junction between the osseous part and the costal cartilage is known as the **costochondral junction**.

Before you start your dissection of the muscles that form the thoracic wall, study the ribs that form the surface landmarks for the **thoracic inlet,** basal **border of the lung and area for lung auscultation, points for punca maxima,** and the **diaphragmatic line of pleural reflection**. Understand the following definitions.

2.3 Thoracic Inlet

Goal: Identify boundaries and list some structures passing through the thoracic inlet.

The term "thoracic inlet" means the entrance to the thoracic cavity. The boundaries of the thoracic inlet include the first thoracic vertebra (T1) dorsally, first pair of ribs laterally, and first sternebra (manubrium)

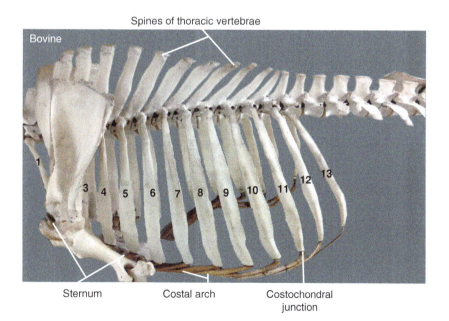

Figure 2.1 Articulated bovine thorax. Rib 2 and part of rib 3 are concealed by the scapula.

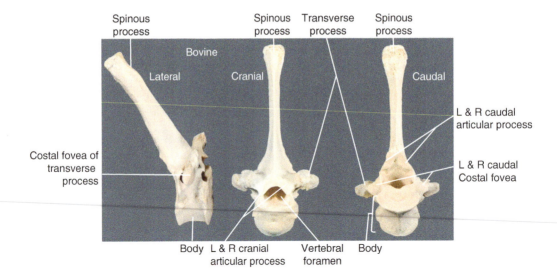

Figure 2.2 Typical bovine thoracic vertebra: lateral, cranial, and caudal views. Each transverse process has a costal fovea for articulation with a tubercle of a corresponding rib. Note the large spinous process of thoracic vertebrae compared with cervical and lumbar vertebrae. The rib head articulates with the cranial and caudal costal fovea of two successive thoracic vertebrae.

ventrally. Many structures pass into or out of the thoracic cavity through the thoracic inlet. Examples include the esophagus, trachea, common carotid arteries, vagosympathetic trunks, longus coli muscles, subclavian arteries, and external jugular veins. Identify the boundaries of the thoracic inlet on a ruminant skeleton.

> Box 2.4
>
> The cupula pleura is vulnerable to puncture by sharp objects leading to a rush of free air into the pleural sac (the condition is known as pneumothorax). This is especially serious in the horse should they run into a sharp object such as a fence post.

2.4 Basal Border of the Lung and Area for Lung Auscultation

Goal: Identify the boundaries for the area used for lung auscultation on the live animal. Consult Boxes 2.4 and 2.5 for clinical applications related to lung applications.

The basal border of the lung is a line that represents the most caudoventral extent of the lung. This line is curved and starts from the costochondral junction of the 6th rib (close to the point of the elbow) to approximately middle of the 10th rib and continues to the vertebral end of the 11th intercostal space dorsally (6-10-11 ribs for short).

The surface **area for lung auscultation** in the live animal is defined by a triangular region (Figure 2.3). The boundaries for this region are as follows:

- **Cranial:** caudal border of the long head of the triceps muscle.
- **Dorsal:** lateral edge of the epaxial muscles.
- **Caudal:** basal border of the lung.

2.5 Diaphragmatic Line of Pleural Reflection

Goal: Identify the line of pleural reflection on the cadaver and the rib numbers that approximate this line on the live animal. Know its clinical significance (Box 2.2).

The **diaphragmatic line of pleural reflection** represents a transition point formed by reflection of the parietal costal pleura on the diaphragm to become

Box 2.5

- Pneumonia is the most clinical problem affecting lungs in cattle.
- Endotracheal intubation is performed after induction of anesthesia. This procedure is best accomplished with the patient in sternal recumbency with the head and neck held in extension. Be cautious not to obstruct the tracheal bronchus when using an endotracheal tube with inflatable cuffs. Inflatable cuffs are important for the creation of a water-tight seal of the tracheal tube to prevent aspiration of saliva and/or ruminal contents. Methods for tracheal intubation include: (i) Use of guided tube/stylet and a laryngoscope; (ii) Blind intubation using a tracheal tube stiffened with a metal rod (known as stick intubation). For more technical information, consult *Farm Animal Anesthesia* edited by Lin and Walz (2014).
- **Lung auscultation**: on a triangular area determined by the following anatomic boundaries:

  Cranial: caudal border of the triceps brachii muscle
  Dorsal: epaxial muscles
  Caudal: the curved line for identification of the basal border of the lungs along the 6-10-11 ribs.

  Auscultation assesses the size of the lung field and the presence of abnormal lung sounds. Emphysema of the lungs can expand the audible airflow beyond the border of the 6-10-11 ribs. Reduced or absent airflow is associated with lung consolidation or atelectasis. In cases of pneumonia, abnormal sounds such as wheezes and crackles signify the presence of inflammation and inflammatory products.

- **Thoracentesis**: a procedure for the removal of excess inflammatory fluid from the chest. Cannulation can generally be performed at the lower seventh intercostal space (7 ICS).
- The lungs of cattle have higher connective tissue contents than those of horses. This renders cattle have a higher respiratory rate (RR) and lower functional residual capacity compared with horses (RR averages 30 breaths/minute in cattle compared with an average of 12 breaths/minute in horses). The smaller chest of cattle (13 ribs) compared with the larger chest of horses (18 ribs) is thought to contribute to the differences in breathing pattern between the two species.

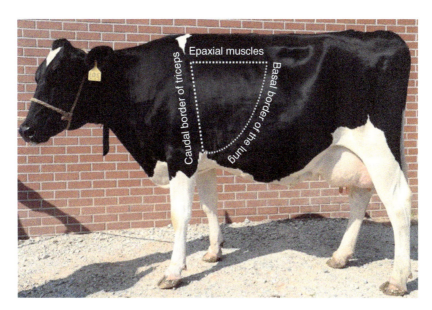

Figure 2.3 Triangular area for lung auscultation on live animal: left lateral view.

the parietal diaphragmatic pleura, or vice versa. The line represents the most caudoventral extent of the pleural cavity.

The ribs that form the surface landmarks for the diaphragmatic line of pleural reflection in cattle include the 8th costochondral junction, middle of the 11th rib, and the dorsal end of the 12th ribs.

In small ruminants (goat and sheep), the diaphragmatic line of pleural reflection extends along the 8th, 9th costochondral junctions to reach the dorsal end of the 12th rib. Like the basal border of the lung, the diaphragmatic line of pleural reflection follows a curved line.

Use a string to draw the basal border of the lung and diaphragmatic line of pleural reflection on a cow or goat skeleton. The space between the two lines drawn is not occupied by the lung and is known as the **costodiaphragmatic recess***.*

2.6 Muscles of the Thoracic Wall

Goal: Identify some of the muscles that cover the thoracic wall (ribs) from superficial to deep. With the exception of intercostal muscles, the muscles of the thoracic wall have either their origin or insertion in the thoracic region.

The muscles of the thoracic wall are best studied when the thoracic limb is removed. They include the thoracic part of the **cutaneous trunci, latissimus dorsi, scalenus (dorsalis, medius,** and **ventralis), thoracic part of the trapezius, thoracic part of the rhomboideus, serratus ventralis (cervical** and **thoracic parts), serratus dorsalis (cranial** and **caudal parts), cranial part (origin) of the external** and **internal abdominal oblique, rectus thoracis, longissimus thoracis, spinalis et semispinalis thoracis, iliocostalis thoracis,** and **external** and **internal intercostal muscles**. Identify select muscles of this group as listed on your laboratory ID list and shown in Figures 2.4–2.7. It is not necessary to dissect all of the aforementioned muscles. Ask your instructor for advice on which muscles of thoracic wall you should identify.

If not already done, skin the thorax as far caudally as the cranial border of the hind limb (Figure 2.5). Remove the fat and fascia to expose the muscles and define their borders. With the help of Figures 2.4–2.7, identify the muscles of the thoracic wall listed on your ID list or as suggested by your instructor.

Your instructor may ask you to preserve the cutaneous muscles (Figure 2.4). To save time you may opt to remove the cutaneous muscles with the skin. The more time you spend cleaning fascia and fat, the more likely

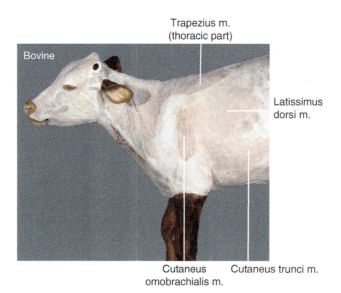

Figure 2.4 Superficial muscles of the bovine thoracic wall: left lateral view.

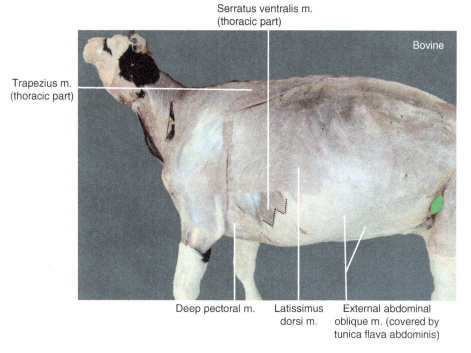

Figure 2.5 Lateral thoracic muscles deep to the cutaneous muscles. Dotted lines show the interdigitation of serratus ventralis thoracis muscle with the origin of the external abdominal oblique muscle.

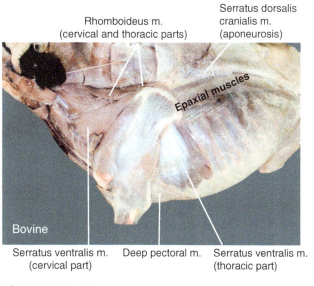

Figure 2.6 Select deep muscles of the thoracic wall.

you will end up with a neat dissection. However, keep in mind that some of the specimens are better than others. Identify the **cutaneous trunci** and **cutaneous omobrachialis** muscles (Figure 2.4).

Next, remove the cutaneous muscles and, with the help of Figure 2.5, identify the **latissimus dorsi,** *thoracic part of the* **serratus ventralis,** *origin of the* **external abdominal oblique,** *and the* **deep pectoral**

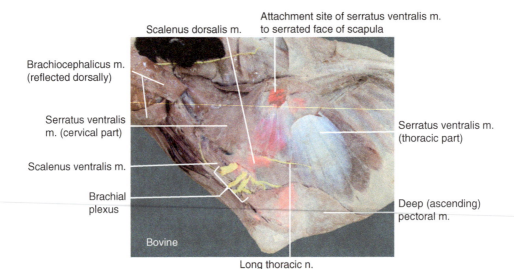

Figure 2.7 Bovine thoracic wall: left lateral view. The left thoracic limb is removed. Note the extent of the thoracic and cervical parts of the serratus ventralis muscle.

muscles. Note the interdigitation of the thoracic part of the serratus ventralis thoracis with the origin of the external abdominal oblique muscle on the ventral surface of the thorax (Figure 2.5).

Next, remove or reflect the latissimus dorsi muscle dorsally to uncover the dorsal part of the thoracic serratus ventralis muscle (Figure 2.6). To expose the rhomboideus muscle, transect the cervical and thoracic parts of the trapezius muscle and reflect them dorsally (Figure 2.6).

Transect some of the superficial neck muscles as shown in Figure 2.6 to uncover the cervical part of the serratus ventralis muscle. Reflect the serratus dorsalis cranialis dorsally to identify the **epaxial muscles** as a group. (There is no need to identify individual muscles; Figure 2.6.)

Remove the thoracic limb by severing several extrinsic muscles. Abduct the limb and, with the use of a long knife, make a circular cut starting from the pectoral muscles ventrally in the area between the thoracic limbs. Cut the axillary vessels and branches of the brachial plexus. Keep abducting the limb until the medial surface of the scapula is separated from the serratus ventralis muscle. Cut the attachment of the dorsal border of the scapula with the trapezius muscle (this may have already been done) and the thoracic and cervical parts of the rhomboideus muscle and remove the limb. You should end up with a view similar to Figure 2.7.

Identify the **long thoracic nerve** coursing caudally on the dorsal border of the scalenus dorsalis muscle. More caudally, the nerve courses on the lateral surface of the serratus ventralis muscle. The long thoracic nerve supplies the serratus ventralis muscle.

Now we are ready to enter the thorax. Remove all of the muscles on the thoracic wall until you uncover the ribs. Care is necessary when removing the intercostal muscles. By making vertical cuts along the cranial and caudal borders of the ribs (watch out for embalming fluid oozing out), being careful not to cut too deep, remove the muscles between all ribs.

Notice the **intercostal vessels** and **nerves** (vein, artery, and nerve) running along the caudal border of each rib. At the costochondral junctions, these neurovascular bundles are present along both the cranial and caudal borders of the ribs. They are more visible inside the thorax deep to the transparent costal pleura.

You may choose one of two methods to expose thoracic viscera.

Method 1: Once you have cleaned the muscles of the thoracic wall, use a large nipper, pruning shears, or saw to cut each of the ribs at their vertebral and sternal attachments and along the costal arch but leave the first two ribs in place. These two ribs will be removed later when you are ready to visualize the vessels and nerves in the cranial thoracic region (Figure 2.8).

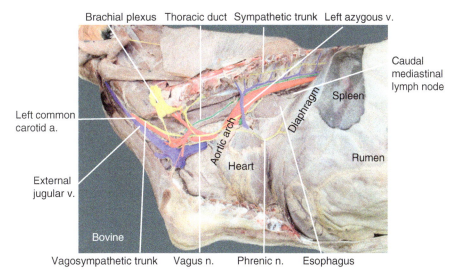

Figure 2.8 Bovine left thoracic and cranial abdominal cavities. Identify the major vessels and nerves on the left thoracic cavity.
* Longus colli m.

Method 2: This method is suitable for small and large cadavers laid on the table. It is described in Appendix A. In this method, reflect the ribs dorsally and cut the diaphragm and abdominal wall ventrally along the dorsal edge of the rectus abdominis muscle. Reflect the ribs and abdominal muscles dorsally as a single flap (see Figure A.2 in Appendix A).

In both methods, use your probe and forceps to perform blunt dissection of intrathoracic structures.

Within the thorax, identify the transversus thoracis muscle fibers coursing on a transverse plane over the dorsal aspect of the sternum. The **internal thoracic artery** and **vein** run deep to this muscle. Remember that these vessels are found on the other side of the body. Dorsally, identify the **longus colli muscle** as it courses from under the body of caudal cervical vertebrae passing through the thoracic inlet to continue along the ventral surface of the bodies of the first few thoracic vertebrae (Figure 2.5).

2.7 Pleura

Goal: Identify left and right lung lobes. Study the different parts of the pleura (parietal pleura [costal, diaphragmatic, and mediastinal], visceral [or pulmonary] pleura, and connecting pleura). Identify the location of the thymus, caudal mediastinal lymph nodes, and major bloods vessels, autonomic ganglia, and nerves (vagus and phrenic nerves, and sympathetic trunk and ganglia). Explain the meaning of the term "mediastinum" and its contents. Study the superficial and internal features of the heart.

Before you disturb or remove any structure, study the **pleura**, and **lung lobes**. The thin transparent serous membrane (mesothelium) that lines the interior of the thoracic cavity and its contents is the pleura. Depending on where it is located or what it covers, the pleura is divided into **parietal, visceral (pulmonary),** or **connecting pleura.**

Again, note the vessels and nerves running at the caudal border of each rib. These are **intercostal arteries, veins** and **nerves**.

2.7.1 Parietal Pleura

The parietal pleura covers interior thoracic walls such as those of the ribs and diaphragm. It is attached to the ribs and diaphragm by a thin layer of connective tissue known as **endothoracic fascia.** Identify the following types of parietal pleura:

- *Costal parietal pleura:* covers the interior wall of the rib cage.

- *Diaphragmatic parietal pleura:* covers the thoracic surface of the diaphragm.
- *Mediastinal parietal pleura:* creates the thin partition (mediastinum) between the left and right pleural cavities.

2.7.2 Visceral Pleura

The visceral pleura is also known as the **pulmonary pleura**. It covers all surfaces of the lungs.

2.7.3 Connecting Pleura

An example of connecting pleura is the **pulmonary ligament** that connects the visceral pleura on the caudal lobe of the lung to the mediastinal pleura (Figure 2.9d). Lift the caudal lobe of the lung cranially to observe the pulmonary ligament. In small animals, this ligament is transected in surgery when the caudal lobe of the lung is removed.

Plica vena cava is another example of connecting pleura. It runs from the ventral surface of the caudal vena cava to the floor of the caudal mediastinum and diaphragm.

The pleural sac on the right side extends through the thoracic inlet beyond the first rib. This cup-shaped extension is known as the **cupula pleura.** The left pleural sac does not extend beyond the first rib.

2.7.4 Content of the Pleural Cavity

The pleural cavity has nothing inside but a small amount of serous fluid. The fluid helps in friction-free movement of the lungs as they expand with air during inspiration.

2.7.5 Lung Lobes

Identify the lung lobes. The **left lung** has **cranial** and **caudal lobes** (Figure 2.9a,b). A notch divides the cranial lobe into **cranial** and **caudal parts**. The **left cardiac notch** typically is located between the third and sixth rib in the live animal. Consult Box 2.5 for clinical applications related to the lungs.

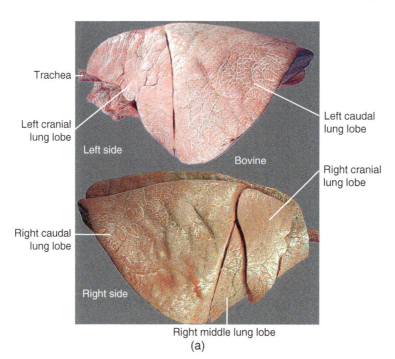

Figure 2.9 (a) Inflated fresh left and right views of bovine lungs; (b) inflated fresh bovine lungs (dorsal and ventral views. 1) right cranial lung lobe, 2) right middle lung lobe.); (c) reflection of the right bovine lung to expose the bronchi on the right side: note the bifurcation of the tracheal bronchus into the cranial and caudal parts of the right lung cranial lobe; (d) medial surfaces of the left (a) and right (b) bovine lungs; (e) dorsal view of lamb lungs. Source: Minnesota Veterinary Anatomy, University of Minnesota.

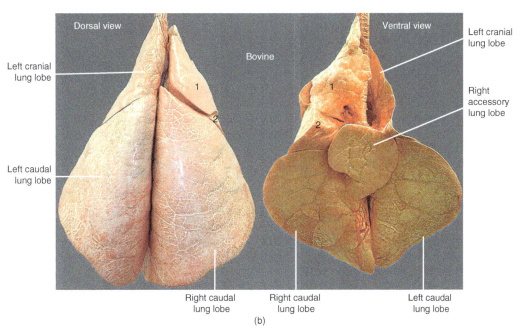
(b)

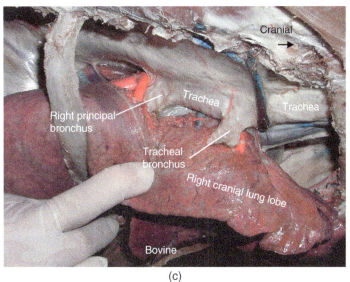
(c)

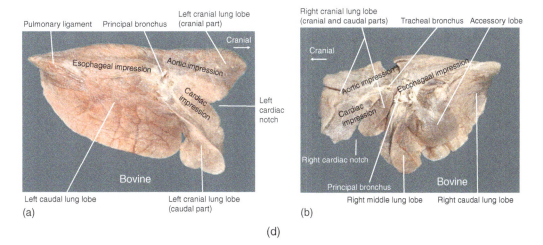
(d)

Figure 2.9 (Continued)

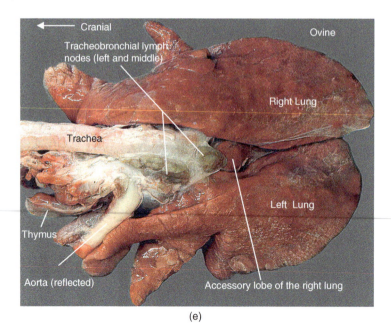

(e)

Figure 2.9 (Continued)

The **right lung** has four lobes: **cranial, middle, caudal**, and **accessory lobes**.

The cranial lobe of the right lung is separately ventilated by a special **tracheal bronchus** that arises directly from the trachea (Figure 2.9c). The trachea then terminates caudally by bifurcating into the right and left principal bronchi (Figure 2.9d). In a fresh lung, you will be able to identify the tracheobronchial lymph nodes at the terminal bifurcation of the trachea (Figure 2.9e).

Remove the lungs by reflecting them dorsally and cutting the vessels at the hilus or root of the lung. Stay close to the root of lung and be careful not to cut the phrenic nerve and branches of the vagus nerve that are close to the surface of the heart.

Study the mediastinum and remove the mediastinal pleura to study the heart, lymphocenters, vessels cranial to the heart, topography of the trachea and esophagus, thoracic duct, pathway of the vagus nerves, and sympathetic trunk (Figure 2.8).

2.7.6 Mediastinum

The mediastinum is the partition between the left and right pleural cavity. It consists of the mediastinal pleurae and organs contained between them including the thymus, heart, trachea, esophagus, and major blood vessels. It is divided into **cranial, middle,** and **caudal mediastinum.** Examples of organs in the three parts of the mediastinum include the thymus in cranial mediastinum, heart in the middle mediastinum, and caudal portion of thoracic aorta and caudal portion of the esophagus in the caudal mediastinum. Other structures traverse the cranial, middle and caudal mediastinum (e.g. phrenic nerve, vagus nerve, and esophagus). Consult Box 2.6 for clinical application related to the mediastinum.

> **Box 2.6**
>
> In ruminants, the mediastinum is relatively thick compared with the relatively thin and perforated caudal mediastinum in horses. This suggests that cattle can sustain a unilateral infection without affecting the other side of the pleural cavity or unilateral pneumothorax.

2.8 Vessels (Arteries and Veins)

Goal: Identify the major vessels and veins on the left and right thoracic cavity. Understand the blood pathway in the pulmonary, coronary, and systemic circulations.

2.8.1 Blood Circulation: An Overview

Before you start identifying blood vessels, it is important to have a broad understanding of blood circulation and the structures (vessels and valves) involved in the regulation of blood within the heart (Figure 2.10).

Briefly, the blood circulation can be divided into **pulmonary, coronary,** and **systemic circulations.**

The pulmonary circulation helps circulate blood between the heart and lungs, and vice versa. The **systemic circulation** distributes oxygenated (arterial) blood from the left side of the heart to the body and brings nonoxygenated (venous) blood back to the right side of the heart (Figures 2.10a,b). **The coronary circulation** circulates blood to and from the heart muscles.

In the systemic circulation, blood returns to the right atrium by the **cranial** and **caudal venae cavae** and the **coronary sinus**.

Venous blood returns to the right side of the heart (right atrium and ventricle) by the caudal (1) and cranial (2) venae cavae. Relatively unoxygenated blood from the right side of the heart (right ventricle) passes to the lungs through the pulmonary trunk (dotted lines) that gives the left and right pulmonary arteries. From the lungs, oxygenated blood passes by several pulmonary veins to the left side of the heart (left atrium and ventricle). Oxygenated blood from the left ventricle is distributed to the body (systemic circulation) by the way of the aorta and named branches. Blood outflow from the pulmonary trunk and aorta is regulated by semilunar valves located in the right and left ventricles, respectively. Blood flow from the atria to the ventricles is regulated by right and left atrioventricular valves (R-AV and L-AV). Venous return from the gastrointestinal tract (GI) is channeled through the portal vein to the liver for detoxification before joining the caudal vena cava by the hepatic veins. Circulatory diseases such as patent ductus arteriosus, persistent foramen ovalae, intra- and extrahepatic shunts are clinically more important in small animals. AV-M, left atrioventricular valve (mitral); AV-T, right atrioventricular valve (tricuspid).

From the right atrium, blood passes into the right ventricle through the **right atrioventricular valve** (right AV or tricuspid valve). The venous blood is then ejected from the right ventricle into the pulmonary trunk through the opening of the **pulmonary semilunar valve.**

From the **pulmonary trunk**, relatively unoxygenated blood passes into the **left** and **right pulmonary arteries** to the left and right lungs, respectively. The left and right pulmonary arteries are the only arteries in the adult body that carry relatively unoxygenated blood.

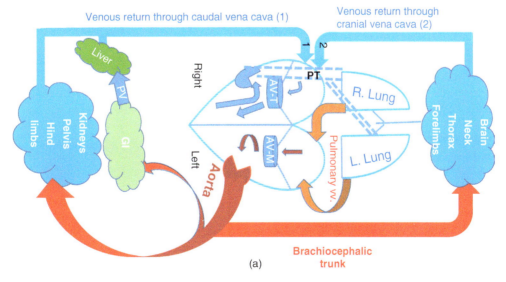

Figure 2.10 (a) Simplified overview of systemic and pulmonary circulations; (b) llama mediastinal dissection showing major vessels of the heart. Source: Minnesota Veterinary Anatomy, University of Minnesota.

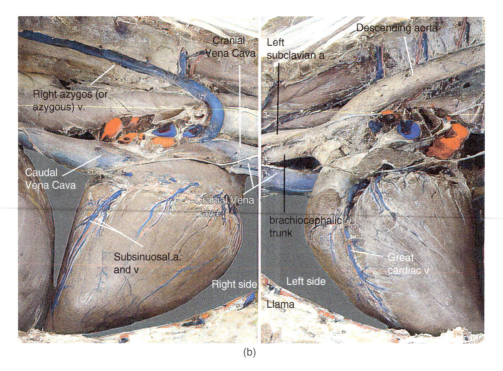

(b)

Figure 2.10 (Continued)

A variable number of **pulmonary veins** carry more oxygenated blood from the lungs to the left atrium. These are the only veins in the adult body that carry oxygenated blood.

The pulmonary trunk, pulmonary arteries, lungs, and pulmonary veins constitute the pulmonary circulation.

From the left atrium, blood passes through the **left atrioventricular valve (left AV or mitral valve)** into the left ventricle. Relatively oxygenated blood from the left ventricle is pumped via the aortic semilunar valve into the ascending and descending aorta for distribution to various parts of the body, including heart muscles as the first tissue to receive oxygenated blood.

The thoracic aorta is generally divided into three topographic regions: **ascending, aortic arch,** and **descending aorta.**

Blood to the head, neck, and thoracic limbs passes cranially in the **brachiocephalic trunk.** The trunk arises from the aortic arch (Figures 2.10a,b and 2.11). Major branches of the brachiocephalic trunk in ruminants are the left subclavian artery, bicarotid trunk, and right subclavian artery (Figures 2.10b and 2.11).

In small animals (dogs and cats), the left subclavian artery originates directly from the aortic arch and the brachiocephalic trunk separately gives rise to the left and right common carotid arteries and the right subclavian artery.

2.9 Major Veins of the Thorax

Goal: Identify the cranial and caudal venae cavae, left and right azygos veins.

2.9.1 Cranial Vena Cava

The cranial vena cava drains the blood from the head and neck region. It empties into the right atrium of the heart. Identify this vessel in the cranial mediastinum (Figure 2.11).

2.9.2 Caudal Vena Cava

The caudal vena cava runs to the right side of the caudal mediastinum to open into the right atrium of the

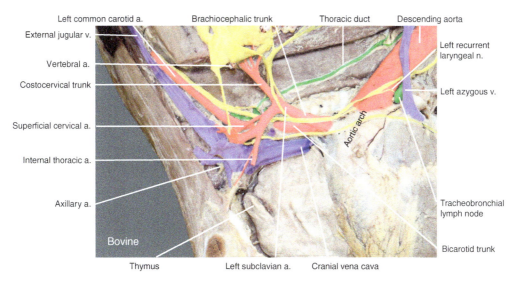

Figure 2.11 Bovine left thorax (cranial part). Figure shows vessels and nerves cranial to the heart. Nerves are labeled in Figure 2.12.

heart. It drains venous blood from the caudal part of the body (abdomen, pelvis, and hind limbs). It passes through the diaphragm via the **caval foramen**. Identify the caudal vena cava and the plica vena cava.

2.9.3 Azygos Veins (Left and Right)

The word "azygos" means "unpaired." The **right azygos vein** is present in ruminants, camelids, horses, dogs, and cats. It drains venous blood from the thoracic wall (intercostal veins) and empties into the **cranial vena cava**. It may not be present in the last few intercostal spaces.

The **left azygos vein** (Figures 2.8–2.11) is present in ruminants and swine but is absent in camelids, carnivores (dogs and cats) and equine (horses and donkeys). In ruminants, the left azygos vein drains into the **coronary sinus** of the right atrium (Figure 2.11).

2.10 Major Arteries of the Thorax

Goal: With the help of Figure 2.11 and the following description, identify some of the major vessels cranial to the heart. These include the brachiocephalic trunk and branches of the subclavian artery. These vessels will be identified on the left thorax.

2.10.1 Brachiocephalic Trunk

The **brachiocephalic trunk** originates from the aortic arch. Unlike in dogs and cats, the brachiocephalic trunk is the only vessel that originates from the aortic arch in ruminants and horses.

In ruminants, the left subclavian is a branch of the brachiocephalic trunk. The brachiocephalic trunk therefore gives rise to all of the arteries in the cranial thorax. (Figure 2.11).

Branches of the brachiocephalic trunk include the **left** and **right subclavian arteries** and the **bicarotid trunk** that gives rise to the left and right **common carotid arteries.**

Identify the **bicarotid trunk** and follow its division into left and right **common carotid arteries** (Figure 2.11).

The left and right **subclavian arteries** give similar branches. Study the branches of the left subclavian artery. Branches of the left subclavian artery include the **costocervical trunk, vertebral, superficial cervical**, and **internal thoracic** arteries. Continuation of the subclavian artery outside the thorax (beyond the medial surface of the first rib) into the thoracic limb is by the **axillary artery**.

There follows a brief description of the four branches of the subclavian artery. Understand that variations in the origin of these arteries are not uncommon.

2.10.2 Costocervical Trunk

The costocervical trunk is the first branch of the subclavian artery. The trunk gives rise to the first few dorsal intercostal arteries. The rest of the dorsal intercostal arteries originate from the thoracic (descending) aorta. The next branch of the costocervical trunk is the deep cervical artery. It supplies the muscles in the dorsal caudal neck region.

No need to identify branches of the costocervical trunk.

2.10.3 Vertebral Artery

The vertebral artery courses deep in the neck to pass through the transverse foramina of C1–C6 cervical vertebrae. It supplies the brain, and in its course through the neck, gives spinal branches to the spinal cord. Identify the vertebral artery (Figure 2.11). It may originate from the costocervical trunk.

2.10.4 Superficial Cervical Artery

The **superficial cervical artery** enters to the caudal neck region by coursing through the thoracic inlet (Figure 2.11). It gives off branches to the craniolateral shoulder region. Find the superficial cervical artery at the thoracic inlet opposite the internal thoracic artery (Figure 2.11).

2.10.5 Internal Thoracic Artery

The **internal thoracic artery** branches from the subclavian artery and runs ventrally toward the sternum. It courses caudally under the transversus thoracis muscle. Reflect this muscle to note the ventral intercostal arteries arising from the internal thoracic artery. The ventral intercostal arteries anastomose with the dorsal intercostal. At the caudal aspect of the sternum, the internal thoracic artery passes out of the thorax and its name is changed to the cranial epigastric artery. Locate the internal thoracic artery at the point where it originates from the subclavian artery opposite the superficial cervical artery.

In ruminants, the cranial epigastric artery gives rise to the cranial superficial epigastric artery that tunnels out of the abdominal wall to course toward the udder in the female or penis in the male. The cranial epigastric artery continues caudally on the dorsal (deep) surface of the rectus abdominis.

The cranial superficial epigastric artery forms an anastomosis with the caudal superficial epigastric artery. Similar arrangements occur with satellite veins (**cranial and caudal superficial epigastric veins**). The combined vein is known as the **milk vein.** The milk vein is very large in lactating cows. The milk vein enters the thorax near the xiphoid cartilage. The point of entrance is known as the **milk well**.

The continuation of the subclavian artery beyond the first rib is the **axillary artery** that supplies the thoracic limb (Figure 2.11).

2.11 Lymphatic Structures

Goal: Identify the thymus and thoracic duct on the left side of the thorax. The lymph nodes of the thorax are variable. Identify the major lymph nodes, especially the tracheobronchial and mediastinal lymph nodes. Pay specific attention to the well-developed caudal mediastinal lymph node and know its clinical significance (Box 2.7).

Box 2.7

Excessive enlargement of the caudal mediastinal lymph node may put pressure on the esophagus and the dorsal vagal trunk in the caudal mediastinum. This could lead to difficulty in the process of swallowing, digestion, and gas eructation.

A condition called vagal indigestion results from irritation of the vagal nerve and results in the disruption of normal rumen motility, rumen tympany (bloat), and abdominal distention.

Esophageal choke: there are four common sites for foreign bodies or food boluses to lodge in the esophagus. These include:

- Over the larynx (at the beginning of the esophagus)
- At the thoracic inlet (due to the sharp angulation of the esophagus and the crowded thoracic inlet)
- Over the base of the heart
- In an area just cranial to or at the esophageal hiatus

2.11.1 Thymus

The thymus is a lymphoid organ important in early life for the process of maturation and programming of T lymphocytes. This process allows T lymphocytes the ability to differentiate self from nonself antigens. Typically, it is located in the cranial mediastinum in front of the heart and dorsal to the cranial part of the sternum (Figure 2.11).

In young animals, the thymus may extend midway into the neck region. The thymus regresses in size in old animals where it is replaced by fat and connective tissue. In some cadavers of old animals, it may be difficult to identify the remnant of the thymus.

2.11.2 Thoracic Duct

The thoracic duct drains lymph from the abdominal, pelvic cavity, hind limb, and left side of the thorax (Figure 2.11).

The thoracic duct originates from a pooling space for lymph caudal to the diaphragm known as **cisterna chyli.** From the cisterna chyli, the thoracic duct passes into the thorax through the **aortic hiatus** of the diaphragm.

In the thorax, the thoracic duct lies initially on the right side, between the right azygos vein and thoracic aorta or dorsal to the aorta. In the mid-thorax, it crosses over to the left side to run below the longus colli muscle toward the thoracic inlet. It drains variably into the large veins at the thoracic inlet; this can include the cranial vena cava or left external jugular vein and left subclavian vein.

Other structures that pass through the aortic hiatus, in addition to the thoracic duct, include the **aorta** and **left and right azygos veins**.

2.11.3 Mediastinal and Tracheobronchial Lymph Nodes

Lymph nodes located in the thorax include **sternal (cranial** and **caudal group), intercostal,** and **thoracic aortic lymph nodes, mediastinal** group **(cranial, middle,** and **caudal),** and **tracheobronchial lymph nodes.** The presence of these nodes is variable. For the sake of time and to avoid confusion in assigning mediastinal lymph nodes to a particular group, identify only the tracheobronchial and caudal mediastinal lymph nodes (Figures 2.8, 2.9e, 2.12, and 2.13a,b).

The tracheobronchial lymph nodes drain the lungs. In the intact animal, they are located at the bifurcation of the trachea into two principal bronchi. They are inspected during meat inspection. They include left, right, cranial, and middle groups. In your specimen, some of these lymph nodes will be transected or removed with the lungs. Look for tracheobronchial

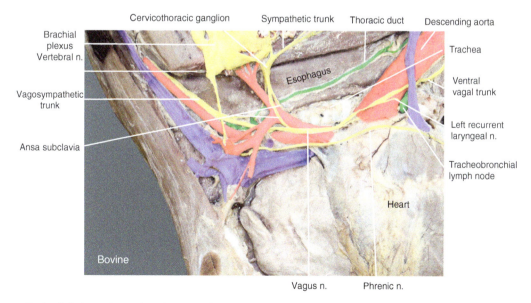

Figure 2.12 Bovine left thorax (cranial part). Figure shows major nerves cranial to the heart.

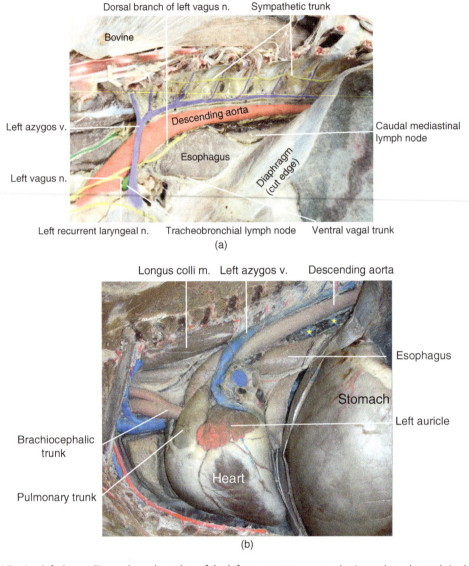

Figure 2.13 (a) Bovine left thorax. Figure shows branches of the left vagus nerve, sympathetic trunk, and vessels in the caudal thoracic region; (b) ovine mediastinal dissection. Yellow stars show the location of the caudal mediastinal lymph node. Source: Minnesota Veterinary Anatomy, University of Minnesota.

lymph nodes at the caudal aspect of the aortic arch (Figures 2.11 and 2.13b).

The **caudal mediastinal lymph nodes** are of clinical interest in ruminants. Typically, a single, large, elongated lymph node is present in the caudal mediastinum between the aorta and esophagus (Figure 2.11). Because of their considerable length (~15 cm or more), the caudal mediastinal lymph node is sometimes likened to a cigar.

2.12 Nerves (Motor Somatic, Sympathetic, and Parasympathetic)

Goal: Identify the phrenic nerve, branches of the vagus nerve, thoracic sympathetic trunk, and associated autonomic ganglia. Know the difference between the origin of the left and right recurrent laryngeal nerves from the vagus. Understand that the nerves of the thorax are bilateral.

You will identify these nerves on the left side (Figures 2.8–2.12).

The nerves within the thorax can be classified as motor somatic nerve (intercostal, phrenic, and recurrent laryngeal nerves), motor (visceral or autonomic) parasympathetic (e.g., thoracic part of the vagus nerve), and motor (visceral or autonomic) sympathetic nerves and ganglia (e.g., thoracic sympathetic trunk, ansa subclavia, and sympathetic chain ganglia). The parasympathetic ganglia are embedded within the target organs and cannot be identified grossly.

2.12.1 Phrenic Nerve

The phrenic nerve innervates the diaphragm (skeletal muscle). It originates from caudal ventral (C6-7) spinal cervical nerves and courses to the diaphragm along the lateral surface of the heart.

Identify the left phrenic nerve and trace with your probe to the diaphragm (Figures 2.8–2.12). The phrenic nerve has somatic motor fibers.

2.12.2 Autonomic Nerves in the Thorax

Goal: With the help of Figures 2.8, 2.12, and 2.13, identify the vagus nerve and follow its divisions on the left side of the thorax (same divisions are present on the right side with the exception of variation in the origin and location of the right recurrent laryngeal nerve).

At the vertebral ends of the ribs, trace the sympathetic trunk from the caudal thorax cranially to the cervicothoracic ganglion at the vertebral ends of the first to third ribs. Identify the cervicothoracic ganglion by tracing the caudal and cranial limbs of the ansa subclavia around the left subclavian artery (Figure 2.12).

2.12.3 Vagus Nerve

The vagus nerve carries motor autonomic parasympathetic fibers to the neck, thoracic, and abdominal viscera. It also carries the fibers of the recurrent laryngeal nerve (somatic motor) fibers that supply the skeletal muscles of the larynx. The vagus also carries sensory fibers from the aforementioned viscera.

With the help of Figures 2.12 and 2.13, identify the left vagus nerve, the dorsal and ventral vagal trunks, and left recurrent laryngeal nerve on the left side of the thorax.

Follow the course of the left vagus nerve from the thoracic inlet caudally until it passes to the abdomen through the esophageal hiatus (an opening on the diaphragm below the aortic hiatus). At the aortic arch, the left vagus gives rise to the **left recurrent laryngeal nerve** (Figures 2.8–2.12). This nerve courses back cranially along the trachea to supply the laryngeal muscles (more will be said about this nerve later).

The **right recurrent laryngeal** nerve originates from the right vagus nerve at the level of the thoracic inlet and right subclavian artery.

The vagus nerve gives parasympathetic cardiac branches to the heart.

Caudal to the heart, each vagus nerve divides into dorsal and ventral branches. The left and right ventral branches of the left and right vagus nerves join together to form a single **ventral vagal trunk.** This trunk courses toward the diaphragm under the ventral surface of the esophagus.

The left and right dorsal branches from the left and right vagus nerves join together more caudally (close to the esophageal hiatus) to form the **dorsal vagal trunk**. This trunk runs toward the diaphragm along the dorsal surface of the esophagus. The ventral and dorsal vagal trunks pass into the abdomen through the **esophageal hiatus**.

The recurrent laryngeal nerve courses cranially through the neck along the ventrolateral surface of the trachea. The nerve terminates in the caudal region of the larynx where it is referred to as the **caudal laryngeal** nerve.

Recall that the left and right recurrent laryngeal nerves innervate all of the laryngeal muscles except the cricothyroideus muscle (supplied by cranial laryngeal nerve from the vagus nerve in the cranial part of the neck).

Of the muscles supplied by the recurrent (caudal laryngeal) nerve, the cricoarytenoideus dorsalis muscle is the only muscle that opens the glottis.

In the horse, damage to the recurrent laryngeal nerve causes laryngeal hemiplegia, a condition known as roaring. This condition mostly involves damage to the left recurrent laryngeal nerve leading to a narrowing of the glottis and generation of a roaring noise during inspiration.

2.12.4 Sympathetic Trunk and Sympathetic Ganglia

Identify **the vagosympathetic trunk** in the neck coursing on the dorsal aspect of the common carotid artery. Follow the trunk caudally to the thoracic inlet. Here the trunk splits into the vagus nerve (coursing toward the heart) and thoracic sympathetic trunk (coursing dorsally toward the longus colli muscle).

Near the separation of the vagus and sympathetic trunk, you **may** see an enlargement. If so, this represents the **middle cervical ganglion**. Extending dorsally from this ganglion, there is a nerve loop around the subclavian artery that connects the middle cervical and **cervicothoracic ganglia**. This loop is known as the **ansa subclavia** (Figure 2.12).

2.13 Heart (Cor)

Goal: Know the atrial and auricular surfaces of the heart. Use the cow skeleton to identify the rib boundaries for listening to the heart sounds. Understand that the heart in the live animal lies between the plane of the third and fifth intercostal space, mostly to the left side of the thorax. The area for heart sounds is therefore mostly covered by the forelimb. Your instructor, depending on your knowledge of the subject, will determine the level of details required.

Build a mental picture of the location of the heart in situ. On an isolated heart, examine the exterior and interior structures of the heart including the fibrous sac covering the heart (pericardium), heart chambers, and heart valves.

The heart lies in the middle mediastinum mostly to the left side of the median plane. The base of the heart faces dorsally and the apex lies ventrally close to the sternum. Within the mediastinum, the heart is surrounded by the pericardium.

2.13.1 Pericardium

The pericardium is the sac that surrounds the heart. It has both **fibrous** and **serous layers,** and a paper-thin **pericardial cavity** that contains a small amount of serous fluid. Superficially, the pericardial sac is intimately surrounded by a serous membrane, the parietal **mediastinal pleura** (Figure 2.14). Consult Box 2.8 for clinical application.

The serous pericardium is sometimes divided into **parietal layer of the serous pericardium** and **visceral layer of the serous pericardium** (Figure 2.14b). The parietal layer of the serous pericardium is adhered to the inner layer of the fibrous pericardium. The visceral layer of serous pericardium is the **epicardium or visceral layer of the serous pericardium**.

With the help of Figure 2.14, study the layers that make up the **pericardium**. As you can see, the fibrous pericardium is interposed between the mediastinal pleura and the parietal layer of the serous pericardium.

From superficial to deep, the pericardium includes the **fibrous pericardium** (the strongest layer of the pericardium), the **parietal layer of the serous pericardium,** and finally the **visceral layer of the serous pericardium** closely adhered to the heart wall. The visceral layer of the serous pericardium is also called the **epicardium.** A space (**pericardial cavity**) lies between the parietal and visceral serous pericardium. It has a small amount of fluid that helps in friction-free contraction of the heart.

Understand that the **mediastinal pleura**, the **fibrous pericardium,** and the **parietal layer of the serous pericardium** are closely fused to each other and are inseparable. Clinicians often refer to these fused layers as the pericardium.

The extension of the fibrous pericardium, **sternopericardial ligament**, anchors the heart to the sternum. This ligament is called **phrenicopericardial ligament** in dogs because it attaches the more obliquely oriented dog heart to the diaphragm instead of the sternum.

2.13.2 External Features of the Heart

Study features of the heart on an isolated fresh or preserved (formaldehyde fixed or plastinated) specimen.

The heart has four chambers (two atria and two ventricles) separated by interatrial and interventricular septa.

Topographically, the left surface of the heart is called the **auricular surface** (the view with two auricles seen hugging the pulmonary trunk). The heart is rotated about its vertical axis to the left side

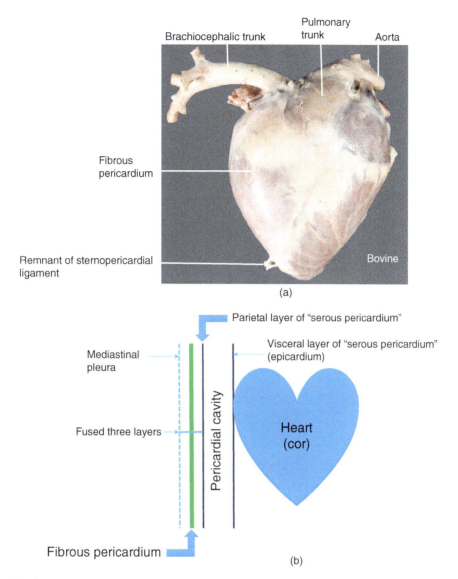

Figure 2.14 (a) Isolated bovine heart (auricular surface). Figure shows fibrous pericardium covering the auricular (left) surface of the heart; (b) schematic illustration of the layers of the pericardium. Understand that the layers of the pericardium form a sac around the heart. The fibrous pericardium extends ventrally from the apex of the heart to form the **sternopericardial ligament** that anchors the heart to the sternum (not illustrated). The outer three layers (with the fibrous pericardium being the thickest) are fused and are inseparable. The pericardial cavity is a very small capillary space filled with a small amount of serous fluid. The visceral layer of the serous pericardium (or the epicardium) adheres closely to the wall of the heart.

Box 2.8
The fibrous pericardium is the strongest layer of the pericardium. Although mild distortion in the pericardium occurs during heart cycle, the fibrous pericardium prevents significant changes or distortion in heart shape that can occur in heart contraction or in heart diseases where excessive fluid could accumulate in the pericardial cavity.

with the right auricle seen on the left side. The right surface is the atrial surface.

The heart has a wide dorsal **base** and a ventral tapering end **apex**. The apex is formed only by the left ventricle.

With help of Figure 2.15, study the following superficial features of the heart:

1) **Atria** (left and right). Use your probe to identify the cranial and caudal venae cavae entering the right atrium. The left atrium receives several pulmonary veins. They bring relatively oxygenated blood from the lungs to the heart.
2) **Auricles** (left and right). The auricles are blind extensions of the atria that provide additional space for blood and have an endocrine function.
3) **Ventricles** (left and right), the left ventricle is thicker and forms the apex of the heart.
4) Grooves:

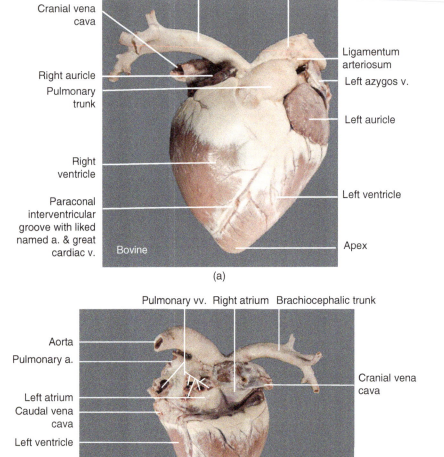

Figure 2.15 Bovine heart. External features of the heart on (a) auricular (left) surface; (b) atrial (right) surface.

- **Paraconal interventricular groove:** lies caudal and parallel to the conus arteriosus on the auricular surface of the heart, hence the name. The paraconal interventricular branch of the left coronary artery and the great cardiac vein course within this groove.
- **(Subsinuosal) interventricular and intermediate grooves:** lies on the caudal aspect of the heart below the coronary sinus, hence the name. The subsinuosal interventricular branch of the left coronary artery and middle cardiac vein course within the subsinuosal groove. An intermediate groove is found in close proximity to the subsinuosal groove in the caudal aspect of the heart in ruminants. The caudal cardiac vein and an intermediate branch of the left coronary artery courses into it.
- **Coronary groove:** separates the atria from the ventricles. The left and right coronary arteries course within the coronary groove.

5) **Conus arteriosus:** The portion of the right ventricle as it approaches the pulmonary trunk is shaped like a cone, hence the name **conus arteriosus** of this region of the heart. Briefly, the conus arteriosus is defined as the outflow tract of the right ventricle.

6) **Pulmonary trunk** and **pulmonary arteries:** The pulmonary trunk carries relatively deoxygenated blood from the right ventricle toward the lungs. It branches into the left and right pulmonary arteries. Identify the **ligamentum arteriosum** between the pulmonary trunk and the aortic arch.

7) **Aortic arch:** The aorta in the thorax is divided into ascending aorta, aortic arch, and descending aorta (Figure 2.11). The left and right coronary arteries that supply the heart wall originate from the ascending aorta. No need to identify the ascending aorta. The aortic arch gives one large vessel, the brachiocephalic trunk.

8) **Brachiocephalic trunk:** The brachiocephalic trunk is the only vessel originating from the aortic arch in ruminants and horses. It gives four vessels (discussed earlier).

9) **Ligamentum arteriosum,** a fibrous structure connecting the pulmonary trunk with the aortic arch. It is the remnant of a fetal shunt that connects these two vessels.

2.13.3 Interior of the Heart

Goal: With the help of Figures 2.16 and 2.17, study the interior of the heart on transverse and vertical sections of the right atrium and right ventricle, respectively. Study the heart valves on a transverse section cut at the level of the coronary groove.

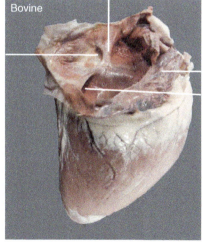

Figure 2.16 Bovine heart. Right atrium opened to show interior structures.

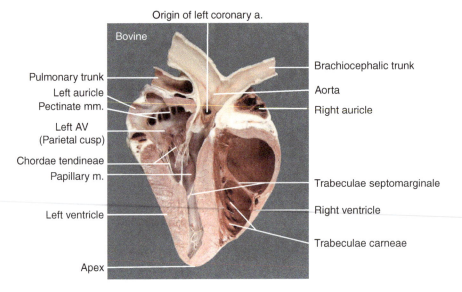

Figure 2.17 Bovine heart: sagittal section. Note the difference in wall thickness of the right (thin) and left (thick) ventricles. The term "trabeculae septomarginale" is plural for trabecula septomarginalis.

With the help of Figure 2.16, open the right atrium by making a transverse incision from the cranial vena cava across the lateral wall of the atrium to the caudal vena cava. Expand the ventral incision to the level of the right atrioventricular valve and to the right auricle.

With the help of Figure 2.16 and the following discussion, identify the **intervenous tubercle, fossa ovalis, coronary sinus, foramina for the cranial** and **caudal vena cava,** and **pectinate muscles** on the right atrium.

2.13.3.1 Structures of the Right Atrium

- **Intervenous tubercle:** a vertical ridge that courses midway between the openings of the cranial and caudal venae cavae (Figure 2.16). The intervenous tubercle is thought to direct the blood from the caval openings ventrally toward the right atrioventricular valves, thus decreasing blood turbulence that might have resulted from the collision of the two blood streams.
- **Fossa ovalis:** a depression behind the intervenous tubercle. It faces the opening of the caudal vena cava. The fossa is a remnant of the *foramen ovalis* in the fetus that connects the right and left atrium (Figure 2.16).
- **Coronary sinus:** look for the coronary sinus opening below the opening of the caudal vena cava (Figure 2.16). The coronary sinus is where the **left azygos,** middle, caudal cardiac, and great cardiac veins empty.
- **The great cardiac vein:** one of the veins that drain the heart muscles. It opens into the coronary sinus. Look for the great cardiac vein coursing in the paraconal interventricular groove and coronary groove on the auricular surface (Figure 2.15a).
- **Pectinate muscles:** long round muscular bands occupying the interior wall of the auricles (Figure 2.17). Some are present in the atrial chamber. They reinforce the wall of the auricle.

2.13.3.2 Structures of the Right Ventricle

With the help of Figure 2.17 and the following discussion, identify the **chordae tendineae, papillary muscles, cusps for atrioventricular valves, right atrioventricular valve, trabecula septomarginalis, interventricular septum,** and **trabeculae carneae.**

Understand that the internal structures in the right ventricle are also present in the left ventricle. We will identify ventricular internal structures on the right ventricle because it has a relatively thin wall and larger cavity compared with the left ventricle. Identify the following structures within the right ventricle:

2.13.3.2.1 Right Atrioventricular Valve

The right atrioventricular valve (R-AV) regulates venous blood flow from the right atrium into the right ventricle where backflow is prevented during systole and permitted during diastole. This valve is also called **tricuspid valve.** Likewise, a **left atrioventricular ventricular (mitral) valve** permits the flow of arterial blood from the left atrium to the left ventricle during diastole and prevents backflow during systole.

2.13.3.2.2 Chordae Tendineae, Papillary Muscles, and Cusps of the Right Atrioventricular Valve

The **chordae tendineae** are thin fibrous cords that anchor the **cusps** of the atrioventricular valves to the tips of **papillary muscles** on the ventricular wall. This arrangement is likened to a parachute (Figure 2.17). The atrioventricular valve has parietal and septal **cusps** (flat connective tissue sheets) that close the atrioventricular opening.

The chordae tendineae help prevent eversion of the cusps dorsally into the atria during heart contraction (systole).

2.13.3.2.3 Trabecula Septomarginalis

The trabecula septomarginalis is a long circular muscular cord that transversely crosses the lumen of the ventricle. It extends from the interventricular septum to the lateral (parietal) wall of the ventricle. The origin on the septal wall is usually from a papillary muscle.

The trabecula septomarginalis contains Purkinje fibers that aid with fast signal conduction (quick detour) across the heart wall.

2.13.3.2.4 Ossa Cordis

The heart skeleton of adult ruminants (cattle, goats, and sheep) has two areas of ossification around the right and left semilunar cusps of the aortic valve known as **ossa cordis** (Figure 2.18). Sheep only have a single os cordis. These small bones support the aortic valve.

2.13.3.2.5 Coronary Arteries

The heart wall receives blood from the **left** and **right coronary arteries**. They are located within the left and right **coronary grooves**, respectively. The branching of the left and right coronary arteries in ruminants is similar to that of the dog but slightly different from the horse.

The substantial left coronary artery originates from the left aortic sinus just dorsal to the aortic valve. The left coronary artery gives rise to septal, **paraconal interventricular**, **circumflex**, **intermediate**, and **subsinuosal interventricular** branches. The septal artery is deeply located at the origin of the left coronary artery from the aorta. The septal artery arborizes

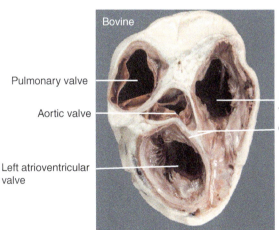

Figure 2.18 Bovine heart valves. Transverse section of the bovine heart at the level of the coronary groove: dorsal view. Singular for the term "ossa cordis" is os cordis.

deeply into the interventricular septum. It will not be identified.

The right coronary artery originates from the right aortic sinus. The right coronary artery is distributed mainly to the wall of the right ventricle with only a **circumflex branch** coursing within the right coronary groove. In general, the distribution of coronary arteries in ruminants is similar to that of dogs, but in horses, the subsinuosal interventricular branch originates from the right rather than the left coronary artery.

Clean the fat from the coronary groove (Figure 2.15a) to identify the left and right coronary arteries and their branches.

On a transverse section of the heart, identify the **aortic** and **pulmonary semilunar valves,** and right (tricuspid) and left (mitral) **atrioventricular valves** (Figure 2.18).

2.14 Point of Maximum Intensity or Puncta Maxima

Goal: You should know the landmarks that approximate the location of the heart valves on the left and right thoracic walls.

The PMI is defined as the location on the thoracic wall that provides maximum accentuation for audible sounds of the heart valves.

Three valves (**pulmonary, aortic,** and **mitral**) are auscultated on the left side, and one valve, the right atrioventricular valve (**R-AV**), is heard on the right side.

The location of the heart sounds on the left side of the thorax can be defined by the acronym PAM 345 low-high-low (**345-LHL**) for the **p**ulmonary, **a**ortic, and **m**itral (**PAM**) valves.

On the left chest, identify the following:

1) The pulmonary (**P**) valve may be best heard when the stethoscope is placed over the third intercostal space low at the costochondral junction (CCJ). (**3L**)
2) The aortic (**A**) valve may be best heard at the fourth intercostal space high just ventral to the shoulder joint. (**4H**)
3) The mitral (**M**) valve may be best heard at the fifth intercostal space low at the CCJ. (**5L**)
4) The **RAV** may be best heard on the right side at the third or fourth intercostal space (ICS) at the CCJ (**R-AV 3–4th ICS, low**). (**3–4 L**)

2.15 Lab ID List for the Thorax

There is no need to identify items in *italics*.

A. **Thoracic wall: bones and muscles**
   1. Boundaries for thoracic inlet
   2. Ribs
      a. Costochondral junction
      b. Costal arch
      c. Basal border of the lung
      d. Line of pleural reflection
      e. Intercostal spaces for listening to heart valves on left and right sides (puncta maxima)
   3. Sternum
      a. Sternebrae
      b. Manubrium
      c. Xiphoid process (with attached xiphoid cartilage)
   4. *Cutaneous trunci m.*
   5. *Cutaneous omobrachialis m.*
   6. Latissimus dorsi m.
   7. Deep pectoral m.
   8. Trapezius m. (thoracic part)
   9. *Intercostal muscles*
   10. *Epaxial muscles*
   11. Rhomboideus m. (thoracic part)
   12. Serratus ventralis m. (thoracic part)

B. **Thoracic viscera, vessels, and nerves**
   13. Thoracic duct
   14. *Intercostal arteries, veins, and nerves* (note location relative to rib margins)
   15. Lung lobes (left and right lungs)
   16. Tracheal bronchus (know clinical significance)
   17. Caudal mediastinal lymph node (know clinical significance)
   18. Phrenic n.
   19. Vagus n. (ventral and dorsal vagal trunks)
   20. Left recurrent laryngeal n.
   21. Tracheobronchial lymph nodes
   22. Sympathetic trunk
   23. Cervicothoracic ganglion
   24. Brachiocephalic trunk (Id branches: left subclavian a., bicarotid trunk, and right subclavian a.)

25. Pulmonary trunk
26. Cranial vena cava
27. Caudal vena cava
28. Left azygos v.
29. Right azygos v.
30. Thymus (young animal)
31. Longus colli m.
32. Trachea (thoracic part)
33. Esophagus (thoracic part)

C. **Heart external and internal structures (optional if done before)**
34. Base
35. Apex
36. Auricular surface (left)
37. Atrial surface (right)
38. Grooves (sulci)
    a. Paraconal interventricular groove (sulcus)
    b. Subsinuosal interventricular groove (sulcus)
    c. Intermediate groove (sulcus)
    d. Coronary groove (sulcus)
39. Right atrium
    a. Sinus venarum
    b. Right auricle
    c. Opening for cranial vena cava
    d. Opening for caudal vena cava
    e. Opening for coronary sinus
    f. Right atrioventricular valve and orifice (tricuspid)
    g. Intervenous tubercle
    h. Fossa ovalis (foramen ovale in fetus)
    i. Pectinate muscles
40. Pulmonary trunk
41. Pulmonary veins (openings in left atrium)
42. Left (mitral) and right (tricuspid) atrioventricular valve
    a. Parietal cusp
    b. Septal cusp
43. Right ventricle (note wall thickness compared with left ventricle)
44. Chordae tendineae
45. Papillary muscles
46. Trabeculae carneae
47. Trabecula septomarginalis
48. *Conus arteriosus*
49. Pulmonary valve (semilunar cusps, *nodule*)
50. Left atrium/left auricle
51. Ligamentum arteriosum (ductus arteriosus in fetus)
52. Aortic valve (semilunar cusps, *nodule*)
53. Right coronary artery
54. Left coronary artery
    a. Paraconal interventricular branch
    b. Circumflex branch
    c. Subsinuosal branch
    d. Intermediate branch
55. Great cardiac vein (or great coronary vein in paraconal interventricular groove or sulcus)
56. Middle cardiac vein (in subsinuosal groove)
57. Caudal cardiac vein (in intermediate groove)

3
The Abdomen

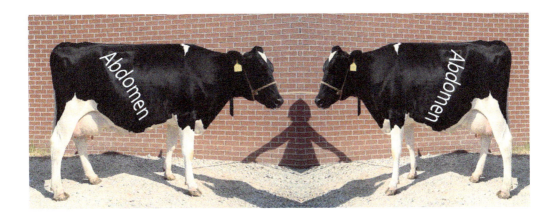

Learning Objectives

- Identify the muscles of the abdominal wall, rectus sheath, inguinal rings and canal, and the tunica flava abdominis that cover the external abdominal oblique muscle and help in supporting the heavy weight of the abdominal viscera.
- Study the innervation of the flank. Know the function and distribution of spinal nerves L1, L2, and T13 that innervate the paralumbar fossa and the rest of the flank region. These nerves are blocked at either the tips of the transverse processes or at the intervertebral foramina of lumbar vertebrae when performing flank anesthesia.
- Identify the greater and lesser omenta and the cavity and slings created by the disposition of the omenta (i.e., omental bursa and supraomental recess).
- Identify and know the topographic location of the different parts of the gastrointestinal tract, especially the complex features and compartments of the stomach and the ascending colon.
- Be able to trace a bolus of food from the mouth to the anus.
- Know the difference in the shape of the bovine and caprine kidneys (e.g., retention of fetal surface lobulation and presence of calyces in cattle and lack of these features in goats). The calyces (singular form is calyx) are cup-shaped terminal branches of the ureter in the bovine kidney.
- Know the topographic relationship of the abdominal viscera on the right and left of the median plane.
- At the end of the abdomen section, watch Videos 12, 13, 14, 15, 16, and 17.

Guide to Ruminant Anatomy: Dissection and Clinical Aspects, Second Edition. Mahmoud Mansour, Ray Wilhite, Joe Rowe, and Saly Hafiz.
© 2023 John Wiley & Sons, Inc. Published 2023 by John Wiley & Sons, Inc.
Companion website: www.wiley.com/go/mansour/dissection2

3.1 Lumbar Vertebrae

Goal: Know the number of lumbar vertebrae and their characteristic features in cattle and small ruminants. In cattle, know the location of paralumbar anesthesia in relation to the intervertebral foramina and the tips of the transverse processes of the thirteenth thoracic (T13) vertebrae, and, first and second (L1 and L2) lumbar vertebrae. There is no need to dissect the ligaments associated with the axial skeleton but study their location on the skeleton.

3.1.1 Bovine Lumbar Vertebrae

Typically, there are six bovine lumbar vertebrae (L1–L6). The lumbar vertebrae have longer transverse processes and larger bodies than the vertebrae in other regions of the body (Figure 3.1a). Study the structure of a lumbar vertebra that consists of a body, arch (composed of ventral pedicle and dorsal lamina), and processes that include left and right transverse processes, spinous process, and cranial and caudal articular processes on each side of the vertebra (Figure 3.1b). The cranial and caudal articular surfaces lie in sagittal planes. Compare these features with cervical and thoracic vertebrae. You do not have to devote time to studying the vertebrae if you have previously studied the bones of the axial skeleton.

3.1.2 Goat and Sheep Lumbar Vertebrae

The number of lumbar vertebrae varies in small ruminants between five and seven (L1–L5–7). Goats typically have six or seven lumbar vertebrae, four pelvic (sacral), and between four and eight caudal

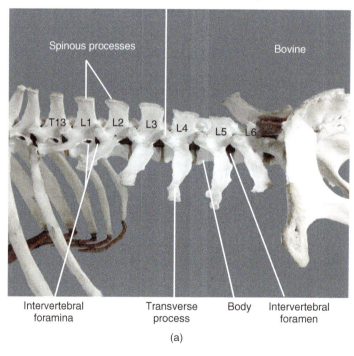

(a)

Figure 3.1 (a) Bovine skeleton showing articulated caudal thoracic and L1–L6 lumbar vertebrae. Note the long transverse processes of the lumbar vertebrae compared, for example, to T12–T13 thoracic vertebrae. Note that the intervertebral foramen between L1 and L2 is divided by a small bone into two foramina. Two intervertebral foramina may be present in some parts of the lumbar region. (b) Typical bovine lumbar vertebra: lateral, cranial, and caudal views. The cranial articular processes are deep and face dorsomedially. The caudal articular processes are cylindrical in shape and fit into the groove (articular surfaces) of the cranial articular processes of the caudally located vertebra. On the lateral view, note the formation of a complete intervertebral foramen on this lumbar vertebra. * Body of vertebra.

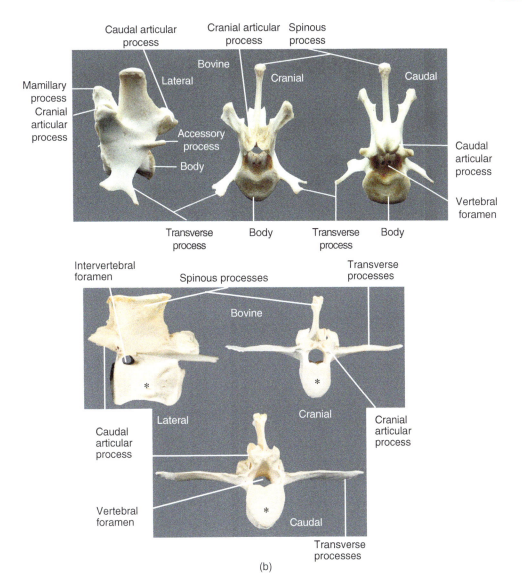

Figure 3.1 (*Continued*)

(coccygeal) vertebrae. Cattle have six lumbar vertebrae, five sacral, and a variable number of caudal (tail) vertebrae (~18–20 vertebrae).

3.2 Ligaments of Lumbar Vertebrae

There are several ligaments associated with the axial skeleton. They give support to the axial skeleton by connecting the vertebrae. Because these ligaments are located deep in the body, it is not necessary to dissect them. Your instructor may ask you to study their general location on the skeleton. With help of Figure 3.1a and the following description, know the general location of the following ligaments in the lumbar region of a bovine or caprine skeleton.

3.2.1 Supraspinous Ligament

The supraspinous ligament courses over the summit of the vertebral spines from T1 coursing caudally to reach the caudal vertebrae.

3.2.2 Interspinous Ligaments

The interspinous ligaments are sheets of connective tissue that occupy the vertical spaces between the spinous processes of adjacent vertebrae.

3.2.3 Intertransverse Ligaments

The intertransverse ligaments fill the spaces between the transverse processes of the lumbar vertebrae.

3.2.4 Yellow Ligaments (Interarcuate or Ligament Flava)

The yellow ligament (ligamentum flavum or interarcuate ligament) fills the dorsal gaps between adjacent vertebral arches along the vertebral column. The yellow ligament is pierced or punctured in caudal epidural anesthesia. This procedure involves the injection of local anesthetic into the epidural space through the yellow ligament in the cranial lumbar region between L1 and L2 (flank anesthesia), at the lumbosacral region between L6 and S1 vertebrae (lumbosacral block), or at the tail region between Cd1 and Cd2 vertebrae (tail block). The epidural space is a fat-filled potential space above the dura mater and below the periosteum lining the vertebral canal. Epidural anesthesia is especially performed under clinical conditions associated with dystocia or injuries related to the udder or female and male external genitalia.

3.2.5 Dorsal and Ventral Longitudinal Ligaments

The dorsal longitudinal ligament courses on the floor of the vertebral canal directly below the spinal cord. In contrast, the ventral longitudinal ligament runs on the undersurface of the vertebral bodies outside the vertebral canal. The dorsal and ventral longitudinal ligaments help stabilize the vertebral column.

3.2.6 Intervertebral Disc

Articulations of adjacent vertebrae consist of synovial joints (between cranial and caudal articular processes) and fibrous joints between the bodies of successive vertebrae with intervertebral discs as the major components of fibrous joints. Each intervertebral disc has an outer fibrocollagenous layer known as the **anulus (or annulus) fibrous** and an inner gelatinous layer known as the **nucleus pulposus** (see Figure 1.50).

Think of the intervertebral disc as a "jelly donut" where the soft jelly material at the center of the donut represents the nucleus pulposus and the outer dough represents the anulus fibrosus. The nucleus pulposus is the material that oozes out in disc herniation (rupture). Anatomy of the intervertebral disc is more clinically relevant in small animals (dogs and cats).

3.3 Abdominal Wall

Goal: Identify the paralumbar fossa and the layers of the abdominal wall. Know the direction of the fibers of the major abdominal muscles. Understand innervation of the flank region (nerves of the paralumbar fossa) and injection sites for proximal and distal paravertebral anesthesia. Understand the clinical significance of the rectus sheath. You should be able to recall how the external and internal laminae of the rectus sheath are formed.

3.3.1 Paralumbar Fossa

The paralumbar fossa is a depression in the upper flank region ventral to the transverse processes of lumbar vertebrae. It can best be appreciated in the live cow (Figure 3.2).

The paralumbar fossa is clinically important in anesthesia of the flank as it is commonly incised to enter the rumen on the left flank (e.g., in rumen cannulation procedure, removal of foreign body), or to access the cecum by incising the skin on the right dorsal flank region. Rumen cannulation, for example, allows for insertion of fistula for long-term studies that require regular rumen sampling.

Take time to study the **boundaries of the paralumbar fossa** that include the last rib (rib 13) cranially, the transverse processes of the lumbar vertebrae dorsally, and the hump or ridge formed by the internal abdominal oblique caudally (Figure 3.2).

The caudal ridge forming the caudal boundaries of the paralumbar fossa is created because much of the internal abdominal oblique muscle is suspended and fans out from the tuber coxae (known as the hook in the live animal). The extreme lateral projection of this process creates the ridge in the middle of the muscle.

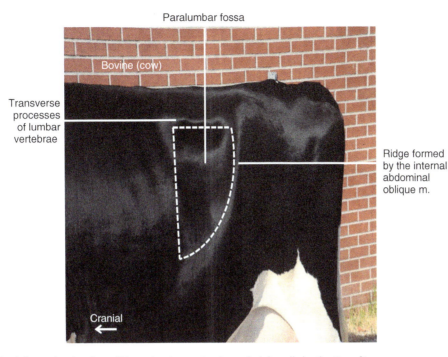

Figure 3.2 Bovine left paralumbar fossa. Triangular depression bounded dorsally by the tips of transverse processes of lumbar vertebrae, caudoventrally by the ridge formed by the internal abdominal muscle, and cranially by the last rib (number 13).

3.3.2 Nerves of the Paralumbar Fossa (Flank Anesthesia)

Spinal nerves **T13** (costoabdominal), **L1** (iliohypogastric), and **L2** (ilioinguinal) of the paralumbar fossa exit the spinal cord through intervertebral foramina and run caudally in an oblique manner on the lateral surface of the transversus abdominis muscle (Figure 3.3a,b).

Once a spinal nerve exits the intervertebral foramen, it immediately divides into the small dorsal branch and the long ventral branch (Figure 3.3b). Cutaneous branches from the dorsal and ventral branches pierce the abdominal wall to supply the skin of the flank. Thus, each spinal nerve carries both somatic motor and cutaneous sensory branches.

The dorsal branches of T13–L1 supply the epaxial muscles and the skin on the dorsal part of the paralumbar fossa down to a plane approximately at the level of the stifle joint. The ventral branches supply the abdominal muscles, peritoneum, and the rest of ventral skin of the flank region.

Dissection of T13, L1, and L2 dorsal and ventral branches is time consuming. Study their location on the skeleton. Your instructor may do a prosection of these nerves or alternatively may ask you to know their general location, function, and clinical significance (Box 3.1).

The **abdominal wall** is formed by several layers of tissues. From superficial to deep, the layers of the abdominal wall include the skin and subcutaneous connective tissue, the cutaneus trunci muscle, the oblique (external and internal) and transversus abdominis muscles, the transversalis fascia deep to the transversus abdominis muscle, and parietal peritoneum as the innermost layer.

You should know the layers and directions of the muscle fibers of the abdominal muscles as this information is important in abdominal surgery through the flank region. Surgical incision techniques that follow the direction of abdominal muscle fibers minimize damage to them. This approach in turns minimizes postoperative surgical complications.

The abdominal muscles are responsible for the abdominal press that helps with forced expiration, defecation, urination, and parturition.

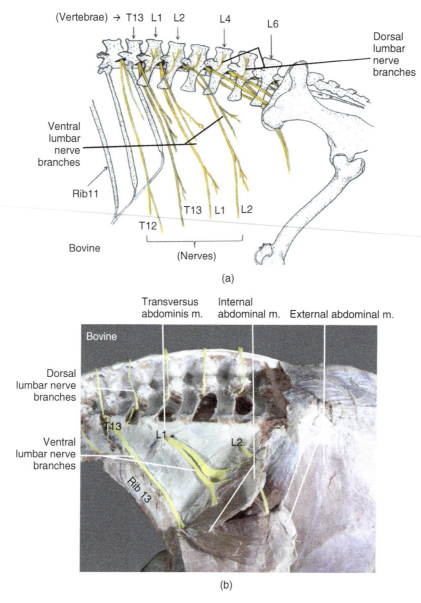

Figure 3.3 (a) Spinal nerves of the left lateral flank in a goat. **T13 (costoabdominal), L1 (iliohypogastric), and L2 (ilioinguinal)** are blocked in flank anesthesia (Box 3.1). Source: Adapted from Garrett (1988). (b) Dissection of the dorsal and ventral branches of spinal nerves **T13 (costoabdominal), L1 (iliohypogastric), and L2 (ilioinguinal)** on a bovine cadaver (suspended on a hanger). The epaxial muscles of the trunk (iliocostalis and longissimus lumborum systems) located dorsal to the transverse processes of lumbar vertebrae have been removed. The dorsal branches run dorsally between the iliocostalis and longissimus lumborum systems. They supply the epaxial muscles and give cutaneous branches. The ventral branches run ventrally between the **internal abdominal oblique (IAO)** and **transversus abdominis (TA)** muscles. They give cutaneous branches and supply muscles of the abdominal wall. (c) Needle placement for anesthesia of the flank using **proximal (P)** or **distal (D) paravertebral nerve blocks in cattle**. In the proximal paravertebral nerve block, the dorsal and ventral nerve roots of T13, L1, and L2 spinal nerves are blocked close to where they emerge from their respective intervertebral foramina. In the distal paravertebral nerve block, ventral and dorsal rami of T13, L1, and L2 are blocked at the distal ends of the transverse processes of L1, L2, and L4, respectively. Because of variations in the pathways of spinal nerves, L2 branches should be blocked at tips of the transverse processes of both L3 and L4 vertebrae. D, distal; P, proximal; T, thoracic, L, lumbar. Source: Holtgrew-Bohling (2016), Elsevier.

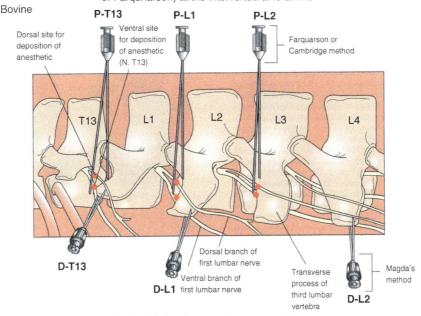

P. Proximal (dorsal) paravertebral nerve block (Cambridge or Farquharson) at the intervertebral foramina

D. Distal (lateral) paravertebral nerve bock (Magda or Cornell) at the tips of the transverse processes

(c)

Figure 3.3 (Continued)

Box 3.1

Abdominal surgery in cattle is most commonly performed using regional local anesthesia of the paralumbar fossa instead of general anesthesia. Typically, surgical procedures in the flank region are performed with the animal in a standing position (e.g., rumenotomy for diagnosis or treatment of foreign bodies or traumatic reticuloperitonitis [hardware disease], correction of gastrointestinal displacement such as abomasal displacement [abomasopexy], intestinal obstruction, and cesarian section). The abdominal wall is innervated by the dorsal and ventral branches of the 13th thoracic (T13) and 1st and 2nd lumbar (L1 and L2) nerves. Three analgesic techniques are among those most commonly used. For an in-depth discussion of local anesthetics and procedures, consult *Farm Animal Anesthesia: Cattle, Small Ruminants, Camelids, and Pigs* edited by Lin and Walz (2014)

1) **Proximal (dorsal) paravertebral nerve block**: desensitizes the dorsal and ventral branches of T13, L1, and L2 spinal nerves close to where they emerge from their respective intervertebral foramina (Figure 3.3c). Other names of this dorsal approach include Cambridge or Farquharson methods. The proximal paravertebral block causes paralysis of the epaxial muscles and bowing of the back (scoliosis toward the desensitized side).

2) **Distal (lateral) paravertebral nerve block**: involves desensitization of the dorsal and ventral branches of T13, L1, and L2 spinal nerves at the tips of transverse processes of L1, L2, and L4, respectively (Figure 3.3c). Other names for the distal paravertebral nerve block include Magda or Cornell methods. This block anesthetizes the ventral rami of T13, L1, and L2.

3) **Inverted L-block or line block**: the anesthetic agent is injected along a line parallel with the transverse processes of the lumbar vertebrae and along the caudal border of the last rib (Figure 3.4). The line block is technically less challenging than the paravertebral anesthesia, which could be more difficult in obese and heavily muscles cattle. In addition, the scoliosis that may develop in the proximal paravertebral block could make closure of the skin much more difficult.

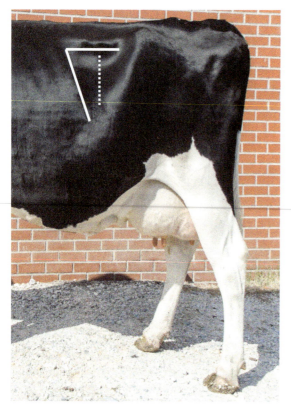

Figure 3.4 **Inverted L-block** is used as an easy alternative to paravertebral blocks. This technique is performed in relatively minor abdominal surgery via flank incision with the animal standing. A local anesthetic is injected along a line parallel to the transverse processes of the lumbar vertebrae and along the caudal border of the last rib (solid lines). The flank incision (dotted line) is ventral and caudal to the injection lines. Nonspecific **line block** can also be used to desensitize the incision site. **Epidural** local anesthesia in cattle is also used for induction of regional anesthesia through anesthetic injections in the interarcuate spaces between L1 and L2, L6–S1, or Cd1–2 vertebrae.

3.3.3 Cutaneus Trunci and Omobrachialis Muscles

As in the horse, ruminants have four cutaneous muscles: the **cutaneus trunci muscle** on lateral thorax and ventral abdomen; the **cutaneus omobrachialis muscle** over the shoulder region; the **cutaneus colli muscle** over the base of the neck; and the **cutaneus faciei muscle** over the lateral surface of the head. Unlike in the horse, the cutaneus colli in ruminants is less developed and arises from the superficial fascia of the neck and not from the manubrium of the sternum.

The cutaneus trunci and cutaneus omobrachialis muscles are discussed here with the abdomen.

The cutaneus omobrachialis muscle covers the lateral shoulder region (lateral scapula and humerus). The cutaneus trunci muscle covers the ventral half of the abdominal wall. Its fibers sweep toward the axilla in a cranioventral direction (Figure 3.5). The cutaneus trunci muscle helps twitch the skin when the animal is repelling flies and insects. The lateral thoracic nerve, from the brachial plexus, innervates the cutaneus trunci muscle.

To save time, it may not be necessary to dissect the cutaneous muscles. Ask your instructor for advice.

3.3.4 Tunica Flava Abdominis

The **tunica flava abdominis** is a yellow elastic layer that covers the **external abdominal oblique** muscle. It helps support the heavy weight of the abdominal viscera. The tunica flava abdominis is present in horses and other food animals (Figure 3.6). Identify it on the surface of the external abdominal oblique before you reflect this muscle. The tunica flava must be sutured in abdominal surgeries in the flank region. This layer tends to curl when incised.

Now move on to identify the abdominal muscles that form the abdominal wall and reflect them down in a sequential order. We will recognize four abdominal muscles and their muscle fiber direction.

3.3.5 External Abdominal Oblique Muscle

Based on the following discussion, identify the fleshy and aponeurotic parts of the external abdominal oblique (EAO) muscle and note fiber direction. There is no need to dissect the inguinal canal, superficial inguinal ring, or the inguinal ligament. The structures that pass through the inguinal canal are discussed here but will be identified with the pelvis and you can skip this part for later study.

At the ventral half of the flank region, the EAO muscle lies deep to the cutaneus trunci muscle. The EAO muscle has both **fleshy** and **aponeurotic parts** and is the most superficial of the abdominal oblique muscles. Fibers of the EAO run in the **caudoventral direction**.

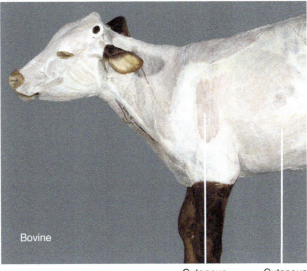

Figure 3.5 Bovine cutaneous muscles over the brachium and ventral thorax and flank regions.

The fleshy part of the EAO muscle is more dorsal than the aponeurotic part and has costal and lumbar parts. The costal part originates from the ventral half of the thorax (6–13 ribs) where it interdigitates with the thoracic part serratus ventralis muscle. The lumbar part originates from the last rib and the thoracolumbar fascia (Figure 3.6a).

The aponeurotic part of EAO continues the fleshy part ventrally. It inserts at two divergent points that include the pelvis dorsally and the midventral part of the abdomen ventrally. On the pelvis, it inserts on the tuber coxae and body of the ilium by what is called the **pelvic tendon** of the EAO. On the ventral abdomen, it inserts on the linea alba and prepubic tendon by an **abdominal tendon**. *Do not look for these tendons.*

Identify the EAO muscle with the help of Figure 3.6a,b. Note the serrated interdigitation with the serratus ventralis muscle (Figure 3.6a). The most dorsal fibers of EAO run horizontally to insert on the tuber coxae.

Close to the medial thigh region and lateral to the ventral midline, the aponeurosis of the EAO muscle has a slit-like opening known as the **superficial inguinal ring**. The superficial inguinal ring is covered by fascia. *Do not look for it now.*

The most caudal part of the aponeurosis of the EAO forms the **inguinal ligament**. This ligament terminates on the iliopubic eminence on the floor of the pelvis. We will identify this ligament later when we study the pelvis.

The superficial inguinal ring is the exit for the inguinal canal, a potential space between the abdominal muscles. The inguinal canal has superficial and deep inguinal rings at each end that allow for structures to pass into and out of the abdomen (Figure 3.7). The vaginal ring is formed by the reflection of the peritoneum to outside the body, and is superimposed on the deep inguinal ring (Figure 3.7).

Review the boundaries of the deep inguinal ring. When drawn, they form a triangle rather than a circular ring:

Caudal: the inguinal ligament.
Medial: the lateral border of the rectus abdominis muscle and prepubic tendon.
Cranial: the caudal border of the internal abdominal oblique muscle.

The structures that pass through the inguinal canal are of clinical interest in domestic animals because castration is one of the more common surgeries performed on male animals (Box 3.2).

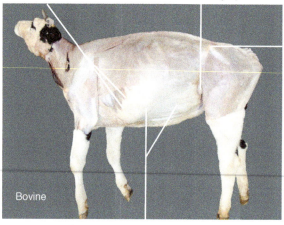

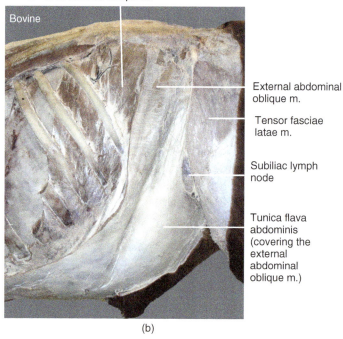

Figure 3.6 (a) Bovine body wall showing the external abdominal oblique (EAO) muscle covered by the yellow elastic deep facial layer, tunica flava abdominis: left lateral view. This tunica helps support the heavy weight of the viscera. (b) Close-up view of the insertion of the EAO muscle. The attachment of the EAO on the ribs is transected and removed. Note the exposure of the internal abdominal oblique fibers caudal to the last rib coursing in a cranioventral direction.

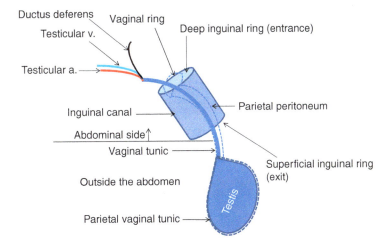

Figure 3.7 Schematic illustration of the inguinal canal in a male ruminant. The inguinal canal is a potential space and pathway for structures located between the abdominal muscles. It is exaggerated for illustration purposes. Other structures that pass through the inguinal canal such as the genitofemoral nerve, lymphatics, and autonomic nerves are not depicted.

Box 3.2
Castration is a common surgical procedure performed in small and large ruminant farm operations. The technical details vary with the procedure used. You will be taught the details in your clinical year (see Box 4.9 for more details).

In male ruminants, the vaginal tunic is a cord-like structure that encloses the spermatic cord. The spermatic cord carries structures from the abdomen to the testes and vice versa through the inguinal canal. The cord is severed during castration.

Structures passing through the **inguinal canal** include the spermatic cord (testicular artery, vein, and ductus deferens), the external pudendal artery and vein, and the genitofemoral nerve.

The vaginal tunic (also called the vaginal process) is a diverticulum of the parietal peritoneum that contains the spermatic cord in the male.

The deep inguinal ring is formed by muscles, in contrast to the vaginal ring that is formed by a reflection of the parietal peritoneum. The superficial inguinal ring is the exit for the inguinal canal formed by a slit in the aponeurosis of the external abdominal muscle.

3.3.6 Internal Abdominal Oblique Muscle

Separate the lumbar part of the EAO muscle from that of the IAO. Reflect the EAO muscle down as shown in Figure 3.8.

The IAO muscle lies deep to the EAO muscle. Like the EAO, it has **fleshy** and **aponeurotic parts**. The fibers of the IAO course to approximately the level of the middle thigh region in a **cranioventral direction**. Note that this direction is opposite to that of the EAO muscle fibers.

The fleshy part of the IAO arises from the tuber coxae in common with the pelvic tendon of the EAO muscle, and from the transverse processes of the lumbar vertebrae. Its attachment on the tuber coxae produces a distinct ridge in the live animal that forms the caudal border of the paralumbar fossa.

The aponeurotic part of the IAO muscle inserts on the last rib and on the linea alba (Figure 3.8). The aponeuroses of the EAO and IAO muscles fuse together on the ventral abdomen to form the external lamina of the **rectus sheath** (read the discussion in Section 3.3.9 on the rectus sheath). This lamina holds the rectus abdominis muscle (Figures 3.8).

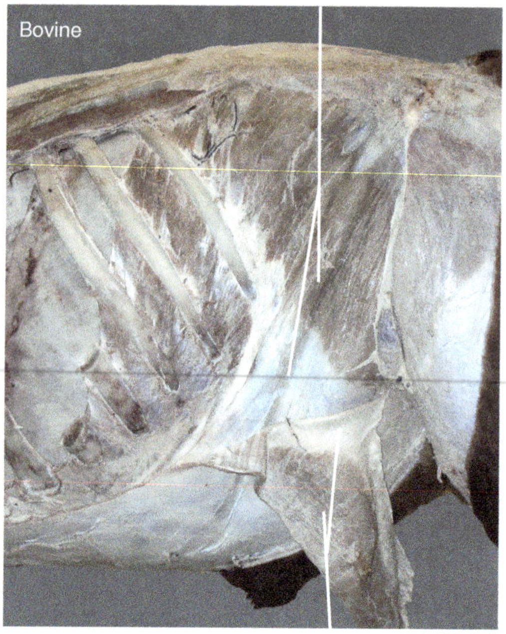

Internal abdominal oblique m.

Bovine

External abdominal oblique m.
(reflected down)

Figure 3.8 Dissection of the bovine internal abdominal oblique (IAO) muscle by transection and reflection of the EAO ventrally: left lateral view. Note the cranioventral direction of the IAO muscle fibers. Distally, the aponeurosis of the EAO and IAO are fused forming the external lamina of the rectus sheath that inserts on the linea alba on the midventral line.

3.3.7 Transversus Abdominis Muscle

The TA muscle lies deep (medial) to the IAO and rectus abdominis (RA) muscles. Its fibers run in the **dorsoventral direction**. The ventral and craniodorsal parts of the TA are tendinous (Figure 3.9). *Transect the dorsal border of the IAO along or ventral to the tips of the transverse processes of lumbar vertebrae and reflect it downward with the EAO muscle.*

The TA muscle arises from the tips of the transverse processes of the lumbar vertebrae and the last rib. Its aponeurotic part inserts dorsal to the RA muscle on the linea alba essentially forming the **internal lamina of the rectus sheath.**

Note that the parietal peritoneum covers the deep (internal) surface of the TA, IAO, and RA muscles (Figure 3.10b). The parietal peritoneum is attached to the abdominal surface of the aforementioned muscles by a thin fascia known as the transversalis fascia. In some specimens, the parietal peritoneum is separated from the transversalis fascia by a layer of fat that varies in thickness depending on the nutritional status of the animal.

3.3.8 Rectus Abdominis Muscle

The fibers of the RA muscle extend from the xiphoid region of the sternum and the external surfaces of the ventral aspects of the final 10 ribs to the cranial ventral part of the pubic ox bone (pectin or pubic brim) (Figure 3.10). The fibers of TA run in a **craniocaudal or caudocranial direction.**

Note the transverse tendinous intersections that interrupt the longitudinal muscle fibers of the RA, giving the muscle fibers a characteristic interrupted appearance (Figure 3.10). The insertion of the RA on the pubic brim is tendinous and is known as the **prepubic tendon.** Other muscles of the medial thigh contribute to the prepubic tendon.

3.3.9 Rectus Sheath

The rectus sheath is formed by the aponeurosis of the EAO, IAO, and TA muscles as they are near the linea alba. This sheath forms a sleeve that wraps around the left and right RA muscles. It has an **external (outer or**

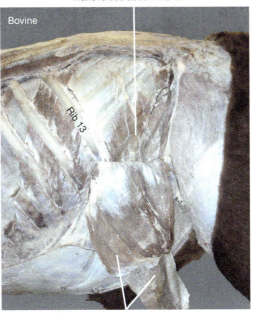

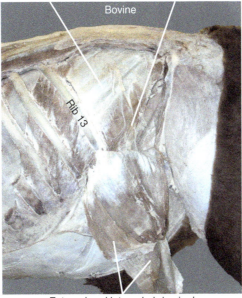

Figure 3.9 Caudal thorax and abdominal flank regions showing the transversus abdominis (TA) muscle and parietal peritoneum: left lateral view. Note the dorsoventral direction of the TA muscle fibers and some of the lumbar spinal nerves running across its surface. The external and internal abdominal oblique (EAO/IAO) muscles are transected and reflected down. Dorsally, the TA muscle is transected and peeled off the transversalis fascia to demonstrate the parietal peritoneum.

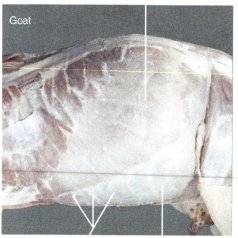

Figure 3.10 (a) Goat abdominal wall with cutaneous trunci muscle removed: left lateral view. The ventrally located RA muscle becomes progressively wider as it courses toward the pubic bone but narrows at its point of attachment on the pubic brim (pectin) to give rise to the prepubic tendon (not visible). Note the distinct transverse tendinous intersections deep to the external lamina of the rectus sheath. The external lamina of the rectus sheath is formed by a fusion of the aponeurosis of the EAO and IAO muscles. (b) The abdominal and pelvic cavities showing the insertion of the RA muscle on the pectin and the disposition of the internal lamina of the rectus sheath: cranial view.

superficial) **lamina** and an **internal (inner or deep) lamina** (Figure 3.10a,b).

The fusion of the aponeuroses of the EAO and IAO muscles forms the external lamina of the rectus sheath. The internal lamina is formed largely by the aponeurosis of the TA muscle that covers the dorsal surface of the RA muscle except for its caudal part, which is covered by parietal peritoneum only.

The rectus sheath is important in paramedian surgical incisions that are not on the midline or through the linea alba (Box 3.5).

3.4 Abdominal Cavity

Goal: Study the abdominal contents in situ and on isolated (extirpated) viscera from bovine and caprine cadavers. Consult Boxes 3.3, 3.4, and 3.5 for clinical applications.

In situ: First, study the disposition of the greater and lesser omenta before you disturb any viscera. Know the difference between the **omental bursa** and **supraomental recess**. Next, identify the abdominal organs residing on the left and right sides of the median plane. Know that the combined rumen and reticulum dominate the left flank, pushing most of the organs to the right median plane except for the spleen and fundic part of the abomasum. At the end of this unit, watch Videos 11, 12, 13, 14, 15, 16, and 17.

On extirpated (isolated) viscera: Study detailed topography of the entire gastrointestinal tract and the interior of the four chambers of the stomach (**reticulum, rumen, omasum,** and **abomasum**). Trace the disposition of the small and large intestines, especially that of the **ascending colon**. Note some of the differences between the abdominal structures in small and large ruminants (e.g., pancreatic ducts, shape, and internal structures of the kidneys).

3.4.1 Dissection Plan

*Refer to the dissection plan in Appendix A and watch **Video 24** on opening the thorax and abdomen. Briefly, remove the thoracic and pelvic limbs. Open the thoracic and abdominal cavities all at once by folding back the rib cage and the entire abdominal wall cranial*

Box 3.3

During abdominal surgery through the paralumbar fossa (paralumbar celiotomy), surgical incisions may be oriented parallel to the direction of muscle fibers at each level to avoid cutting nerves and muscle fibers more than necessary.

Left flank surgery: Because the rumen dominates the left abdomen, left flank exploratory surgery is not performed. Procedures typically done on the left include rumenotomy and C-section.

Right flank surgery: Right flank surgery can be performed for abdominal exploration following an abnormal sign on ultrasound. Several organs can be accessed on the right. These include the kidneys, abomasum, liver, duodenum, cecum, and small intestine.

Box 3.4

Rupture of the prepubic tendon is reported in cows with heavy belly weight, resulting from twin pregnancy, which is an undesirable and rare situation. The rupture of the prepubic tendon is likely to be more common in mares than in cows.

Box 3.5

The external and internal laminae of the rectus sheath have strong holding power and can be sutured during the closure of abdominal incisions (paramedian celiotomy) or through the linea alba on the midventral line (recumbent ventral midline celiotomy).

---

to the pelvic limb (Figures 3.11, 3.12, 3.13, 3.14, and 3.15). Study the peritoneal cavity, omenta, and the contents of the abdominal cavity.

3.4.2 Peritoneum

The peritoneum is the serous membrane that lines the walls of the abdominal and pelvic cavities, covers most surfaces of the abdominal organs, and connects abdominal organs together. On the interior of the abdominal wall (TA and RA muscles), the surrounding peritoneum is known as the **parietal peritoneum** (Figure 3.10b). The part of the peritoneum found on

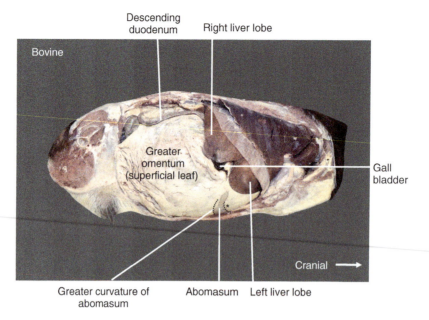

Figure 3.11 Bovine thoracic and abdominal cavities (limbs removed): **right** lateral view. The **greater omentum** is composed of a **superficial leaf or wall** (visible) and a deep leaf or wall (directly deep to the superficial leaf; not visible in this view). The deep leaf can be exposed by gently lifting up the superficial leaf on the right flank. Note the line of attachments of the superficial leaf along the greater curvature of the abomasum and the ventral border of the descending duodenum. Trace this leaf ventrally to the abdominal floor where it passes to the left side under the ventral sac of the rumen. On the left side, it attaches to the left longitudinal groove of the rumen (Figure 3.12). The **lesser omentum** (*) covers the right lateral surface of the omasum and attaches along the lesser curvature of the abomasum, pylorus, beginning of the duodenum, and visceral surface of the liver (porta hepatis). See Figure 3.13.

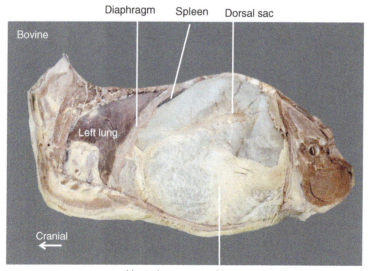

Figure 3.12 Bovine abdominal and thoracic viscera (limbs removed) to show the **superficial leaf (or wall)** of the greater omentum on the left side: **left** lateral view. Note the attachment of the superficial leaf of the greater omentum on the **left longitudinal groove** of the rumen passing cranially to the reticulum. Dotted line shows left longitudinal groove.

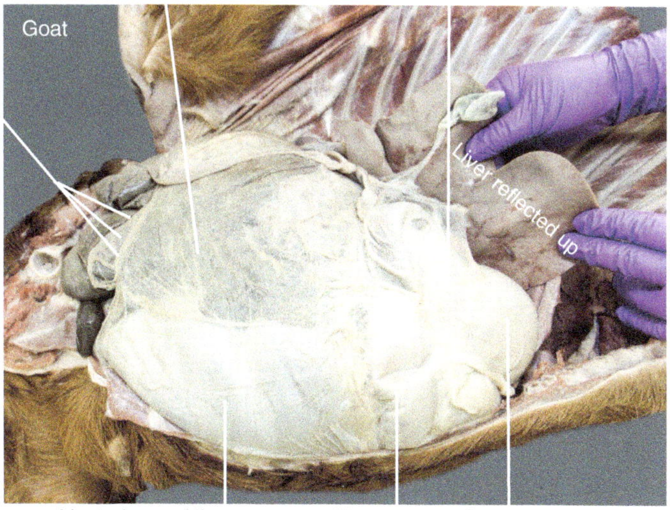

Figure 3.13 The abdominal cavity of the goat showing the **lesser omentum** coursing from the visceral surface of the liver to the lesser curvature of the abomasum (dotted line): right lateral view. The omental bursa, between the superficial and deep leaves of the greater omentum, is opened caudally (see also Figure 3.24a). No organ is present in the omental bursa.

the surface of abdominal organs is the **visceral peritoneum.** The space between the parietal and visceral peritoneum is the **peritoneal cavity.**

The peritoneal cavity contains no organs but normally has a small amount of serous fluid that allows for friction-free movement of abdominal organs against each other and against the interior of the abdominal wall.

3.4.3 Omentum

Goal: Study the disposition and arrangement of the **greater** and **lesser omenta** on the left and right flank before disturbing any of the abdominal organs.

The omentum (plural form is omenta) is an extremely fatty and vascular double-layered, serosal sheet of peritoneum that attaches various parts of the stomach to the dorsal body wall or to other organs. It consists of **greater** and **lesser omenta** (Figures 3.11, 3.12, and 3.13). The omenta contain fat deposits with amounts that vary between different animals.

In fetal development, the greater and lesser omenta are called **dorsal** and **ventral mesogastrium**, respectively. The dorsal mesogastrium suspends the greater curvature of the small and simple primordium of the ruminant stomach to the roof wall of the developing embryo. Following the development of the rumen, reticulum, and large part of the abomasum, the dorsal mesogastrium forms the greater omentum.

The ventral mesogastrium suspends the lesser curvature of the developing stomach to the floor of the abdominal cavity of the developing embryo. It forms the lesser omentum following the differentiation of omasum and the remaining part of the abomasum.

The **greater omentum** has both **superficial** and **deep leaves or walls** (Figures 3.12 and 3.13). The **superficial leaf** of the greater omentum can be identified on the right and left sides of the abdomen. It lies against the floor of the abdominal cavity beneath the ventral sac of the rumen and between the left and right walls of the abdomen. It encloses the ventral sac of the rumen. The **deep leaf** lies deep to the superficial leaf on the right side of the abdomen. It attaches to the right longitudinal groove of the rumen and encloses the intestines. You should understand the complex disposition of the omenta by reading the following detailed description along with studying relevant figures.

With the help of Figures 3.11, 3.13, and 3.14, trace the line of attachments of the **superficial leaf of the**

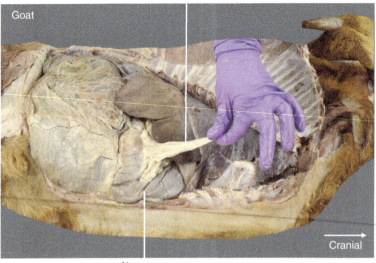

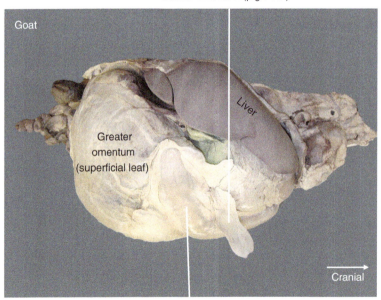

Figure 3.14 (a) Abdominal and thoracic cavity of the goat showing what is colloquially known as "**pig's ear**" in the lesser omentum: right lateral view. Dotted line shows the location of the lesser curvature of the abomasum. (b) Lesser omentum "pig's ear": right lateral view of isolated bovine abdominal viscera. In small ruminants, the pig's ear is a feature of the lesser omentum.

greater omentum on the right flank. Note that it has a wide area of attachments along the greater curvature of the abomasum, pylorus, and descending duodenum. Ventrally, it courses down to the abdominal floor (Figure 3.11). It then passes from the right side to the left side of the abdomen under the ventral sac of the rumen. On the left flank, it attaches along the **left longitudinal groove** of the rumen (Figure 3.12).

To identify the **deep leaf**, return to the right side and follow the superficial leaf along the ventral surface of the descending duodenum to where it reflects medially upon itself forming the **deep leaf.** Note that the deep leaf courses ventrally to run below the intestines and then turns medially to attach on the **right longitudinal groove** of the rumen (Figure 3.15a). Consult Boxes 3.6 and 3.7 for clinical applications related to the omentum.

The sling around the intestines formed by the reflection of the deep leaf and its attachment along the right longitudinal groove of the rumen is the **supraomental recess** (Figure 3.15a,b). The cavity created by the supraomental recess is akin to a holding hammock. The supraomental recess suspends different segments of the intestines: jejunum, ileum, cecum, and the spiral part of the ascending colon (Figure 3.15a).

With help of Figure 3.15b, gently insert your gloved fingers in the supraomental recess and examine how this recess confines the intestines away from the body wall, a feature touted as helpful in keeping the intestines tucked away from surgical incisions made on the right side of the flank.

To demonstrate the **omental bursa**, gently lift the superficial leaf of the greater omentum with your finger and separate it from the underlined deep leaf. The space

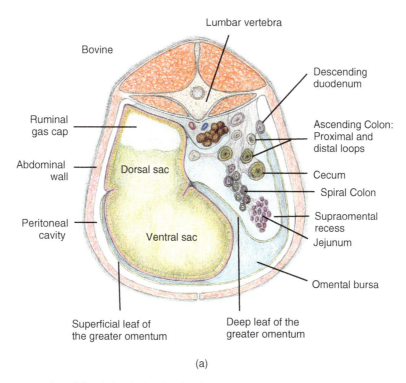

(a)

Figure 3.15 (a) Schematic cross section of the abdominal cavity that illustrates the disposition of the **superficial** and **deep layers of the greater omentum**. The **omental bursa** (enlarged for demonstration purposes) is a paper-thin space between the superficial and deep layers of the greater omentum. The ventral sac of the rumen projects into the omental bursa. The **supraomental recess** is a sling formed by the deep leaf of the greater omentum. It suspends the intestinal mass. (b) Thorax and abdomen in a goat showing the **supraomental recess:** right lateral view. Fingers are inserted medial to the superficial and deep leaves of the greater omentum to demonstrate the supraomental recess.

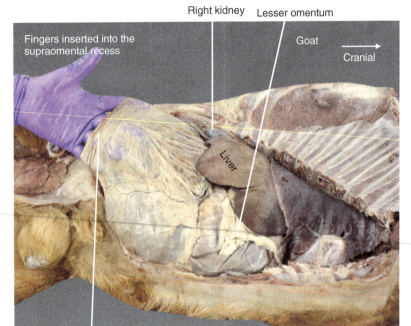

Greater omentum: Superficial and deep layers

(b)

Figure 3.15 *(Continued)*

Box 3.6
The omenta have a unique ability to promote hemostasis and healing because of their pronounced angiogenic activity and rich leukocyte cellular contents. Because of their ability to adhere to adjacent structures, they are frequently used in abdominal surgery to seal off gastrointestinal defects and promote healing in various types of abdominal surgery.

Box 3.7
The supraomental recess helps keep the intestines away from the incision site in right flank laparotomy (right paralumbar celiotomy). The omentum provides storage sites for visceral abdominal fat. Clinically, the omentum helps in tissue repair when sutured over surgical wounds (Box 3.5). It readily adheres to sites of inflammation and provides vascularization and leukocytes for local immune defense. Omentopexy is a surgical procedure whereby the greater omentum is sutured to the body wall to prevent displacement of organs from their normal position (e.g., left abomasal displacement).

between the superficial and deep leaves is the omental bursa (Figures 3.13 and 3.15). The bursa communicates with the peritoneal cavity via the **epiploic foramen** deep to the visceral surface of the liver (Figure 3.16).

Lift the liver dorsally to identify the **epiploic foramen** (Figure 3.16). The foramen is located between the caudate liver lobe and caudal vena cava dorsally, and the right lobe of the pancreas (mesoduodenum) and the portal vein ventrally. You should be familiar with these boundaries.

To study the **lesser omentum** in more detail, expose the visceral surface of the liver by lifting the right

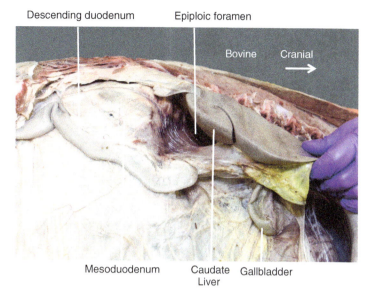

Figure 3.16 The bovine abdominal cavity: right lateral partial view. The **epiploic foramen** is seen ventral to the **caudate process of the caudate lobe of the liver** and dorsal to the **mesoduodenum**. The liver is pulled dorsally to demonstrate the epiploic foramen. Study the complete boundaries of the epiploic foramen from the text.

border dorsally as seen in Figure 3.13. Trace the attachment of the lesser omentum from the visceral surface of the liver to the lesser curvature of the abomasum. Additionally, the lesser omentum courses dorsocaudally along the pyloric part of the abomasum and the beginning of the descending duodenum (Figure 3.13).

The lesser omentum covers the right surface of the omasum (Figure 3.13).

A free slip of the lesser omentum has the appearance of an ear of a pig and is colloquially known as the "**pig's ear**" (Figure 3.14a,b). The pig's ear can be used in omentopexy, and in identifying the abomasum in cases of left abomasal displacement. The "**pig's ear**" in the bovine is usually associated with the greater omentum near the pyloric region. However, the presence of this structure in the bovine can vary and may even be absent. As indicated earlier, the pig's ear is a feature of the lesser omentum in small ruminants.

3.4.4 Ruminant Stomach

The stomach of ruminants (cattle, sheep, and goats) is composed of four complex chambers or compartments: (i) **reticulum,** (ii) **rumen,** (iii) **omasum,** and (iv) **abomasum,** from proximal to distal, respectively (Figures 3.17a,b and 3.18a–d). Camelids such as camels, alpacas, and llamas have a stomach with three compartments (discussed later at the end of this chapter). *Identify each of these organs in situ and study the exterior and interior features of each on an extirpated viscera.*

The abomasum is the true (glandular) stomach and is found like that in monogastric animals (equine and carnivores).

In situ, the rumen dominates the left side of the abdomen (Figure 3.17a,b). The dorsal and ventral sacs are proportionally similar in size in cattle (Figure 3.18a,b). In contrast, the dorsal sac and ventral sacs are asymmetrical in sheep and goats, with the caudoventral blind sac extending more caudally than the caudodorsal blind sac (Figures 3.17a and 3.18c). The following is a detailed description of each of the four chambers of the stomach.

3.4.4.1 Reticulum

Goal: You should be able to identify the **parietal** and **visceral** surfaces of the reticulum. Understand the clinical significance of the proximity and the close topographic relationship of the reticulum, diaphragm, and heart. In the interior, identify the shape or appearance of the **reticular mucosa,** the

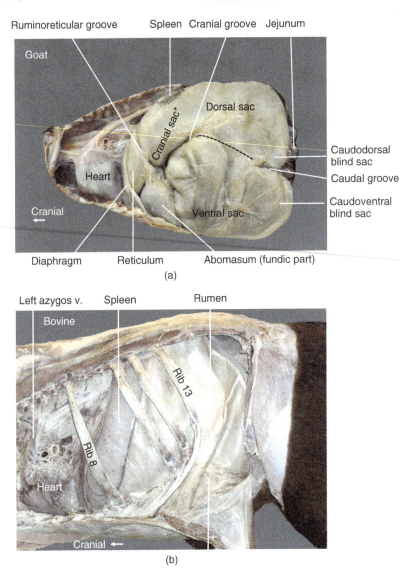

Figure 3.17 (a) The abdominal and thoracic cavities in a goat cadaver: **left** lateral view. The **rumen, reticulum,** and **the fundus of the abomasum** are the major occupants of the left side of the abdominal cavity with the ruminoreticular compartment dominating most of the left flank in situ. In a live animal, the dorsal sac of the rumen occupies the left paralumbar fossa. Note that the fundic part of the abomasum lies between the reticulum and ventral sac of the rumen. * Cranial sac is also called the ruminal atrium. Dotted line, left longitudinal groove. (b) Bovine thoracic and abdominal cavities: **left** lateral view. The **rumen** extends from the cardia (eighth rib or seventh intercostal space) to the pelvic inlet. The **spleen** is relatively enlarged in this cadaver and covers the lateral wall of the reticulum.

ruminoreticular fold, cardia, reticular groove, and **reticulo-omasal orifice.**

The reticulum forms the first part of the **forestomach** (reticulum, rumen, and omasum). It is located largely on the left side of the median plane cranial to the rumen, caudal to the diaphragm, and dorsal to the xiphoid process of the sternum (Figure 3.17a). The surface of the reticulum close to the diaphragm and left lobe of the liver is called the **parietal surface.** The surface in contact with the rumen is the **visceral surface.**

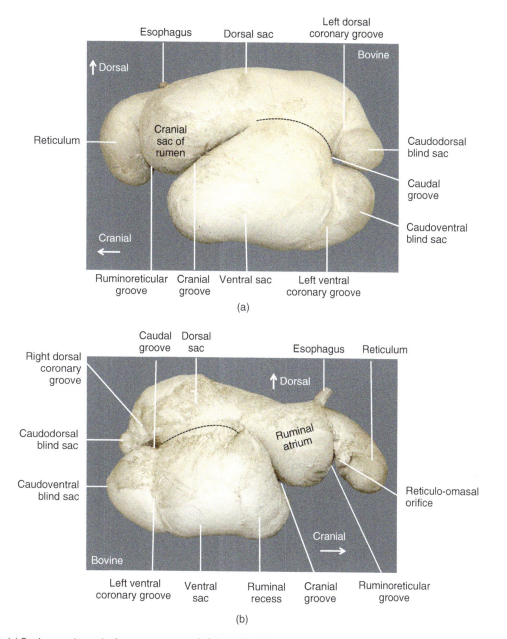

Figure 3.18 (a) Bovine ruminoreticular compartment: **left** lateral surface. Dotted line is the left longitudinal groove. The cranial, caudal, left, and right longitudinal grooves encircle the rumen dividing the rumen into dorsal and ventral sacs. The coronary grooves define the caudodorsal and caudoventral blind sacs. (b) Bovine ruminoreticular compartment: **right** lateral view. Dotted line is the right longitudinal groove. The right longitudinal groove gives off a right accessory groove with a bulge, insula ruminis, in between the two grooves. (c) Goat's stomach: **left** lateral view. Note that the caudoventral blind sac extends more caudally than the caudodorsal blind sac. Dotted line is the left longitudinal groove. (d) Goat's four-chamber stomach: **right** lateral view. Chambers are the reticulum, rumen, omasum, and abomasum. Dotted line is the right longitudinal groove. Schematic illustrations of the left (e) and right (f) views of a **goat's stomach.**

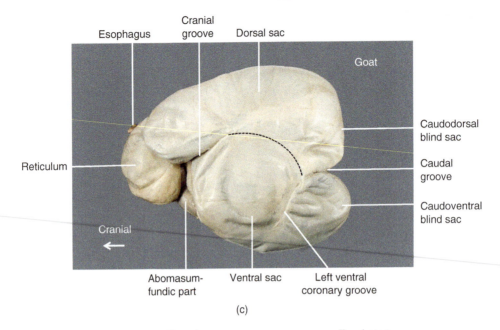

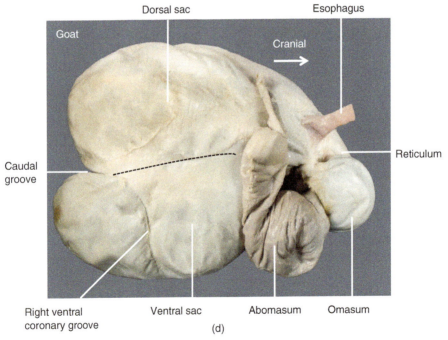

Figure 3.18 (*Continued*)

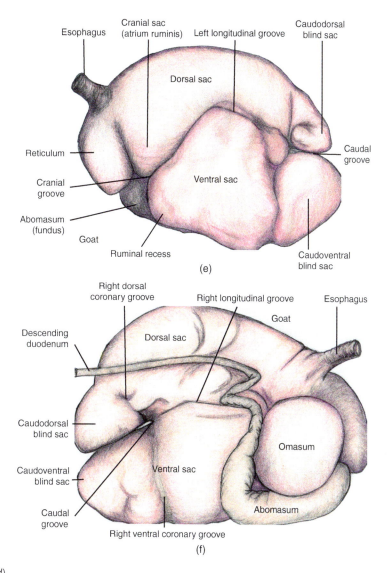

Figure 3.18 (Continued)

The lumen of the reticulum and rumen are more or less continuous with each other, hence the term **ruminoreticular compartment**. The ruminoreticular compartment is a site for fermentation (more details about fermentation in the rumen shortly).

The interior of the reticulum has a characteristic **honeycomb appearance** (Figure 3.19a–d) allowing for easy identification of this compartment in an open gastrointestinal tract.

To understand the clinical significance of the close topographic relationship of the reticulum, diaphragm, and heart, review Figure 3.17(a).

Identify the **reticular groove** on the interior of the reticulum. The reticular groove is similar to the human mouth, with cranial and caudal lips (Figure 3.19b–d). The reticular groove is the first part of a long channel called the **gastric groove**. The **gastric groove** comprises three successive grooves: the **reticular, omasal,** and **abomasal grooves**.

Identify the **cardia** at the proximal end of the reticular groove and the **reticulo-omasal orifice** at the distal end (Figure 3.19d).

Pharyngeal nerve stimulation by suckling causes the lips of the reticular groove to come together with sub-

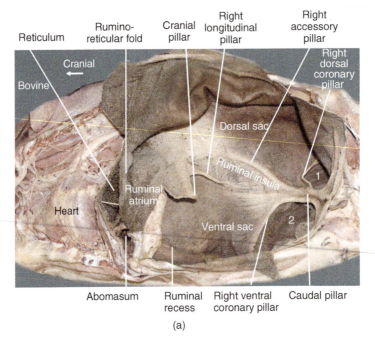

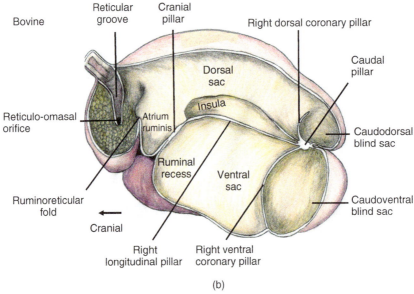

Figure 3.19 (a) Bovine rumen opened in situ to demonstrate **chambers of the rumen** and internal **pillars** on the right interior wall of the rumen. 1, caudodorsal blind sac; 2, caudoventral blind sac. The reticulum is held open by a small stick. Note that the right accessory pillar coursing dorsal and parallel to the right longitudinal pillar. (b) Illustration of the **pillars** in the interior of the bovine stomach: left sagittal view. Practice drawing this sketch on your own. In the ox, the right longitudinal pillar reaches the caudal pillar (the left longitudinal pillar does not). (c) Bovine stomach: left sagittal view. Star 1, cranial sac (ruminal atrium); star 2, ruminal recess; star 3, dorsal sac; star 4, ventral sac; star 5, caudodorsal blind sac; star 6, caudoventral blind sac. (d) Opened bovine rumen: left sagittal view (insert on the left) with a close-up view of the reticular groove (insert on the right). (e) Close-up view of the interior of the caudodorsal and caudoventral blind sacs and dorsal (right and left) and ventral (right and left) coronary pillars. The dorsal and ventral coronary pillars separate between the dorsal and ventral blind sacs and dorsal and ventral ruminal sacs, respectively.

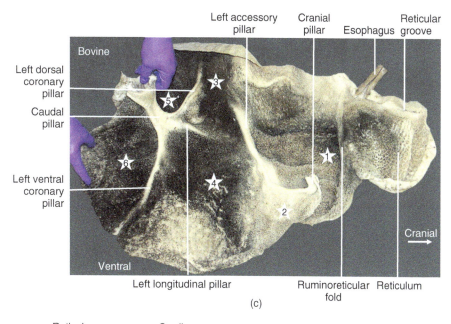

(c)

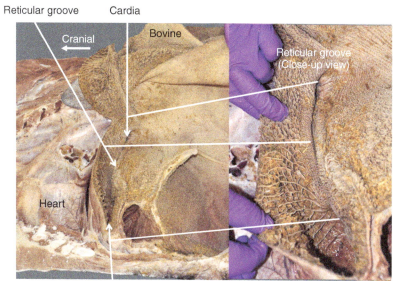

(d)

Figure 3.19 (*Continued*)

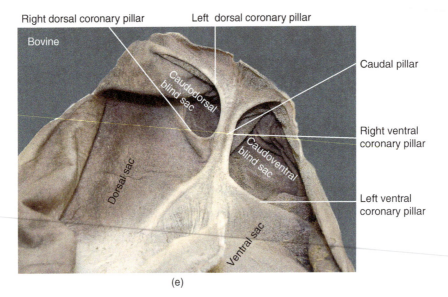

(e)

Figure 3.19 (Continued)

sequent closure of the entire gastric groove (Box 3.8). The closure of the gastric groove in nursing calves allows the channeling of swallowed colostrum and milk directly to the true stomach (abomasum) avoiding bacterial fermentation in the rumen. Thus, the gastric groove forms a continuous passage from the **cardia** (opening of esophagus in the ruminoreticular compartment) directly to the abomasum, bypassing the interior of the rumen, reticulum, and omasum.

Several factors stimulate closure of the gastric groove (Box 3.8).

3.4.4.1.1 Cardia

In the live animal, the cardia (opening of the esophagus into the ruminoreticular compartment) is located at the level of the seventh intercostal space or eighth rib (Figure 3.19d). This information is useful in determining the length of an esophageal feeder in nursing calves or gastric tube in yearling steers or adult cows. The distance can be marked on the tube by measuring the distance from the mouth to the seventh intercostal space or point of the shoulder.

3.4.4.2 Rumen

> **Goal:** On the exterior of the rumen, identity the **dorsal, ventral, cranial, caudodorsal,** and **caudoventral blind sacs.** The **dorsal** and **ventral sacs** are demarcated by the left and right longitudinal grooves that are continuous with cranial and caudal grooves. The blinds sacs are demarcated by the coronary grooves. Consult Boxes 3.8, 3.9, and 3.10 for clinical applications related to the ruminoreticular compartment.

In the interior of the rumen, the outer grooves will be reflected inside the cavity of the rumen as pillars. In cattle, the interior features of the rumen are more developed than in small ruminants. Identify the **ruminoreticular fold, cranial, caudal,** and **left** and **right longitudinal pillars.** The **coronary grooves** will be reflected inside the rumen as **dorsal (right** and **left),** and **ventral (right** and **left) coronary pillars.**

The rumen is the largest compartment of the ruminant's stomach and is composed of dorsal, ventral, cranial, and caudal (caudodorsal and caudoventral) blind sacs. It dominates the abdominal topography on the left side of the median plane where it extends from the cardia to the pelvic inlet (Figure 3.17a,b).

With the help of Figures 3.17 and 3.18(a–f), identify the **cranial, caudal, left** and **right longitudinal,** and **coronary grooves** on the exterior of the rumen.

Note that the cranial, caudal, and longitudinal (left and right) grooves divide the rumen into **dorsal** and **ventral sacs.** The coronary grooves outline the left and right **caudodorsal** and **caudoventral blind sacs** (Figure 3.18a–f).

The ruminoreticular compartment forms a large fermentation vat for microbial digestion and

Box 3.8

The muscular lips of the **reticular groove** and the rest of the **gastric groove** can be stimulated to form a continuous channel by the act of suckling in young calves. This effect can be mimicked by drugs containing copper and/or nicotine sulfates. These chemicals stimulate the pharyngeal nerve endings that reflexly induce closure of the gastric groove.

Drench intended for the treatment of abomasal worms contains copper and/or nicotine sulfates to induce closure of the gastric groove and avoid dilution in the rumen.

In calves affected by a condition called "ruminal drinker," milk passes into the rumen where it ferments, causing lactic acidosis. The condition is caused by using improperly mixed milk replacements, high rates of milk administration, or failure of the gastric groove to close due to disease conditions.

Box 3.9

Hardware disease: This condition is also known as traumatic reticulopericarditis or traumatic reticuloperitonitis. Note the close proximity of the reticulum to the diaphragm and heart (Figure 3.17a). Cattle use their tongues to graze and in doing so they may ingest sharp objects such as nails and wires. Metal objects could drop to the bottom of the reticular floor and become lodged within the reticulum. Contraction of the stomach could cause sharp objects to penetrate the wall of the reticulum and diaphragm and reach the heart. This can lead to a condition known as traumatic reticulopericarditis or reticuloperitonitis (commonly known as hardware disease).

In some farms, magnets are introduced into the reticulum to reduce the incidence of hardware disease. Additional preventive measures include installation of magnets in feed mills and forage harvesting equipment.

A firm push with the knee or palm of the hand on the xiphoid process can be used as a quick diagnostic test for hardware disease. The pressure on the sternum could elicit a grunt suggestive of pain.

A test known as the **withers pinch test** is used in physical diagnosis to detect pain in a cow with traumatic reticuloperitonitis (hardware disease). In a healthy cow, pinching the withers with both hands causes the animal to dip and make a shrug-like action. In a cow with hardware disease, the cow may not dip or may grunt while dipping. A moderate amount of force is needed to elicit a dip from a cow with good body condition.

Box 3.10

Rumen acidosis resulting from lowered pH and the increased concentration of volatile fatty acids could lead to ruminal parakeratosis, a condition characterized by the hardening and enlargement of the papillae of the rumen.

Bloat is another condition that could result from excessive gas buildup in the rumen, resulting from fermentation. Temporary relief can be achieved by passing an orgogastric tube into the rumen or by ruminal trochar in the left paralumbar fossa, which should only be performed as a last resort. Administration of mineral oil or other antifoaming agents can eliminate the foam that traps gases. Bloat (also known as rumen tympany) is typically described as free gas or frothy bloat. Severe distension of the left paralumbar fossa could be evident. Free gas is typically associated with esophageal obstruction or interference with eructation secondary to vagal nerve dysfunction. In contrast, frothy gas (more common) is generally associated with pasture feeding of legumes, such as alfalfa, clover, or green chop.

Rumen hypomotility occurs with stress, pain, or specific disease conditions, such as grain overload.

generation of volatile fatty acids. Ruminants void gases, principally methane, produced by the process of fermentation in the rumen. This process is called eructation (belching).

Make a sagittal incision in the rumen and remove the contents. Clean the interior with running water in order to identify the internal structures of the reticulum and rumen (Figure 3.19a–c,e). In the live animal, the ingesta are stratified with a gas cap and coarse food material occupying the dorsal aspect of the rumen while fine, relatively heavy food particles sink down in the ventral aspect. The dorsal coarse material covering the cardia is usually regurgitated to the mouth for further mastication. This process is called chewing the cud.

On a left sagittal view, identify the **ruminal pillars** that project into the interior surface of the right ruminal wall (Figure 3.19a,b). Note that the same pillars could be identified on the internal surface of the left ruminal wall (Figure 3.19c). The left accessory pillar and insula are vague and will not be identified.

Note that the mucosa of the rumen has small papillae that give the interior of the rumen a carpet-like appearance. The development of these papillae is stimulated by the production of volatile fatty acids in the ruminoreticular compartment.

The cranial, caudal, and left and right longitudinal grooves on the exterior wall of the rumen correspond to internal **pillars** that carry similar names to the grooves.

With the help of Figure 3.19a–c,e, identify the **ruminoreticular fold, cranial** and **caudal pillars, right** and **left longitudinal pillars, dorsal (right** and **left),** and **ventral (right** and **left) coronary pillars.**

The **ruminoreticular fold** forms a U-shaped partition between the reticulum and **cranial sac** (also known as **ruminal atrium**) of the rumen. The ruminal atrium (or atrium ruminis) is the space between the ruminoreticular fold and the cranial pillar. The opening across the U-shaped partition between the reticulum and atrium ruminis is known as the ruminoreticular orifice.

The **cranial pillar** runs obliquely between the ruminal atrium and the ventral sac (specifically the cranial part of the ventral sac or **ruminal recess**) of the rumen. Do not confuse this pillar with the ruminoreticular fold (Figure 3.19b).

Identify the **atrium ruminis** and **ruminal recess** as the most cranial parts of the dorsal and ventral sacs of the rumen, respectively. The cranial pillar is located between these two chambers.

The **left** and **right longitudinal pillars** extend from the cranial pillar toward the caudal pillar along the right and left walls of the rumen. They are continuous with the cranial pillar but may not reach the caudal pillar (e.g., in cattle, the right longitudinal pillar extends caudally to reach the caudal pillar, whereas the left longitudinal pillar does not reach the caudal pillar). In small ruminants, the left longitudinal pillar is described as indistinct. The left and right longitudinal pillars define the dorsal and ventral sacs.

Caudally in the ruminal cavity, identify the **dorsal (right** and **left),** and **ventral (right** and **left) coronary pillars** that define the caudodorsal and caudoventral blind sacs (Figure 3.19a–c,e). The caudodorsal and caudoventral blind sacs are separated by a thick **caudal pillar.**

Keep in mind that there are differences among animals in the development of the dorsal and ventral coronary pillars. In sheep for example, the dorsal coronary pillars (left and right) are absent.

3.4.4.3 Omasum

Goal: You should be able to identify the **parietal** and **visceral** surfaces of the omasum. Appreciate the differences in the shape of the omasum in the ox (round and firm) compared with small ruminants (bean-shaped). In the interior, identify the shape or appearance of the **omasal laminal** mucosa, the **reticulo-omasal orifice,** and **omasal groove** (less distinct when compared with the reticular groove), **omasoabomasal orifice,** and **vela abomascia** at omasoabomasal orifice (Figures 3.20 and 3.21a).

The omasum lies right to the reticulum on the right side of the median plane. The right surface is covered by the **lesser omentum** (Figure 3.13a). The parietal surface faces the diaphragm while the visceral surface is located toward the reticulum, rumen, and abomasum.

In cattle, the omasum has a firm consistency and an approximately round shape similar to that of a basketball. It is bean-shaped in small ruminants.

To study the interior, make a longitudinal cut along the lesser curvature of the omasumabomasum (abomasal groove) and remove the contents. Use running water to clean the interior of the walls.

The interior of the omasum has **long laminae** dotted with **small papillae** (Figure 3.20) with some species having both long and short laminae. The disposition of the laminae is similar to the pages of a book and hence the common name "**butcher's bible**."

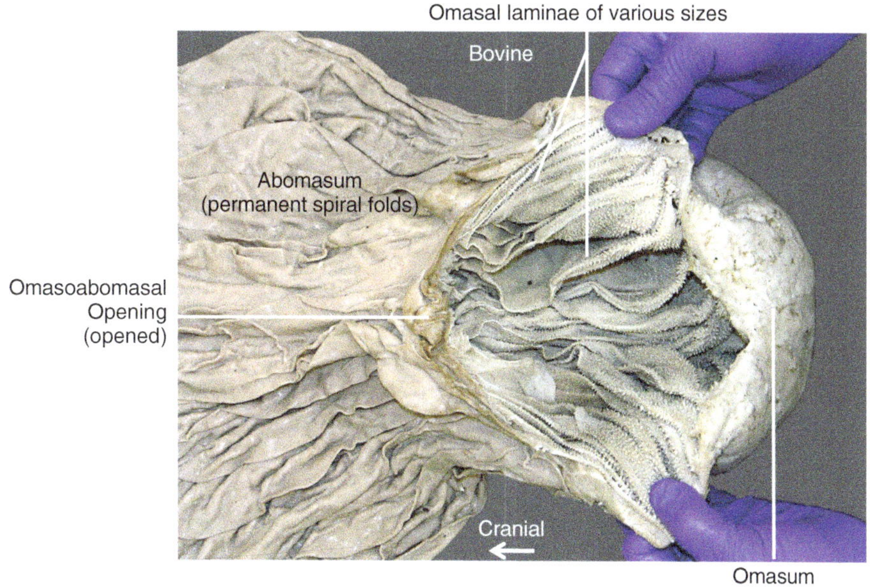

Figure 3.20 **Omasum** and **abomasum** opened along the lesser curvature (the cut is along the omasal and abomasal grooves). Note the small variable omasal papillae dotted on the large flat **omasal laminae.** The laminae are stacked together giving an appearance of the pages of a book. The two folds at the omasoabomasal orifice form a valve known as the **vela abomascia**.

Identify the long thin laminae arising from the greater curvature of the omasum.

The function of the omasum is to press food between the laminae and absorb water. The shallow straight passageway on the lesser curvature between the reticulo-omasal orifice and omasoabomasal orifice is the **omasal groove**. The omasal groove is devoid of laminae and is continuous with the reticular and abomasal grooves. The omasal groove is less distinct than the reticular groove. *Do not look for it.*

3.4.4.4 Abomasum

Goal: You should be able to identify the abomasum and its various regions (**fundus, body**, and **pyloric region**). Identify the parietal and visceral surfaces. Know the difference between the pyloric region and **pylorus** (sphincter). Understand that the abomasum can be displaced to the right or left of the median plane, especially in the late stages of pregnancy and in the postpartum period. You should be able to identify the **torus pyloricus**, a tissue prominence at the pylorus.

The abomasum has a thin wall and is J-shaped in appearance (Figures 3.14 and 3.18d). It lies on the floor of the abdomen mostly to the right of the median plane. The fundic part of the abomasum, however, can be seen on the left side of the median plane between the reticulum cranially, and ventral sac of the rumen caudally (Figure 3.17a). The parietal surface of the abomasum faces the floor of the abdomen while the visceral surface faces the omasum and rumen.

Grossly, the abomasum is divided into **fundus, body,** and **pyloric** regions. The pyloric region joins the duodenum, the first segment of the small intestine.

Open the abomasum along the greater curvature where the superficial leaf of the greater omentum attaches or along the lesser curvature where the lesser omentum attaches. Empty the ingesta and rinse the interior with running water to study the interior (Figure 3.21a).

The pylorus contains the pyloric sphincter that regulates food passage to the duodenum. A tissue projection at the pylorus is known as the **torus pyloricus**. The torus pyloricus adds strength to the pyloric sphincter but is sometimes mistaken for tumor in

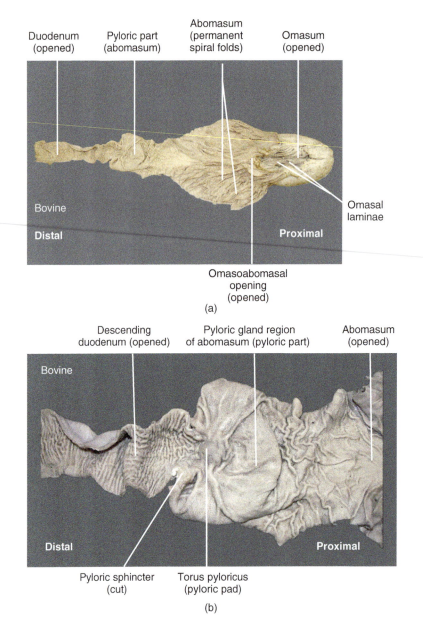

Figure 3.21 (a) Bovine omasum, abomasum, and proximal part of the duodenum (opened along the lesser curvature). The muscular projection at the pylorus is the **torus pyloricus** (see also Figure 3.21b). The mucosa of the abomasum contains **cardiac glands** (at the omasoabomasal orifice), **proper gastric glands** (in the fundus and body), and **pyloric glands** (at the pyloric region). (b) The distal part of the abomasum, and proximal part of the duodenum. The abomasum and duodenum are opened and reflected along the lesser curvature.

necropsy exams. Identify the torus pyloricus at the pyloric region of the abomasum (Figure 3.21a,b).

The interior of the abomasum has permanent **spiral folds** (Figure 3.21a). The abomasum has a glandular mucosa equivalent to the true stomach of monogastric animals (dogs, cats, horse, and pigs).

At the omasoabomasal orifice note the mucosal folds that form a valve near this orifice. This valve is

> **Box 3.11**
>
> **Abomasal displacement and abomasal volvulus:** several factors, such as hypomotility and gas production, contribute to this condition. Typically, the abomasum can be displaced from its normal position to the left or right side of the body (LDA or RDA). Volvulus occurs when the abomasum rotates on its mesenteric axis. Several surgical procedures can be performed to correct an LDA or RDA, including the abomasopexy, performed via a left paralumbar incision or the pyloropexy and omentopexy, which are performed via a right flank celiotomy.

called **vela abomasica**. The vela abomasica is more developed in small ruminants (sheep and goats) than in cattle.

The narrow interior area of the abomasum along the lesser curvature is the **abomasal groove**. Like the **omasal groove**, it is less distinct. The abomasal groove is the third part of what is known as the **gastric** (or **esophageal**) **groove**. As discussed earlier, this groove is formed by the **reticular, omasal**, and **abomasal grooves**. The gastric groove is more developed in young ruminants. *Identify the reticular groove only.*

When excessive gas accumulates in the abomasum, it can cause it to rotate from its normal location on the right ventral part of the abdomen. Both left and right abomasal displacements (LDA and RDA) are reported, with LDA occurring more frequently (Box 3.11).

Stomach of camelids: Cattle, sheep, and goats are considered true ruminants with four stomach compartments. Camelids, such as Dromedary and Bactrian camels, alpacas, llamas, vicunas, and guanacos have only three stomach compartments and considered by some as pseudoruminants. The stomach of alpacas for example has three compartments known as C1 (equivalent to the rumin with cranial and caudal sacs), C2 (equivalent of the reticulum), C3 (equivalent of the abomasum or true stomach). Fermentation takes place in the C1 compartment.

3.5 Intestines

Goal: You should know that the intestinal tract lies to the **right** of the median plane within the **supraomental recess**. Identify the regions and structures associated with the small intestine (**cranial part of the duodenum, sigmoid flexure, descending duodenum, caudal duodenal flexure, ascending duodenum, duodenocolic fold, duodenojejunal flexure, jejunum, mesojejunum, ileum, ileocecal fold,** and **ileal orifice**). Identify regions and structures associated with the large intestine (**cecum, cecocolic orifice, ascending colon [has proximal, spiral, and distal loops], transverse colon,** and **descending colon**). Identify regions of the spiral loop (**centripetal coils, central flexure,** and **centrifugal coils**). Know the difference between small and large ruminants in the disposition of large centrifugal coils.

The intestinal tract comprises the **small** and **large intestines**. It lies mostly to the right of median plane because the large ruminoreticular compartment dominates the left side of the abdomen. Use Figure 3.22 to study a global view of the various parts of the intestinal tract before you start studying the details of each segment.

With help of Figure 3.22 and the following description, use goat cadavers to identify regions of the small and large intestines in situ and on isolated viscera. In situ, begin by studying the regions of the duodenum. Pull the intestines from the supraomental recess and trace the terminal part of the jejunum to the colon. Identify the ileocecal fold. Next, study regions of the ascending colon. Finally, identify the transverse and descending colon. It will be difficult to identify the transverse colon in situ.

3.5.1 Small Intestine

The small intestine has three parts: (i) **duodenum,** (ii) **jejunum,** and (iii) **ileum.** The ileum joins the large intestine at the junction between the cecum and the beginning of the proximal loop of the ascending colon.

3.5.1.1 Duodenum

The duodenum has five identifiable parts: (i) **cranial part**, having near its end a **sigmoid flexure**, (ii) **descending part**, (iii) **caudal duodenal flexure**,

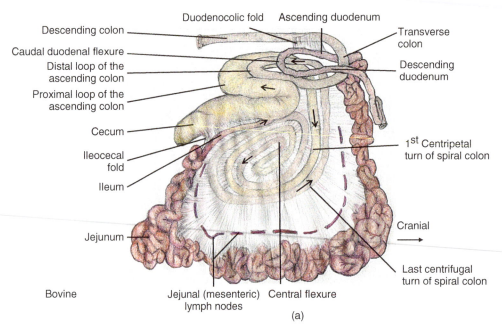

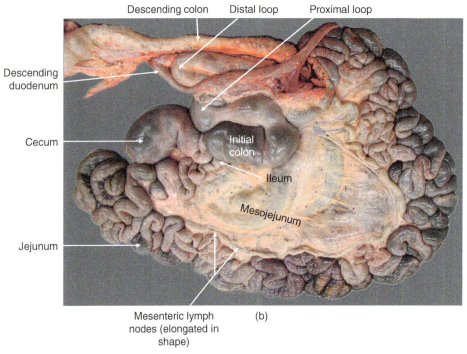

Figure 3.22 (a) Overview of the bovine intestinal tract: right lateral view. The small intestine includes the duodenum (has several parts), jejunum (the longest part), and ileum (defined by the ileocecal fold). The large intestine consists of the cecum, ascending, transverse, and descending colons. The ascending colon is more complex. Trace the three loops of the ascending colon (**proximal**, **spiral**, and **distal loops**). The spiral loop has **centripetal turns**, **central flexure**, and **centrifugal turns**. The last centrifugal fold of the spiral colon in goats lies close to the jejunum and is adhered to the great mesentery (mesojejunum). Its appearance has been likened to that of a "pearl necklace." (b) Right side view of bovine intestines from a lean animal. Source: image was obtained with permission from the University of Minnesota. (c) Left side view of bovine intestines from a lean animal. Source: image was obtained with permission from the University of Minnesota.

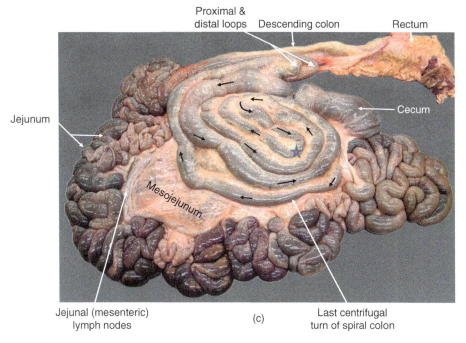

Figure 3.22 (Continued)

(iv) **ascending duodenum**, and (v) **duodenojejunal flexure**.

Find the beginning of the duodenum on the right side of the abdomen beneath the visceral surface of the liver. The **cranial part** (pars cranialis) of the duodenum begins at the pylorus and courses caudodorsally over the distal loop of the ascending colon. (Figure 3.23). Next, it forms a **sigmoid flexure** (still part of the pars cranialis). The distal bend of the sigmoid flexure is called the **cranial flexure**. This is where the **descending part** (pars descendens) begins.

Reflect the liver dorsally to observe the sigmoid flexure. Trace the descending part of the duodenum toward the pelvic cavity.

Near the pelvic inlet and caudal to the root of the mesentery, the duodenum turns from right to the left of the median plane to form the **caudal duodenal flexure**. On the right side, it courses cranially to form the **ascending duodenum**. Note that the ascending duodenum is connected to the descending colon with a peritoneal fold known as the **duodenocolic fold** (Figures 3.22 and 3.23).

The duodenum terminates by joining the jejunum at the **duodenojejunal flexure**. There is no need to identify the duodenojejunal flexure.

3.5.1.2 Mesoduodenum

Identify the peritoneum that suspends the duodenum. This is the **mesoduodenum** (Figure 3.23). The right lobe of the pancreas is enclosed by the double serosal layers of the mesoduodenum.

3.5.1.3 Duodenocolic Fold

The **duodenocolic fold** attaches the ascending duodenum to the descending colon. Identify this fold at the beginning of the ascending colon on the right side of the median plane (Figures 3.22 and 3.23).

3.5.1.4 Jejunum

The **jejunum** is the longest part of the small intestine. Its coils are suspended by the **mesojejunum** around the root of the mesentery. The mesojejunum is also called the **great mesentery** (Figure 3.24b).

Note that the presence of elongated **jejunal (mesenteric) lymph nodes** within the double layers of the mesojejunum (Figure 3.22). Understand that most the jejunal coils are contained within the **supraomental recess** (Figure 3.24a–c) although some coils may migrate out and can be seen on the left side of the median behind the blind sacs of the rumen (Figure 3.24d,e).

Advanced pregnancy and fullness of the rumen influence movement of the jejunum.

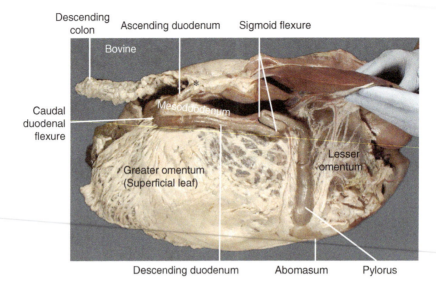

Figure 3.23 Isolated bovine abdominal viscera showing the course of the duodenum: right lateral view. Trace the cranial part of the duodenum off the pylorus, the sigmoid flexure, cranial duodenal flexure (distal part of the sigmoid flexure), descending duodenum, caudal duodenal flexure, and ascending duodenum. The liver is pulled dorsally to expose the lesser omentum and the origin of the duodenum from the distal part of the pylorus. * Duodenocolic fold.

3.5.1.5 Ileum

The gut segment next to the jejunum is the **ileum**. It forms the terminal part of the small intestine and is the shortest part of the small intestine. It is readily identifiable by its mesenteric attachment to the cecum by the **ileocecal fold** (Figures 3.22 and 3.24a).

3.5.1.6 Ileal Orifice

The ileum enters the large intestine and terminates at the **ileal orifice**. Authors disagree as to where in the large intestine the ileum opens. Some authors are of the opinion that the ileum opens into the proximal part of the cecum, some suggest the ascending colon, and others suggest a "no man's land" at the junction between the cecum and the beginning of the ascending colon (i.e., at the beginning proximal loop). In any case, the disagreement does not have any clinical implications. Opening at the junction between the cecum and the beginning of the ascending colon is a safe bet and the name of the opening (ileal orifice) does not indicate a preference.

3.5.1.7 Ileocecal Fold

Different landmarks define the ileum in domestic species. The **ileocecal fold** defines the location of the ileum in ruminants (Figures 3.22 and 3.24a).

In horses, the ileum is distinguished by both the **ileocecal fold** and by its **thicker wall** that gives the impression of a water hose. In ruminants, the ileum has a softer consistency similar to that of the jejunum.

In dogs, the ileum is defined by the presence of **antimesenteric vessels** that are uniquely located on the opposite side of the mesentery.

3.5.2 Large Intestine

Identify the three regions of the large intestine: (i) **cecum**, (ii) **colon (ascending, transverse,** and **descending parts),** and (iii) **rectum** (Figures 3.22 and 3.24a–c).

Of these three parts, the ascending colon is the most complicated in large domestic animals. The simplest form is found in humans and carnivores.

In ruminants, the ascending colon has (i) **proximal**, (ii) **spiral**, and (iii) **distal loops** (Figures 3.22 and 3.24b). Further, three parts form the spiral loop: (i) **centripetal coils** or **turns**, (ii) **central flexure**, and (iii) **centrifugal coils** or **turns** (Figures 3.22 and 3.24b).

3.5.2.1 Cecum and Cecocolic Orifice

In the live animal, the **cecum** is accessed in the right dorsal flank. It continues cranially as the **proximal loop of the ascending colon** without an appreciable

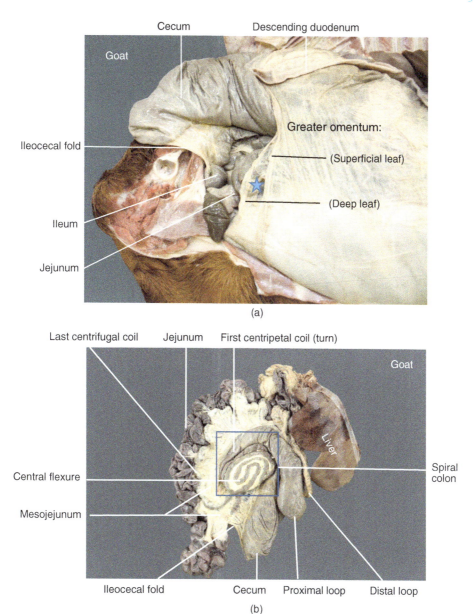

Figure 3.24 (a) Goat isolated abdominal viscera: right lateral view. The cecum and intestine are pulled out of the supraomental recess. The superficial leaf is incised to open the omental bursa. (* – omental bursa). (b) Small and large intestines of the goat: left view of the cecum and ascending colon. The cecum and ascending colon are pulled cranially. In a normal arrangement, the part of the spiral colon shown here faces the right wall of the rumen. (c) Isolated goat abdominal viscera: lateral right view. The intestines are pulled caudally from the supraomental recess. (d) Abdominal and thoracic viscera in a goat: left lateral view. Note the spillover of the jejunum from the right side to the left side residing behind the blind sacs of the rumen. (e) Abdominal and thoracic viscera in a goat: left lateral view. Note spillover of the jejunum and the spiral colon (left surface) from the right side to the left side because of a relatively empty ruminal compartment. This spill could also be a postmortem event.

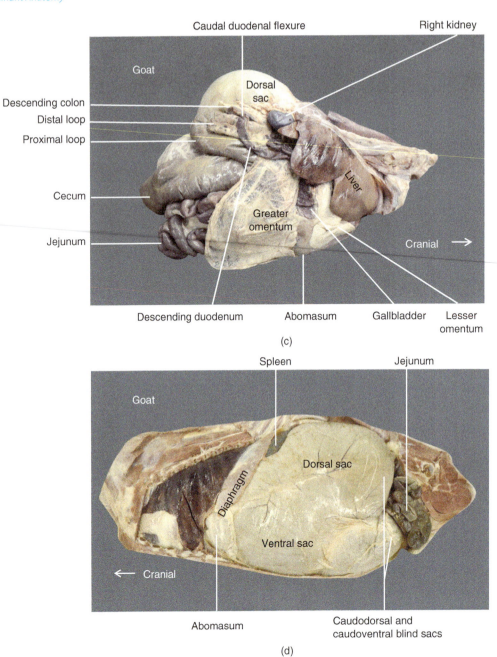

Figure 3.24 (*Continued*)

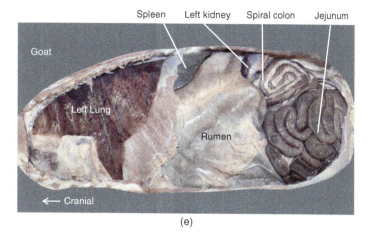

Figure 3.24 (Continued)

sphincter or change in tubular diameter (Figures 3.22 and 3.24a). Consequently, the cecolic orifice is a less-defined site. It is generally located at the point where the ileum enters the large intestine at the junction between the cecum and ascending colon (Figure 3.22). From the ileum, ingesta travels to the colon.

The cecolic orifice is much more well defined in the horse and dog.

3.5.2.2 Ascending Colon

The ascending colon is the more extensive part of the colon. It is divided into the **proximal**, **spiral** (which has **centripetal**, **central flexure**, and **centrifugal turns or coils**), and **distal loops** (Figures 3.22 and 3.24b). The spiral loop is sometimes called the spiral colon. The next segments of the colon, transverse and descending colon, are relatively simple.

3.5.2.2.1 Proximal Loop

The **proximal loop** begins where the ileum enters the cecum. From there, it continues cranially, turns in a caudal direction, and turns again in a cranial direction before making a final turn ventrally where it is identified as the spiral loop or spiral colon. The diameter of the proximal loop is similar to that of the cecum (Figures 3.22 and 3.24c), but the spiral loop is of a smaller diameter.

3.5.2.2.2 Spiral Loop

To identify the parts of the spiral loop, pull the jejunum, cecum, and ascending colon cranially out of the supraomental recess. With the help of Figures 3.22 and 3.24b,c, trace the proximal loop to the beginning of the spiral colon. The spiral colon has three parts where it first turns inward as **centripetal coils or turns**, folds upon itself as **central flexure**, and finally it spirals outward as **centrifugal coils**. In cattle, there are two centripetal turns followed by two centrifugal turns. In goats, there are three or four turns in each direction.

In goats, the last centrifugal coil lies close to the jejunum. It is adhered to the mesojejunum. This coil has the appearance of a "**pearl necklace**" as it often contains small round fecal balls (Figure 3.24b). In cattle, the last centrifugal coil remains close to the rest of the spiral colon (Figure 3.22).

While reviewing the parts of the spiral colon, identify the long **jejunal (mesenteric) lymph nodes** embedded within the double layers of the mesojejunum.

3.5.2.2.3 Distal Loop

The final segment of the ascending colon is the **distal loop** (Figures 3.22 and 3.24b,c). It is a single bend of intestine situated slightly dorsal to the second turn of the proximal loop. From the terminal part of the distal loop, the colon crosses from the right to the left of the median plane as the **transverse colon**. The transverse colon turns caudally and continues as the **descending colon** on the left side of the median plane (Figures 3.22 and 3.24c).

Note that in small ruminants (goats and sheep), the last centrifugal coil of spiral colon, the distal loop, and the descending colon may have small fecal pellets that are covered with fat (Figure 3.24c).

For easy identification, note the order of the proximal loop, distal loop, and caudal duodenal flexure from ventral to dorsal (study Figure 3.24c).

Identify this arrangement on the right flank or on isolated whole viscera (Figure 3.24c). The proximal loop is largest and similar in size to the cecum. The caudal duodenal flexure and distal loop are similar in size but the distal loop is covered by fat deposits while the caudal duodenal flexure is not (Figure 3.24c).

3.6 Other Abdominal Organs

Goal: Identify the liver lobes and associated ligaments of the liver, and the location of the gallbladder. Know the location of the spleen in relation to the rumen. Know the anatomical differences between the kidney of the ox and that of small ruminants (goat and sheep). Identify the lobes of the pancreas, and know that in the ox, the accessory pancreatic duct is the main duct, whereas the pancreatic duct is the major duct in small ruminants.

3.6.1 Liver

The liver in adult ruminants lies entirely within the rib cage on the right side of the median plane behind the diaphragm. The overwhelmingly large compound stomach pushes the liver to right side of the median plane (Figure 3.25a,b). Consult Box 3.12 for clinical applications related to the liver.

In adult ruminants, the liver has four lobes, some of which can be difficult to identify (e.g., quadrate lobe). On the visceral surface, identify four liver lobes: **left, right, quadrate**, and **caudate lobes**.

The caudate lobe has caudate and papillary processes. The caudate process has an indentation that embraces the cranial pole of the right kidney. In horses, the papillary process is absent.

The hepatorenal ligament attaches the caudate process of the liver to the right kidney. There is no need to identify this ligament.

The papillary process is covered by the lesser omentum and is located near the lesser curvature of the abomasum.

Unlike the horse, ruminants have a **gallbladder** that lies between the right and quadrate liver lobes.

The **round ligament of the liver** (ligamentum teres) courses from the umbilicus cranially. Find this peritoneal ligament between the quadrate and left lobes of the liver.

Triangular ligaments and coronary ligaments anchor the liver to the diaphragm. The triangular ligaments include left and right triangular ligaments. The coronary ligament encircles the caudal vena cava. There is no need to identify these ligaments.

With the help of Figure 3.25a,b, identify the left, right, quadrate, and caudate liver lobes.

3.6.2 Spleen

The spleen is located on the cranial sac of the rumen on the left side of the median plane. Only a small part of its parietal surface is attached to the diaphragm while its visceral surface is attached to the cranial sac of the rumen (Figures 3.26 and 3.27).

The shape and size of the spleen vary among species. It is relatively small in small ruminants compared with the ox. It is triangular in sheep, quadrilateral in goats, and oblong in cattle.

The spleen in your cadaver may be enlarged if barbiturates were administered for euthanasia. Consult Box 3.13 for additional clinical information.

3.6.3 Pancreas

The pancreas has **right** and **left lobes** that connect with a **body**. Identify the right lobe within the mesoduodenum (Figure 3.23) along the medial edge of the descending duodenum. It is relatively larger than the left lobe.

Find the left lobe of the pancreas medial to the right lobe of the pancreas in the proximity of the dorsal sac of the rumen and the left crus of the diaphragm. The right and left lobes join the narrow body near the porta of the liver.

The **accessory pancreatic duct** is the major pancreatic duct in the ox. It opens at the **minor duodenal papilla.** In contrast, the **pancreatic duct** is the major duct in small ruminants. In small ruminants, the pancreatic duct joins the **bile duct** and the shared duct opens on the **major duodenal papilla**.

3.6.4 Kidney

The bovine kidney has 12–20 small lobes (**multipyramidal kidney**). In contrast, the kidney of a small ruminant (goat or sheep) has a smooth surface similar to that of the dog (**pseudounipyramidal**).

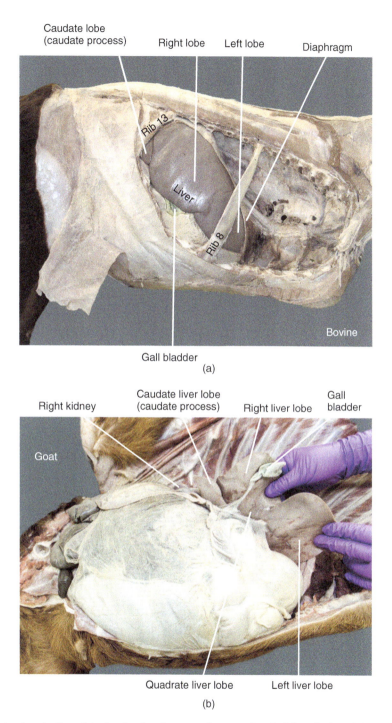

Figure 3.25 (a) Right lateral projection of the bovine liver between the ventral end of the 6th rib and dorsal aspect of the last (13th) rib. (b) Goat in situ abdominal viscera: right lateral view. Liver lobes as they are seen from the visceral surface of the liver. The papillary process of the caudate lobe is not visible.

Box 3.12

Liver biopsies in cattle are obtained on the right side at the 10th or 11th intercostal space at the level of an imaginary line between the tuber coxae and the olecranon. In clinical practice, liver biopsies are often collected using ultrasound guidance, which allows easy visualization of the liver and avoids puncturing hepatic vessels.

Liver abscesses are common in feedlot and dairy cattle. Generally, it is associated with rumen acidosis and can lead to caudal vena cava thrombosis.

Additionally, differences also exist in the interior of the kidney in cattle and small ruminants. After passing the hilus, the ureter in cattle divides into cranial and caudal principal branches that travel toward the opposite poles of the kidney (embedded in fat and can be hard to identify). Each of these principal branches further divides into several secondary branches (estimate is 18–22), each of which carries a funnel-shaped structure known as the **calyx**. Calyces can be defined as major or minor.

Cortical and medullary regions are easily identifiable when the kidney is sectioned (Figure 3.28a,b).

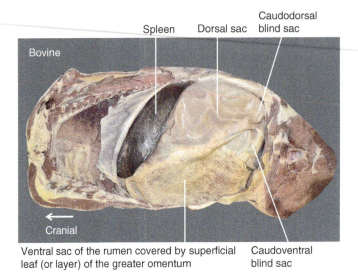

Figure 3.26 The bovine thoracic and abdominal cavities: **left** lateral view. Note the long and oblong-shaped spleen on the craniodorsal surface of the rumen (ribs are removed).

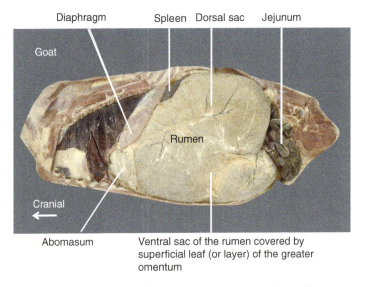

Figure 3.27 Thoracic and abdominal cavities in a goat: **left** lateral view. Note the small quadrilateral spleen in goats compared with the large oblong-shaped spleen in cattle (compare with spleen in Figure 3.26).

Box 3.13

Excessive presence of fibrous tags at the splenic attachment to the rumen could be suggestive of traumatic reticulopericarditis. Collection of abdominal fluid (**abdominocentesis**) is typically taken to the right of midline and just above the udder to avoid the rumen at the left of the midline. If available, ultrasound is helpful in localizing fluid pockets.

Identify the medullary pyramids on a cross section of the bovine kidney. The apex of each pyramid is known as the papilla (Figure 3.28b). The apex of each papilla projects into a minor calyx. Small papillary ducts open into the minor calyx. Urine passes from the minor calyces into one of two major calyces that join to form the ureter. The two major caylces are sometimes called the principal branches of the ureter.

In small ruminants (goat and sheep), the kidney has a **renal pelvis** and **renal crest** similar to that of the dog and cat. No renal pelvis is present in cattle (Figure 3.28a).

The renal artery, vein, and ureter in goats and cattle can be identified at the **hilus**, an indentation where the renal vein and ureter leave the kidney and the renal artery enters (Figure 3.28).

Identify the **renal cortex, renal medulla, renal crest, renal pelvis**, and **renal sinus** on median and sagittal sections of the goat or sheep kidney (Figure 3.29a,b). No calyces are present in small ruminants.

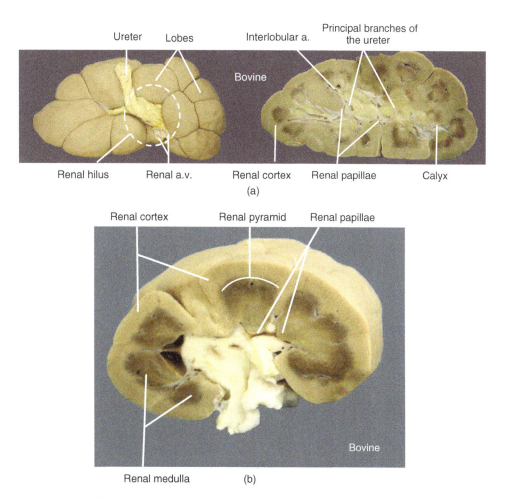

Figure 3.28 (a) Bovine kidney. Figure shows intact (left) and sagittal section (right). (b) Sagittal section of the bovine kidney showing renal pyramids and renal papillae.

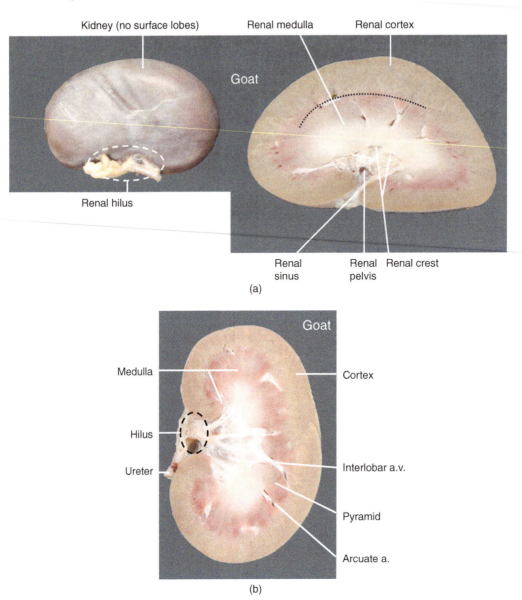

Figure 3.29 (a) Goat kidney: intact kidney (left) and median section (right). (b) Goat kidney: a dorsal plane section (off the center) of a caprine kidney showing the renal pyramids and interlobar vessels.

3.7 Vessels

Vessels are best identified when injected with colored latex (red for arteries and blue for veins). Uninjected medium and small-sized vessels can be hard to identify. Generally, arteries are best identified on target structures supplied.

3.7.1 Arteries

Goal: Identify the aorta, celiac, and cranial mesenteric arteries.

Arteries that supply the abdominal viscera comprise **paired** and **unpaired vessels** that originate from the abdominal aorta.

The unpaired arteries include (i) **celiac,** (ii) **cranial mesenteric**, and (iii) **caudal mesenteric** arteries. Paired arteries include (i) **lumbar**, (ii) **phrenicoabdominal**, (iii) **renal**, (iv) **gonadal (testicular or ovarian)**, and (v) **deep circumflex iliac arteries.** Your instructor may ask you to identify some of these arteries. Apart from the aorta, celiac, cranial mesenteric, and renal arteries, we tend not to trace other arteries of the abdomen if they are not injected.

A brief discussion of the abdominal arteries follows.

The **celiac artery** gives three major branches: **splenic, left gastric**, and **hepatic arteries**. Their names indicate their target organs. Each of the aforementioned three branches of the celiac artery gives several named branches.

There are usually variations in the origin of branches from the celiac, left gastric, and hepatic arteries. Thus, there is little practical benefit in identifying these branches or tracing their origin. However, you can easily identify the right ruminal artery (from the splenic) coursing on the right longitudinal groove of the rumen. Likewise, the left ruminal artery (from the left gastric) runs in the left longitudinal groove.

Arteries running on the greater curvature of the abomasum are the right and left gastroepiploic arteries that anastomose end-to-end about midway along the greater curvature. They originate from the hepatic and left gastric arteries, respectively. The left and right gastric arteries anastomose on the lesser curvature of the abomasum. The right gastric artery is a branch of the hepatic artery.

The **cranial mesenteric artery** supplies the small and large intestines except for the most caudal segment of the transverse and descending colon, which are supplied by the caudal mesenteric artery. Branches of the cranial mesenteric artery include caudal pancreaticoduodenal, middle colic, ileocolic, right colic, colic branches, mesenteric ileal branch, and cecal arteries. There is no need to identify these branches.

The **caudal mesenteric artery** gives rise to the left colic and cranial rectal arteries. The left colic artery supplies the descending colon. The cranial rectal artery supplies the first part of the rectum.

Paired arteries include phrenicoabdominal, renal, gonadal (testicular or ovarian), lumbar, and deep circumflex iliac arteries. The renal arteries could be identified on isolated kidney or a dorsal view of the aorta. The gonadal arteries are discussed with the pelvis. There is no need to identify these arteries.

Identify the **celiac, cranial mesenteric**, and **renal arteries** by making a longitudinal incision of the dorsal wall of the abdominal aorta (Figure 3.30). Insert

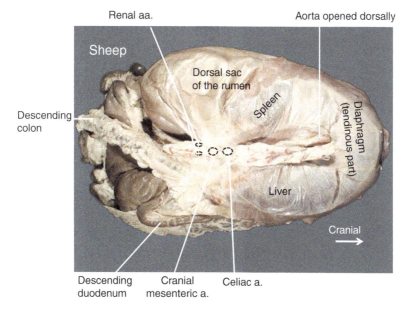

Figure 3.30 Isolated sheep abdominal viscera: dorsal view. The dotted circles indicate the location of the origins of the celiac, cranial mesenteric, and renal arteries on the floor of the abdominal aorta.

your probe on the closely associated celiac, cranial mesenteric, and renal arteries from proximal to distal, respectively.

3.7.2 Veins

Goal: Identify the caudal vena cava and portal vein.

Venous return from the abdominal viscera (stomach, small intestine and the majority of large intestine, and the spleen) is high in fat and toxic contents. It drains into the **portal vein** that carries venous blood from the gastrointestinal tract to the liver for detoxification.

It is important to understand that blood from the gastrointestinal tract traverses two capillary beds, one in the gastrointestinal tract and the other in the liver. From the liver, detoxified blood reaches the **caudal vena cava** via the **hepatic veins**.

You have identified the cauda vena cava in the thorax and could do so on the visceral surface of the liver. Follow its termination into the right atrium of the heart. The caudal vena cava drains blood from the pelvis, hind limbs, and from paired organs (kidney, adrenal, and gonads.)

Hepatic veins that drain into the caudal vena cava can be demonstrated by opening the dorsal portion of the caudal vena cava that traverses the liver.

Your instructor may ask you to identify the portal vein and or its branches. It is formed by the merger of the **cranial mesenteric, caudal mesenteric, splenic,** and **gastroduodenal veins.**

3.7.3 Lymphatics

Goal: Understand the major lymph centers of the abdomen. Identify the jejunal (mesenteric) lymph nodes (Figure 3.22).

The function of the lymphatic system is to carry large particles that are too bulky to be drained by the veins. Lymphatic vessels start as small lymph capillaries and ultimately merge to form large lymphatic vessels (e.g., thoracic duct, intestinal, lumbar, and other trunks). The thoracic duct joins the large veins near the thoracic inlet.

Lymph passes through lymph nodes for filtration before joining the venous system. **Lymphocenters** consist of a single lymph node or multiple nodes.

Lymph from the abdomen is drained by three large lymphocenters: (i) **celiac,** (ii) **cranial mesenteric**, and (iii) **caudal mesenteric lymphocenters**.

Large numbers of lymph nodes are associated with each of the centers. Note that each of these lymphocenters drains an area supplied by similarly named unpaired arteries (celiac, cranial, and caudal mesenteric arteries).

Lymph nodes of the celiac lymphocenter receive lymph from organs and lymph nodes associated with the celiac artery. The nodes include **gastric (in ruminants, these are referred to as the various ruminal, reticular, etc. nodes), hepatic, splenic,** and **pancreaticoduodenal lymph nodes that drain to the colic or intestinal trunk.**

The nodes of the cranial mesenteric lymphocenter receive lymph from the **cecal, colic,** and **jejunal lymph nodes.** The jejunal lymph nodes (also called mesenteric lymph nodes) are very long and are in the mesojejunum close to the mesenteric border of the jejunum (Figure 3.22).

The caudal mesenteric lymph nodes are associated with the descending colon and caudal mesenteric artery.

3.8 Palpation of the Live Animal

Goal: Understand that rectal palpation is a useful technique in the diagnosis of pregnancy and evaluation of the health of bull accessory sex glands. In the abdominal region, you can palpate the abdominal organs that lie close to the pelvic cavity (e.g., apex of the cecum, dorsal blind sac of the rumen, and left and right ovaries). You need to develop the ability to visualize the location of abdominal organs on the left and right flanks based on your anatomical knowledge. Several bony prominences (e.g., transverse processes of lumbar vertebral spines), vessels, and soft structures can be palpated by hand on the surface of the body. The lobulated left and right kidneys are palpable to the right of midline (the right kidney is pushed slightly more cranial than the left kidney and may be unreachable by some examiners with short arms).

Example of organs on the left flank are the rumen and the spleen. The spleen is normally not palpable.

> **Box 3.14**
>
> Examples of organs that can be palpated per rectum in an average sized cow are caudal blind sacs of the rumen, left kidney, apex of cecum, uterus, and ovaries and accessory sex glands in mature bulls that include vesicular, bulbourethral, and prostate glands.

The intestinal mass, including the cecum, occupies the caudal part of the right half of the abdomen. The liver, abomasum, and descending duodenum are located on the right side of the median plane. Note that the paralumbar fossa is well developed in the cow.

Palpation per rectum is a valuable diagnostic technique that you need to master to become a skilled practitioner. In bovine practice, palpation per rectum is one of the most frequent procedures performed by veterinarians. The size of the animal and length of the arms of the examiner can influence the outcome.

Rectal palpation in cattle can be used for the manual determination of pregnancy or, by using transrectal ultrasonography, to examine a fetus. In pregnancy diagnosis by rectal palpation, the examiner will look to feel (depending on the stage of pregnancy) one or more of the following: (i) a fetal membrane slip; (ii) the amniotic vesicle; (iii) placentomes; (iv) pulsation in the uterine artery (on the ipsilateral side of pregnant horn); (v) the presence of corpus luteum; or (vi) a fetus. In males, it may be used for the evaluation of accessory sex glands in bulls as part of the bull soundness examination (BSE) and in diagnosis of diseases and pelvic bone fractures.

Skill and clinical acumen in rectal palpation is built by practice and by sound knowledge of the anatomy and physiology of ruminants (read Box 3.14 for examples of organs palpable per rectum).

3.9 Lab ID List for the Abdomen

There is no need to identify items in *italics*. Abdominal wall and segments of the gastrointestinal tract

1. Know muscles of the abdominal wall and the direction of their fibers
   a. *Cutaneous trunci m.*
   b. *Cutaneous omobrachialis m.*
   c. External abdominal oblique (EAO)
   d. Internal abdominal oblique (IAO)
   e. Transverse abdominis (TA)
   f. Rectus abdominis (RA)
2. Tunica flava
3. Paralumbar fossa
4. Understand the innervation of the abdominal flank (local anesthesia)
5. Stomach
6. Spleen
7. Cardia
8. Reticular groove
9. Reticulum
10. Rumen
    a. Right and left longitudinal grooves
    b. Cranial groove
    c. Caudal groove
    d. Blinds sacs (caudodorsal and caudoventral blind sacs)
    e. Ventral and dorsal sacs
    f. Ruminoreticular fold
    g. Cranial sac (ruminal atrium)
    h. Ruminal recess
    i. Cranial pillar
    j. Caudal pillar
    k. Coronary pillars (in sheep, the left dorsal coronary pillar is absent)
    l. Right or left longitudinal pillar (depending on the wall you cut into)
11. Omasum
12. Reticulo-omasal orifice
13. Omasoabomasal orifice
14. Abomasum
    a. Torus pyloricus
    b. Vela abomasica
15. Greater omentum (superficial and deep leaf)
16. Omental bursa
17. Lesser omentum
18. Supraomental recess
19. Duodenum (cranial part of the duodenum beginning at the pylorus and cranial duodenal flexure)
    a. Sigmoid flexure
    b. Descending duodenum
    c. *Duodenojejunal flexure*
    d. Caudal duodenal flexure
    e. Ascending duodenum
20. Jejunum

21. Ileum
22. Ileocecal fold
23. Cecum
24. Colon (ascending transverse and descending)
25. Ascending colon
    a. Proximal loop
    b. Spiral loop (centripetal turns, central flexure, and centrifugal turns)
    c. Distal loop
26. Transverse colon
27. Descending colon
28. Kidney (know the term "calyx")
29. Liver lobes (ID left, quadrate, right, caudate [caudate and papillary processes] lobes)
30. Gallbladder (know location between liver lobes)

4

The Pelvis and Reproductive Organs

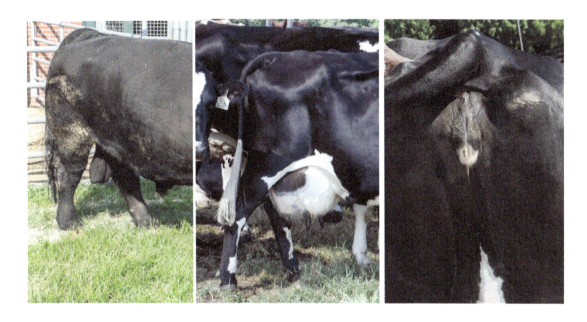

Learning Objectives	
• Identify the bones and major muscles of the pelvis. Some of the pelvic bones have features that are palpable in the live animal (e.g., ischial, coxial, and sacral tubers). • Understand the meaning of the terms "pelvic inlet and pelvic outlet" and the bony boundaries for the inlet and outlet. Understand how to determine the size of the pelvic cavity in heifers prior to breeding using pelvimetry. This information is used by breeders to predict dystocia.	• Identify the major nerves of the lumbosacral plexus and terminal branches of the abdominal aorta that supply the bladder and reproductive organs. Know the clinical significance of some of the major nerves and arteries (e.g., peculiar pulsation in the uterine artery during pregnancy, obturator nerve compression during calving, and damage of dorsal nerve of the penis in bulls intended for breeding services). • Identify and know the clinical significance of the different parts of the male and female reproductive

Guide to Ruminant Anatomy: Dissection and Clinical Aspects, Second Edition. Mahmoud Mansour, Ray Wilhite, Joe Rowe, and Saly Hafiz.
© 2023 John Wiley & Sons, Inc. Published 2023 by John Wiley & Sons, Inc.
Companion website: www.wiley.com/go/mansour/dissection2

systems. Pay specific attention to the anatomy of the urethra in male and female and what makes catheterization difficult in male ruminants (penile sigmoid flexure, urethral process [vermiform appendage], and dorsal urethral recess). Understand that female ruminants have a suburethral diverticulum that you should avoid when passing a catheter.
- Know the clinical significance of the penile sigmoid flexure, the pudendal and dorsal nerves of the penis in the male.
- Understand the structures associated with breeding soundness evaluation (BSE) in breeding bulls. In addition to evaluation of sperm motility and libido, the BSE includes a physical examination and inspection of the external (testis, prepuce, and penis) and internal (accessory sex glands) reproductive organs.
- You should be familiar with the anatomy of the female reproductive tract for physical diagnosis and palpation of the ovary, pulsation in the uterine artery during pregnancy, identification of the cervix when performing artificial insemination (AI), and detection of pregnancy as early as 35 days by slipping of the fetal membranes (chorioallantois) through the fingers in a pregnant uterine horn.
- Identify the mammary duct system and know the innervation, blood supply, and the laminae of the suspensory apparatus of the udder.
- Identify and know the clinical significance of the mammary lymph nodes or superficial inguinal lymph nodes (mastitis).
- At the end of the pelvis section, watch Videos 18, 19, and 20.

4.1 Bones of the Pelvis

Goal: Start by identifying the bones of the pelvis. Understand the terms pelvic inlet and pelvic outlet. Study male and female reproductive organs, urinary bladder, peritoneal pouches, vessels, and nerves within the male and female pelvis.

4.1.1 Os Coxae (Pelvic Bone)

The pelvic bone (os coxae) comprises three major fused bones: the **ilium**, **ischium**, and **pubis**. Identify the major features of the pelvic bones that are palpable in the live animal (Figure 4.1): tuber coxae (coxal tuber), tuber sacrale (sacral tuber), and tuber ischium (ischial tuber).

Cattlemen call the coxal tuber the "**hook**" and the sacral tuber the "**pin**." With help of Figure 4.1, identify the ischiatic spine, **body (shaft) of the ilium**, **pecten**, **obturator foramen**, **ischiatic arch**, and the **pelvic symphysis**.

The **pelvic inlet** is bounded dorsally by the **promontory** and wings of the sacrum, laterally by the left and right bodies of the ilia, and ventrally

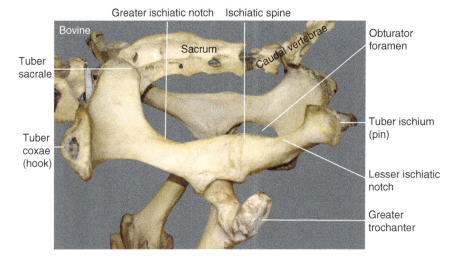

Figure 4.1 Bones of the bovine pelvis. Note the vertical and horizontal diameters of the pelvis. They are important measurements used for predicting calving difficulties. Differences in pelvic inlet and outlet exist between the male and female pelvis (Box 4.1).

Box 4.1
Because the **vertical diameter** of the pelvic inlet and birth canal is larger than the **transverse diameter**, it is possible to twist a large fetus vertically to ease its birth in cases of dystocia (difficult birth). A pelvimeter is an instrument used for measurement of vertical and horizontal dimensions of the pelvis. These measurements can be used in eliminating heifers with a small pelvis from breeding.

by the pubic **pecten** or pubic brim. Note that the vertical diameter of the pelvic inlet is relatively larger than the transverse diameter.

The pelvic outlet is bounded by the **sacrosciatic (broad sacrotuberous) ligament** laterally, the **ischiatic arch** ventrally, and 3–4 **caudal vertebrae** dorsally.

The space between the pelvic inlet and outlet is the **pelvic canal**.

4.2 Sacrosciatic Ligament (Broad Sacrotuberous Ligament)

Goal: Identify the sacrosciatic ligament (forms the non-osseous lateral wall of the pelvic cavity) and the neurovascular structures that are located on its lateral and medial surfaces. Know the major and lesser ischiatic foramina and what structure passes through each.

The sacrosciatic ligament is a broad sheet of connective tissue that forms the dorsal softer part of the lateral wall of the pelvic cavity (Figure 4.2). The ventral part of the lateral wall of the pelvis is formed by the body of ilium and ischium. Consult Box 4.2 for clinical application.

As in the horse, the course of the sacrosciatic ligament on the ischiatic spine and over the greater and lesser ischiatic notches of the bovine pelvis allows for the formation of the greater and lesser ischiatic foramina, respectively. Identify the ischiatic spine and the greater and lesser ischiatic notches on a bovine or caprine skeleton (Figures 4.1 and 4.2).

The **sciatic (or ischiatic) nerve, cranial gluteal vessels (artery** and **vein)**, and **cranial** and **caudal gluteal nerves** pass through the **greater ischiatic foramen**. The **caudal gluteal artery** and **vein** pass through the **lesser ischiatic foramen.**

In horses, the tendon of the internal obturator muscle passes through the lesser ischiatic foramen but no vessels or nerves pass through it. With the help

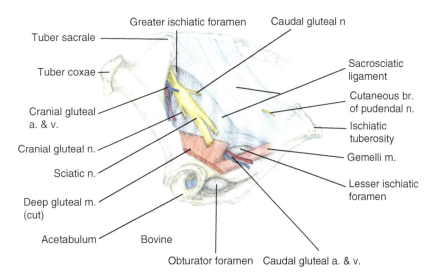

Figure 4.2 Schematic illustration of the bovine sacrosciatic ligament and the structures passing through the greater and lesser ischiatic foramina: left lateral view.

> **Box 4.2**
>
> Slackening (softening) of the sacrosciatic ligament is an indication of an impending parturition. The softening is thought to be caused by secretion of the hormone relaxin from both the ovary and placenta.

of Figure 4.2, identify the sacrosciatic ligament, the greater and lesser ischiatic foramina, and the structures that pass through these foramina.

4.3 Pelvic Peritoneal Pouches

Goal: Know that the reflection of the peritoneum in the pelvic cavity forms four peritoneal pouches or fossae. From dorsal to ventral, identify the pararectal fossa, rectogenital pouch, vesicogenital pouch, and pubovesical pouch. Know the dorsal and ventral boundaries for each pouch. Consult box 4.3 for clinical significance.

Before you start learning the pelvic viscera, take a moment to study the pelvic peritoneal pouches on a median sagittal section of a female or male pelvis or on a complete pelvis looking caudally onto the pelvic inlet (Figure 4.3).

The pouches are created by continuations of abdominal parietal peritoneum into the pelvic cavity. They project in and around the digestive, genital, and urinary organs. They represent the most caudal extent of the parietal peritoneum.

From dorsal to ventral, four pouches are recognized: the **pararectal fossae, rectogenital pouch, vesicogenital pouch,** and **pubovesical pouch.**

The **pararectal fossae** are the peritoneal spaces on either side of the mesorectum. They continue ventrally to merge with the rectogenital pouch.

The **rectogenital pouch** is the peritoneal space between the rectum and genital tract (uterus and cranial part of the vagina in the female or ductus deferens and genital fold in the male).

The **vesicogenital pouch** is the peritoneal space between the genital tract (uterus and cranial part of the vagina in the female or genital fold in the male) dorsally and the urinary bladder ventrally. The prefix "vesico" in vesicogenital means bladder.

The peritoneal space between the bladder and the pubic floor is the **pubovesical pouch**. With the help of Figure 4.3, identify each pouch by inserting your gloved fingers or probe between the structures that form the boundary for each pouch.

In male cadavers, note the peritoneal fold located on the dorsal surface of the bladder containing the ampullae of the deferent ducts. This is the **genital fold.** As discussed earlier, the peritoneal space between the genital fold and the bladder in the male is the vesicogenital pouch.

4.4 Urinary Bladder, Ureters, and Ligaments of the Bladder

Goal: Identify the ureters, the three peritoneal ligaments that suspend the bladder in the pelvic cavity: the lateral, medial, and median ligaments of the bladder. Identify the round ligaments of the bladder (remnant of the fetal umbilical arteries) that are located within the lateral ligaments.

The urinary bladder is positioned in the pelvic cavity when it is empty. The bladder in your embalmed cadaver may be stiff in texture and contracted. If you are working on a cadaver with abdominal contents present, follow the **ureters** from the hilus of the kidney to the dorsal wall of the urinary bladder to

> **Box 4.3**
>
> The peritoneal pouch determines the caudal extent of the peritoneum. Vaginal and rectal tears caudal to these pouches carry more favorable prognosis compared with tears involving the pouches and therefore the possibility of peritonitis.
>
> Rectovaginal fistula is a complication of dystocia that results from a difficult birth when a malpresented or oversized calf tears through the rectovaginal septum (perineal body), a musculofibrous tissue that separates the rectum from the vagina.

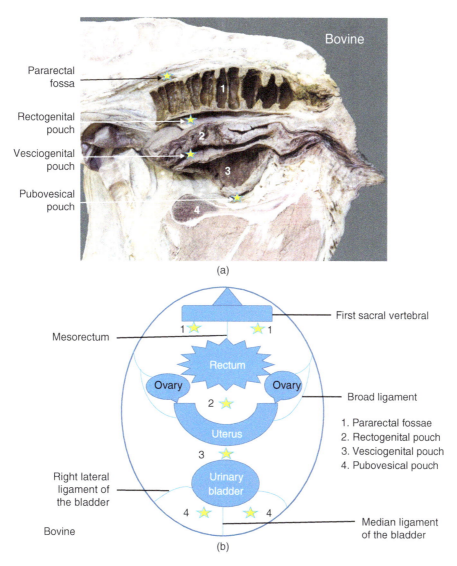

Figure 4.3 (a) Pelvic peritoneal pouches. Female bovine pelvis: midsagittal section. 1, rectum; 2, uterus; 3, vagina; 4, bladder; 5, pubic bone; dotted line, pelvic symphysis, black star, rectovaginal septum or perineal body; (b) cranial view of the pelvic bovine (cow) pouches and ligaments of the bladder.

where they terminate close to the neck of the bladder. If you are working on an isolated pelvis, look for the stump of the ureter on the dorsal aspect of the urinary bladder near the neck.

Three peritoneal ligaments suspend the urinary bladder in the pelvic cavity (Figure 4.3b): **left** and **right lateral ligaments** and the **median ligament of the bladder.** The median ligament extends from an area caudal to the umbilicus on the dorsal surface of the linea alba and parietal peritoneum to the midventral surface of the urinary bladder. The lateral ligaments extend from the lateral walls of the urinary bladder to the left and right pelvic walls. They carry the **round ligaments of the bladder** on their peripheral borders. Identify the ligaments of the bladder on an intact pelvis.

4.5 Male Genitalia

Goal: You should be able to identify the major male reproductive structures, including the testes and their adnexa, penis, prepuce (sheath), and accessory sex glands. These structures are examined in the BSE of bulls. At the end of this unit, watch **Video 18**.

The male genitalia comprise the paired **testes** and their **adnexa, penis and urethra, prepuce,** and **accessory sex glands**.

4.5.1 Penis

Goal: Know that male ruminants have a fibroelastic penis compared with the musculocavernous type of penis of the equine. Dogs have bone (os penis) incorporated in the distal part of the corpus cavernosum penis. Bulls, bucks (billy), and rams have no bone in their penises.

Identify the **corpus cavernosum penis** (CCP), **corpus spongiosum penis** (CSP), and **tunica albuginea (TA) penis** surrounding the CCP. Identify the **sigmoid flexure** and its proximal and distal bends.

Note the post-scrotal position of the **sigmoid flexure** in small and large male ruminants.

Identify the urethral process in the bull and small ruminants. In small ruminants, the urethral process is also known as "vermiform process or vermiform appendage" because of its resemblance to a small worm in shape. Know where the penis has a weak TA that could rupture from increased blood pressure in the CCP.

Understand that a major contributor to the thinness of the TA on the inside of the distal bend is the stretching when the sigmoid flexure straightens upon erection, similar to a glove thinning if you pull it tight over your finger.

Identify regions where the urethral diameter becomes small (potential location for urethral calculi). Understand the importance of the dorsal nerve of the penis, the size of the testes, physical conditions, and accessory sex glands in the BSE in bulls.

The penis of male ruminants is of the **fibroelastic type**. It is rigid in a non-erect state. It is characterized by the presence of a sigmoid flexure and well-developed retractor penis (Figure 4.4). The penis is topographically divided into **root**, **body**, and **glans** (Figure 4.4). Clinically sound anatomy of the penis is very important for bull breeding soundness and must be examined for any bruises and injuries.

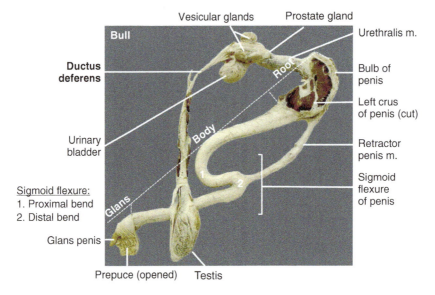

Figure 4.4 Isolated urogenital tract of the bull (urinary bladder, penis, accessory sex glands, and testis). Note the post-scrotal position of the sigmoid flexure. Keep this location in mind when palpating the sigmoid flexure in the live animal. 1 and 2, the proximal and distal bends of the sigmoid flexure, respectively.

4.5.1.1 Root of the Penis and Cavernous Tissue

The root of the penis is composed of two lateral (left and right) **crura** and a midline located **bulb of the penis**. The crura attach the root of the penis to the left and right **ischiatic tuberosities** (**pins**) on the os coxae.

The penis is also attached to the ischial arch and pelvic symphysis by a pair of collagenous sheets known as the suspensory ligament of the penis (Figure 4.5). There is no need to dissect this ligament.

Each **crus** is composed of cavernous tissue known as CCP, surrounded by a layer of dense collagenous connective tissue, **TA penis**. A short **ischiocavernosus muscle** covers each crus (Figure 4.5).

The **bulb of the penis** is the enlarged middle portion of the root. The bulb is an expansion of the proximal end of the corpus spongiosum penis (CSP). This expansion is covered by the **bulbospongiosus muscle** (Figure 4.4). Study the structures that make

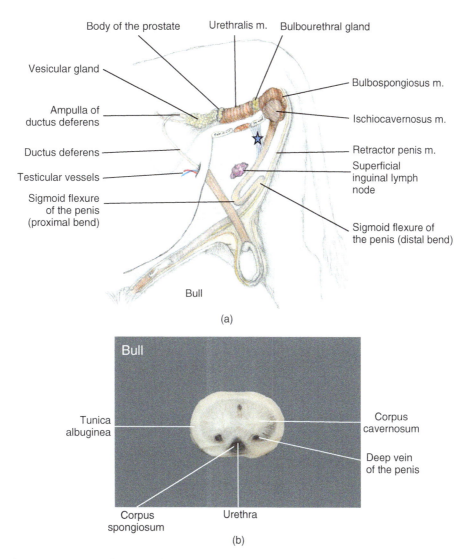

Figure 4.5 (a) Schematic illustration of the reproductive tract of the bull in situ. Note the location of the superficial inguinal lymph nodes that are also known as scrotal lymph nodes. They drain the scrotum, prepuce, and penis but not the testes. Star, suspensory ligament of the penis (bilateral). (b) Cross-section of the bovine penis at the level of the sigmoid flexure.

up the root of the penis with the help of Figures 4.4 and 4.5.

The body of the penis is the region between the root and the glans (Figure 4.4). It is characterized by the presence of an S-shaped **sigmoid flexure,** a clinically important feature. In the non-erect penis, the sigmoid flexure is situated caudal to the neck of the scrotum (post-scrotal position).

The post-scrotal location of the sigmoid flexure in the bull is different from that in the boar where the sigmoid flexure has a prescrotal position. In boars, the testicles have a perineal position, whereas in ruminants the testicles are vertically suspended below the pelvic floor.

4.5.1.2 Free Part of the Penis and Glans Penis

The free part of the penis and the glans are the regions of the penis distal to the attachment of the internal lamina of the prepuce (Figure 4.6b). The glans is the most proximal enlargement at the tip of the penis (Figures 4.4, 4.6a,b, and 4.7a,b). It asymmetrical in shape. Push the prepuce backward to expose the free part of the penis and glans penis (Figure 4.7a,b).

A shallow ridge of skin along the ventral surface of the free part of the penis is called the raphe of the penis (Figure 4.7b). The raphe of the penis is a thickening of the skin on the midventral line of the free part of the penis. It extends from the preputial fornix to the tip of the glans on the right side (Figure 4.7b).

Note that in small male ruminants (rams and bucks), the glans has a long **urethral process** that extends a few centimeters beyond the glans. In contrast, the bull urethral process does not extend beyond the glans (Figure 4.7b). The **external urethral orifice** is located at the tip of the urethral process.

4.5.1.3 Retractor Penis Muscle

The **retractor penis** comprises well-developed, paired smooth muscles that are separated at their origin but come together at their insertion on the ventral surface of the distal bend of the sigmoid flexure and beyond (Figures 4.4 and 4.5a).

The retractor penis muscle originates from the caudal vertebrae dorsally. It passes on each side of the external anal sphincter muscle (where a few fibers from external and internal sphincter muscles are added), and inserts distally at the ventral surface of the distal bend of the sigmoid flexure in small ruminants. In the bull, the muscle continues distally to insert on the free part of the penis.

The retractor penis muscle is innervated by sympathetic fibers that are thought to travel through branches of the pudendal nerve that include the caudal rectal, or deep peroneal nerves to reach the muscle. Relaxation of the retractor penis muscle is essential for attainment of full erection and straightening of the sigmoid flexure. Relaxation of the penis for clinical examination can be accomplished by blocking the pudendal nerve within the pelvis or through the ischiorectal fossa.

Make cross sections of the body of the penis proximal and distal to the sigmoid flexure and compare the size of the urethral lumen in the two cross sections. Note that the urethra is narrower at the distal bend than its diameter in cross sections proximal to the sigmoid flexure. In general, the sigmoid flexure of the penis is a typical site for obstruction by urinary calculi, especially at the distal bend. In small ruminants, both the sigmoid flexure and urethral process are potential sites for calculi.

The penile urethra runs on the midventral urethral groove of the penis. It is surrounded by CSP. Identify the CCP and CSP on cross sections of the body of the penis (Figure 4.5b). In small male ruminants (bucks and rams), note that the urethra extends beyond the glans penis through the vermiform urethral process.

4.5.1.4 Apical Ligament

Identify the **apical ligament** on the dorsum of the distal portion of the penis of the bull (Figure 4.6). The apical ligament typically arises from the dorsal midline of the TA approximately eight inches from the penile tip (Figure 4.6b). The fibers are shorter but more firmly attached on the left and longer and more easily undermined on the right side. Defects of the length, strength, or attachment of the apical ligament can lead to pathological penile deviations. Consult Box 4.4 for clinical application of the apical ligament.

Male goats and sheep have apical ligaments, but unlike the single apical ligament of the bull's penis, these animals have two lateral ligaments situated on each side of the apex of the penis with no outward connection over the dorsal surface of the penis. Do not attempt to dissect these ligaments.

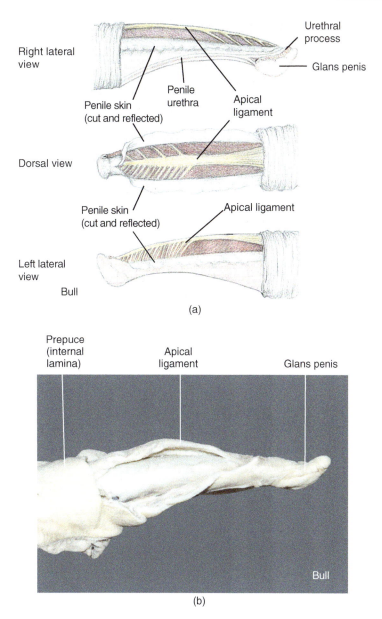

Figure 4.6 (a) Right lateral, left lateral, and dorsal views of the apical ligament in the penis of the bull. Source: Garrett (1988). (b) Dissection of the apical ligament on the dorsum of the bull penis: right lateral view. The apical ligament is a feature of the TA covering corpus cavernosum penis (CCP). It arises distal to sigmoid flexure from the dorsal midline and left side, with thinner fibers on the left side. (c) The dorsal apical ligament can be used to help hold the penis in extension during clinical exam. Note the placement of a towel clamp under the apical ligament to hold penis in extension. Source: Hopper (2021). (d) Spiral deviation during breeding attempt. According to some reports misshapen dorsal apical ligament may prevent the fully erect penis from assuming its normal straight orientation and the bull may be unable to control the penis sufficiently to locate the vulva of the cow. Source: Hopper (2021). Figures reprinted with permission of John Wiley & Sons, Inc. From Bovine Reproduction, Richard M. Hopper, second edition 2021.

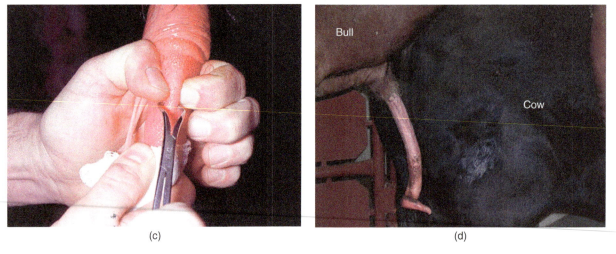

(c) (d)

Figure 4.6 (*Continued*)

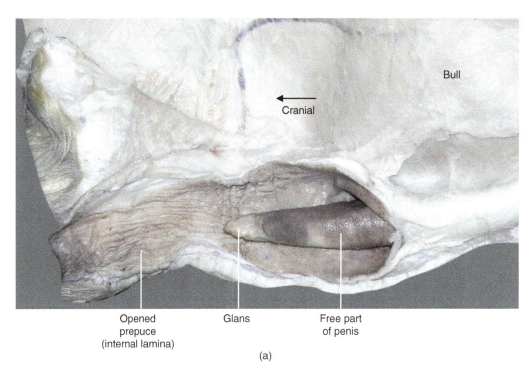

Opened prepuce (internal lamina) Glans Free part of penis

(a)

Figure 4.7 (a) The **free part** and glans of the penis: right lateral view. The right lateral wall of the prepuce is transected longitudinally and removed to expose the **preputial cavity** and the **free part of the penis**. (b) The glans penis in the bull and small male ruminants (buck and ram): right lateral view. Note the extension of the **urethral process** beyond the glans in the penis of small ruminants (2–4 cm). The internal lamina of the prepuce is peeled backward. (c) Pathology: Persistent frenulum causing phimosis (short penis). Source: Hopper (2021). (d) Preputial prolapse on presentation. Note the "elephant trunk" appearance. Source: Hopper (2021). (e) Paraphimosis secondary to preputial laceration. Source: Hopper (2021).

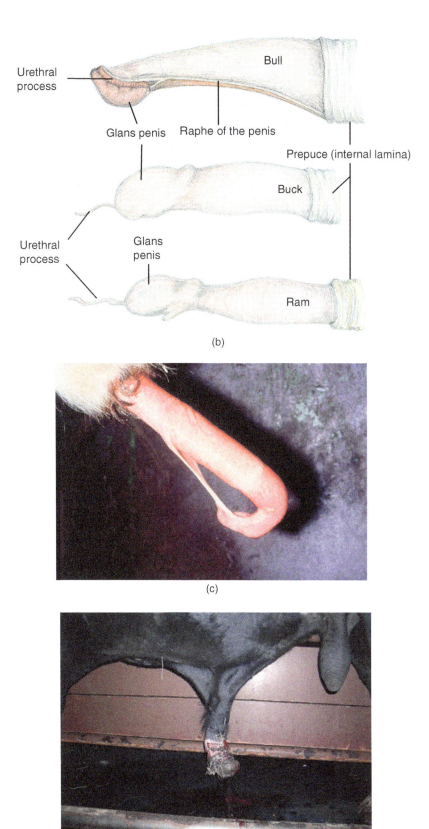

Figure 4.7 (*Continued*)

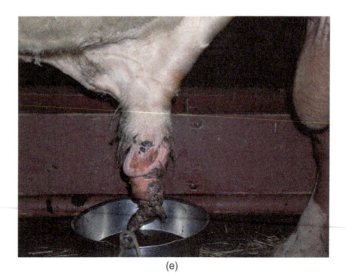

(e)

Figure 4.7 (*Continued*)

Box 4.4

Abnormalities in the strength of the apical ligament can cause spiral, ventral, and S-shaped deviations of the penis (Figure 4.6d). The ligament can be dissected out and reinforced surgically. Two surgical procedures have been described: (i) apical ligament splitting and interweaving and (ii) fascia lata auto-grafting. Sexual rest for two months is recommended.

The apical ligament can be used to facilitate extraction and handling of the penis during some surgeries (e.g., preputial injuries such as prolapse abscesses, papilloma, persistent frenulum (see Figures 4.6c and 4.7c,d,e), and fractured penis). Typically, the penis is extended and grasped with a gauze pad. A penetrating towel forceps is placed deep to the dorsal apical ligament in the area proximal to the glans penis (Figure 4.6c).

4.5.1.5 Dorsal Nerve of the Penis

Identify the dorsal nerve, artery, and vein of the penis coursing distally on each side of the dorsal wall of the penis (all are paired structures) (Figure 4.8).

The **dorsal nerve of the penis** is a branch (continuation) of the **pudendal nerve.** The nerve supplies important sensory fibers to the glans penis. The integrity of the pudendal nerve and the dorsal nerve of the penis are critical for breeding soundness of the bull and its ability to inseminate a cow (Box 4.5).

4.5.2 Male Urethra

The male urethra is technically divided into **pelvic urethra** (within the pelvic cavity) and **penile urethra** (within the penis). It transports urine from the urinary bladder to the exterior. The urethra is a potential site for calculi deposition and bacterial infections. Consult Box 4.6 on clinical relevance of the urethra and the sigmoid flexure.

As discussed earlier, the urinary bladder is located within the pelvic cavity when is empty. It extends further cranial in the abdomen when distended.

Make a midventral incision on the ventral wall of the bladder and locate the openings of the ureters inside the bladder cavity. Note that the ureters' tunnel for short distance inside the dorsal wall of the bladder before they open inside the urinary bladder. This helps prevent backflow of the urine to the kidneys when the urinary bladder is full.

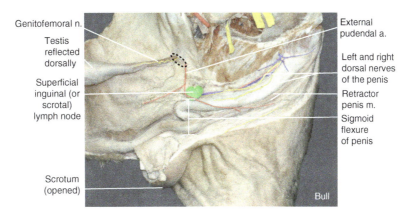

Figure 4.8 In situ dissection of the bull reproductive tract showing the dorsal nerves of a bull penis and the sigmoid flexure. The black circle indicates the position of the superficial inguinal ring.

Box 4.5
The dorsal nerve of the penis can be blocked on the exterior dorsal wall of the penis. Alternatively, the pudendal nerve can also be blocked inside the pelvic cavity along the inner surface of the sacrosciatic ligament or as it crosses the ischiatic arch. Pudendal nerve block leads to the relaxation of the retractor penis and hence facilitates clinical examination.

Make a note of the relationship of the ureters and ductus deferens. Note that the left and right ductus deferens course from the inguinal canal and pass caudally and dorsally to reach the roof of the bladder. Here they course medial (i.e., below) to the ureters. Because of this relationship, it is recommended that you avoid excessive pulling of the ductus deferens in castration procedures. Forceful pull on the ductus deferens could result in tearing of the ureters, a disastrous outcome.

The triangular area on the inner dorsal wall of the neck of the urinary bladder defined by the two openings of the ureters in the bladder and opening of the bladder into the urethra is called the **trigone of the bladder** (Figure 4.9a,b).

The male urethra forms a **dorsal recess or diverticulum** deep to the **bulb of the penis** (the area between the left and right crus of the penis). The diverticulum can be demonstrated by making a

Box 4.6
Penile sigmoid flexure
In the bull, **the dorsal surface of the distal bend** of the sigmoid flexure is a frequent site for penile rupture and hematoma, a condition that may require surgical intervention. This condition is a common injury in breeding bulls during mating when there is a sudden bend of an erect penis during breeding. A serious injury left unattended can lead to hematoma, infection, and possible retirement of the affected bull. The sigmoid flexure is also a frequent site for calculi (obstructive urolithiasis), especially in young male pet ruminants (bucks and rams) that have been castrated at a young age for marketing. The condition can also be secondary to feeding pet goats inappropriate diets. For example, hay containing high amounts of oxalates promotes oxalate stone formation. Ruminants have evolved to consume mainly forages and browse. Feeding too much grain can result in the formation of struvite or calcium apatite stones. Similarly, a diet composed of high amounts of calcium-containing grains, legumes, or clover hay promotes the formation of calcium carbonate calculi. The urethral process in small male ruminants can also be a potential site for urolith obstruction (obstructive material formed from mucus, proteins, and minerals). Surgical amputation of the urethral process is sometimes employed as part of the treatment of small ruminants affected by obstructive urolithiasis.

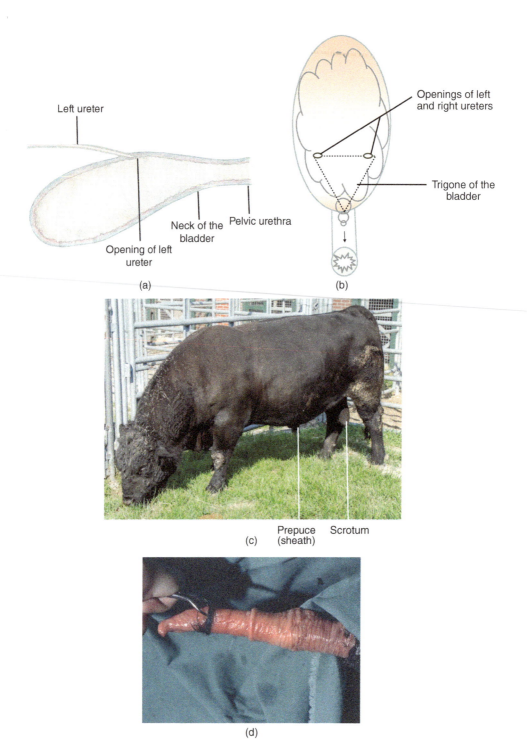

Figure 4.9 (a) Schematic illustration of a longitudinal section of the urinary bladder to show an opening of the ureter on the caudodorsal surface of the urinary bladder. (b) Schematic illustration of the inner dorsal surface (roof) of the urinary bladder showing the **trigone of the bladder:** ventral view. (c) The **testes** and **prepuce (external lamina)** of the bull: left lateral view. Note the vertically suspended (pendulous) testicles. **Rudimentary teats** may be present on the scrotum. The **external lamina of the prepuce** is very long and extends from the scrotum to the **umbilicus**. Note the preputial hair ring around the external **preputial orifice**. The external lamina is continuous with the skin of the abdominal wall dorsally. (d) Penile hair ring. Source: Hopper (2021). Figures reprinted with permission of John Wiley & Sons, Inc.

Box 4.7
The presence of the dorsal urethral diverticulum or recess and the sigmoid flexure make it difficult to catheterize a male ruminant.

vertical cut through the midline of the bulb of the penis down to the lumen of the urethra.

Note the dorsal recess formed at the junction of the pelvic and penile urethra in the most proximal part of your cut. Insert the tip of your probe in the lumen of the proximal penile urethra and move it dorsally until the tip of the probe becomes trapped in the recess at the point where the penile urethra turns cranially toward the pelvis to become the pelvic urethra. Note the clinical significance of the dorsal urethral recess in male ruminants (Box 4.7).

4.5.3 Prepuce

You should be able to identify the external and internal **laminae of the prepuce**, **preputial orifice**, **preputial cavity**, and **free part of the penis**. Clinicians call the prepuce "**the sheath**." With the help of Figures 4.7a and 4.9c, identify these parts.

The prepuce consists of an **external preputial lamina** (has hair; Figure 4.9c) and **internal preputial lamina** (without hair; Figure 4.7a).

The external lamina is continuous with the skin of the abdomen. The internal lamina of the prepuce lines the **preputial cavity** in the non-erect state. The preputial cavity houses the **free part of the penis** (Figure 4.7a).

The **preputial orifice** (opening at the junction of the external and internal laminae) is surrounded by a preputial hair tuft that helps divert the urine away from the skin (Figure 4.9c).

Clinically, preputial injuries are common especially during breeding seasons (e.g., preputial lacerations and preputial prolapse). Consult Box 4.8 on persistent frenulum and penile hair ring.

4.5.4 Superficial Inguinal (Scrotal) Lymph Nodes

The **superficial inguinal lymph nodes** (also called **scrotal** or **mammary lymph nodes**) are located on each side of the body of the penis above the sigmoid flexure (Figure 4.8) or above the base of the udder in the female. In the male, they drain the scrotum, prepuce, and penis but not the testes. Lymph from the testicles is drained through independent lymphatic vessels coursing within the spermatic cord. In the female, these nodes drain the udder and skin of the medial thigh region.

Lymph from both the superficial inguinal lymph nodes and the testicles drain into the medial iliac lymphocenter. This center is located at the terminal branches of the abdominal aorta.

4.5.5 Blood Supply to the Pelvic Viscera and Male Genitalia

In ruminants, the penis receives blood from the **artery of the penis**, a terminal branch of the **internal pudendal artery** (Figure 4.10a). The arterial distribution of blood to the penis in male ruminants is similar to that of the dog but differs from that of the stallion.

Box 4.8	
Persistent frenulum	**Penile hair ring**
Separation of the internal lamina of the prepuce from the free part of the penis occurs at puberty. Failure of this process, when the internal lamina remains attached to the free part of the penis, is known as **persistent frenulum** (Figure 4.7c). Persistent frenulum causes the penis to bend and prevent full extraction of the penis during erection. Persistent frenulum is a heritable condition. The frenulum can be removed surgically.	Hair at the preputial orifice occasionally becomes entrapped, forming a tight ring around the penis in bulls (Figure 4.9d). It can be a source of serious penile and preputial injuries. Hair rings occur in young bulls exhibiting homosexual behavior when they mount each other. Hair rings are also thought to form during attempts at mounting females and rubbing of the penis on loose skin hair. The presence of tight hair rings at the proximal free part of the penis may prevent erection (phimosis).

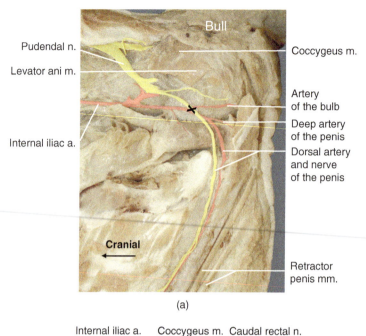

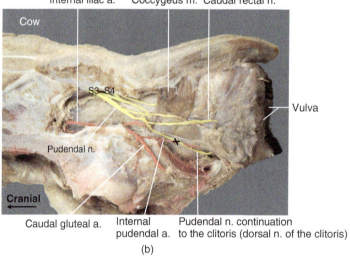

Figure 4.10 (a) Sagittal section of the pelvis of a bull showing arterial supply of the penis. Note that the **internal pudendal artery** and **pudendal nerve** make a cross (X) intersection close to the ischial arch. (b) Nerves and vessels located medial to the sacrosciatic ligament (cow). The cross sign (X) represents the intersection of the internal pudendal artery with the pudendal nerve. Curved dotted line=pelvic symphysis.

At the root of the penis, the artery of the penis terminates by giving rise to the **artery of the bulb of the penis** (supplying the bulb and CSP), the **deep artery of the penis** (supplying the CCP), and **dorsal artery of the penis** (supply the glans and prepuce). The dorsal artery of the penis follows the dorsal vein and dorsal nerve of the penis.

Using a sagittal section of the pelvis, follow the terminal branches of the aorta. Note that the aorta gives rise to two **external iliac arteries** and then terminates by trifurcating into two **internal iliac arteries** and a median sacral. The **internal iliac artery** is relatively very long in ruminants when compared with the equine species.

In female ruminants, the **umbilical artery**, a branch of the **internal iliac artery**, gives the clinically important **uterine artery**. Beyond the umbilical artery, the internal iliac gives the vaginal artery and terminates close to the lesser ischiatic foramen by dividing into **caudal gluteal artery** (passes outside the pelvis through the lesser ischiatic foramen) and **internal pudendal artery** that courses toward the vulva in the female or the penis in the male (Figure 4.10). Note that the internal pudendal artery and **pudendal nerve** makes an "X" intersection close to the pelvic outlet (Figure 4.10).

Identify the **internal iliac artery** and its terminal branches, **internal pudendal** and **caudal gluteal arteries.**

Because of time constraints and the complexity of this area of the pelvis, your instructor may opt to use a prosection for a quick demonstration of the major blood vessels and nerves. Understand that many of the vessels (e.g., prostatic, iliolumbar, obturator) have no clinical significance in ruminants. Ask your instructor which vessels and nerves you need to identify. Check the lab ID list at the end of this chapter for more details.

4.5.6 Testes

Goal: Identify testicular layers from superficial to deep (skin–tunica dartos, spermatic fascia–parietal vagina tunic–vaginal cavity and visceral vaginal tunic). Do not cut into the TA testes that forms the testicular capsule deep to the visceral vaginal tunic. Identify the scrotal septum that separates the left and right testes.

Identify the ligaments of the testis (proper ligament of the testis and ligament of the tail of the epididymis) and understand the process of thermoregulation and testicular descent.

Study the location of the testes in situ and its relation to the sigmoid flexure of the penis. Identify the pampiniform plexus, the mesoductus deferens, and mesorchium. Identify the head, body, and tail of the epididymis.

A bull with larger testicular circumference is desirable for breeding as the size of the testes is positively correlated to sperm production. Measurement of testicular diameter is part of BSE for bull selection.

Start by studying the testicular layers. Identification of testicular layers is important when performing castration. Remove one testicle for close in vitro inspection.

Using a sharp scalpel, cut through the skin and peel the testis out of the scrotal sac. Using scissors, open the vaginal tunic longitudinally and spread the components of the spermatic cord on the table.

Note that the **skin**, **tunica dartos** (whitish smooth muscle deep to the skin), and **scrotal (spermatic) fascia** form the scrotal sac. The scrotal fascia is technically divided into external and internal spermatic fascia. There is no need to make this distinction.

The tunica dartos muscle is involved in thermoregulation of the testes. It involuntarily draws the testicles close to the body in cold weather. Other structures that contribute to thermoregulation include the pampiniform plexus and cremaster muscle (these will be discussed in more detail later).

Deep to the scrotal fascia, note the relatively tough fibrous layer covering the surface of the testis (Figure 4.11). This is the **parietal vaginal tunic**. Incise this layer and peel the testis out. This will not be complete as you will discover later that the parietal vaginal tunic remains attached to the testes by the **ligament of the tail of the epididymis** (Figure 4.11c). This ligament must be severed in an open castration method (Box 4.9). Consult Box 4.10 on castration methods.

At this point, identify the epididymis, the large tubular structure wrapped tightly around the surface of the testis. The epididymis is composed of three identifiable regions: **head, body**, and **tail** (Figure 4.11b). The tail is ventrally located and is the site for storage of spermatozoa. The head is proximal to the tail and is where the testicular vein and artery leave or enter the testis, respectively.

Box 4.9

In open surgical castration, the parietal vaginal tunic must be incised to expose or "exteriorize" the testicle. Additionally, the ligament of the tail of the epididymis must be severed to pull the testicle away from the parietal tunic.

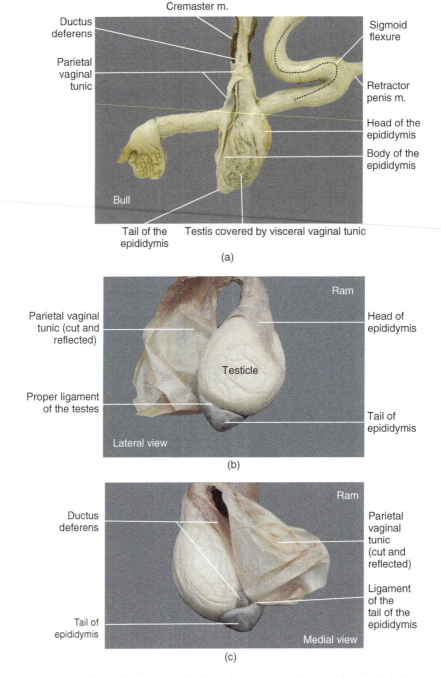

Figure 4.11 (a) Reproductive tract of the bull: distal parts. Testicular layers deep to the scrotal sac include the parietal and visceral vaginal tunics with a vaginal cavity in between. The figure shows the proper ligament of the testis and ligament of the tail of the epididymis (in b and c, respectively). Ram testis: (b) lateral and (c) medial views. The testicular parietal vaginal tunic is incised to show ligaments of the testis. Identify the proper ligament of the testis and ligament of the tail of the epididymis. The body of the epididymis is out of sight (Figure 4.11b).

> **Box 4.10**
>
> Ruminants are usually castrated when they are young (less than 3 months of age). Several procedures are used in small and large ruminants. Broadly speaking, castration can be accomplished by surgical or nonsurgical methods. In most cases, surgical methods are preferred and cause less stress and pain than nonsurgical methods.
>
> Nonsurgical procedures, such as banding (or elastrator), are commonly used on male goats and sheep where a rubber ring is placed around the scrotum proximal to the testicles for 2–3 weeks after testicular descent. Often mistakingly thought to be less painful than surgical castration methods by animal owners, banding causes significant long-term pain and stress, especially in older animals. Additionally, band castration predisposes the animal to tetanus. In cattle and small ruminants, a handheld Burdizzo clamp (crushing pincher) can be applied proximal to the testicles to crush the contents of the spermatic cord without cutting into the skin. These procedures are among several nonsurgical methods.
>
> In surgical castration, the skin of the scrotum is incised at the ventral aspect to expose the testicles and the spermatic cord. Next, the spermatic cord can be crushed and severed using an emasculator.
>
> The difference between "open vs closed" surgical castration refers to whether the vaginal tunic is opened to remove the testicles (open) or whether the tunic is removed with the testicles (closed). At Auburn University Veterinary Teaching Hospital, closed castrations are typically performed. The word "surgical castration" should be used to differentiate it from other methods of castration.

Sperm are produced in the seminiferous tubules within the testicular parenchyma. They next travel through several microscopic ducts (straight tubules, rete testis, and efferent ductules) to reach the head of the epididymis. You will study these structures in microanatomy of the testes in histology classes.

The tail of the epididymis is attached to the testes by the **proper ligament of the testis** and to the parietal vaginal tunic by the **ligament of the tail of the epididymis** (Figure 4.11b,c). Both ligaments are remnants of the **gubernaculum testis**, a gelatinous mesenchymal structure responsible for testicular descent into the scrotal sac.

The tubular structure that carries the sperm from the tail of the epididymis to the pelvic urethra caudal to the neck of the bladder is the **ductus deferens**.

Next, study the **vaginal tunic** and **spermatic cord**. The term vaginal tunic includes all of the peritoneal structures that have descended out of the abdominal cavity (through the inguinal canal) with the testicle. It is divided into parietal and visceral layers. These two layers are frequently called the parietal vaginal tunic or common tunic and the visceral vaginal tunic. The spermatic cord consists of the visceral vaginal tunic and all of its contents that lead to and from the testicle including the visceral layer of the vaginal tunic, testicular artery, vein, lymphatics, sympathetic autonomic nerves, and the ductus deferens with very small artery and veins of the ductus deferens.

The double layer of mesothelium that suspends the ductus deferens is called **mesoductus deferens**. The testicular vein and artery are suspended by a similar peritoneal fold known as the **mesorchium**. The mesoductus deferens and mesorchium are continuous with each other.

Identify the **pampiniform plexus**. This is formed by the torturous bends of the **testicular vein** that wrap around the testicular artery. The function of the pampiniform plexus is to cool the blood in the testicular artery before entering the testis (Figure 4.11c).

Thermoregulation, where the temperature in the testicles is lowered by at least 2–3°C, is critical for spermatogenesis (production of sperm).

The **cremaster muscle** is a ribbon-like strip of skeletal muscle that originates from the caudal boundary of the internal abdominal oblique muscle (Figure 4.12). It courses on the superficial surface of the parietal vaginal tunic lightly covered by spermatic fascia. The muscle is not part of the spermatic cord. Like the tunica dartos muscle, the cremaster muscle is involved in testicular thermoregulation. It voluntarily draws the testicle close to the body when it contracts.

The **genitofemoral nerve** innervates the cremaster muscle in the male and the udder in the female. It can

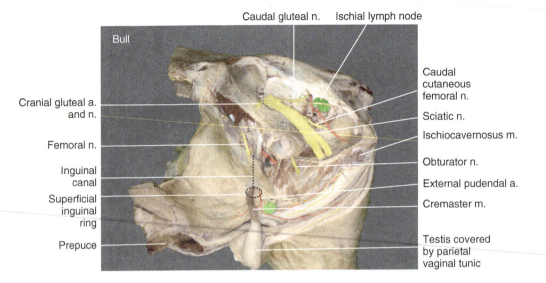

Figure 4.12 Bovine male (bull) reproductive tract and major pelvic nerves. Dissection of cremaster muscle and pelvic nerves. Note the testicles are oriented vertically. * Medial circumflex femoral artery.

be found coursing through the superficial inguinal ring (Figure 4.12).

The double layer of mesothelium that suspend the ductus deferens is called **mesoductus deferens**. The testicular vein and artery are suspended by a similar peritoneum known as the **mesorchium**. The mesoductus deferens and mesorchium are continuous with each other.

4.5.7 Male Accessory Sex Glands

Goal: Identify the major accessory sex glands in the bull (ampullary glands, vesicular glands, prostate [body and disseminate part], and bulbourethral glands) and compare them with small ruminants (buck or ram). Know that the prostate glands in small ruminants (buck and ram) are entirely of the disseminate type (embedded within the pelvic urethral wall) whereas bulls have both compact and disseminate types. Consult Box 4.11 on clinical application.

Understand that accessory sex glands are palpated per rectum as part of a BSE to diagnose any inflammatory processes (e.g., seminal vesiculitis of the vesicular glands).

The accessory sex glands in the bull include the **ampullary glands** (ampullae of the ductus deferens), **vesicular glands, prostate (compact and disseminate parts),** and **bulbourethral glands.**

Identify these glands on a dorsal view of the pelvis where the caudal vertebrae and rectum have been removed or on an isolated penis and pelvic urethra (Figures 4.5 and 4.13).

Box 4.11

The accessory sex glands are palpable per rectum in the intact bull. They are usually palpated as part of a BSE in the bull. The prostate is said to feel like a ring on a finger. The finger in this case is the pelvic urethra surrounded by the urethralis muscle (Figure 4.13).

A cow-calf enterprise requires healthy breeding bulls. Emphasis should be placed on evaluating the size of the vesicular glands during transrectal palpation of bulls in the breeding soundness exam (BSE). Pathology of these glands (seminal vesiculitis) is common and could affect BSE. Typically, seminal vesiculitis stems from infectious bacteria circulating in the bloodstream (originating from either rumen acidosis or body abscesses). Signs may include increased vesicular gland size and the presence of purulent material in the semen. Young bulls may respond to antibiotic treatment; however, the infection is usually chronic and unresponsive to treatment in older bulls.

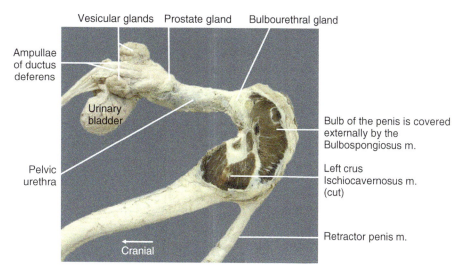

Figure 4.13 Close-up view of the accessory sex glands of the bull.

In small ruminants, the prostate is present only as a disseminate part and so you will not be able to see a grossly visible body of the prostate. The other accessory sex glands in small ruminants are similar to those of the bull.

The **ampullary glands** are found within the walls of the terminal parts of the ductus deferens (Figure 4.13). They are located on the dorsal surface of the urinary bladder on each side of the genital fold.

4.6 Female Reproductive Tract

Goal: Know the major components of the female reproductive organs. Identify the suburethral diverticulum in females and know its clinical significance. Know the palpable reproductive structures (ovaries, uterine body, cervix, uterine horns, and intercornual ligaments). Understand some of the changes associated with pregnancy (increased size of one of the uterine horns, presence of fetal membranes, and peculiar pulsation in the uterine artery known as the thrill or fremitus). Know the type of placentation in ruminants (cotyledonary placenta). Clinical applications associated with the female reproductive tract include diagnosis of pregnancy and mastitis and management of dystocia and retained placenta. At the end of the female section, watch Video 19.

The female ruminant reproductive tract is composed of the **ovary**, **uterine tube**, **uterus (uterine horn, uterine body**, and **uterine cervix)**, **vagina**, **vestibule**, and **vulva.** The more cranial components of the reproductive tract are suspended to the pelvis and lateral body wall by the **broad ligament**, a bilateral sheet of peritoneal fold (Figures 4.14a,c and 4.16a). Identify the parts of the reproductive system in situ as shown in Figure 4.14.

In the live animal, the uterine horns curls ventral toward the abdominal floor, then course caudally toward the pelvis, and finally head in a dorsal direction where they connect with the uterine tube close to the ovary.

4.6.1 Ovaries

The **ovaries** of the cow are oval in shape. They are relatively large and lie close to the pelvic inlet in the live animal. Being close to the pelvic inlet, they are easily palpable per rectum.

Using an isolated female (cow or goat) reproductive tract, pass your fingers over the surface of the ovary to palpate any irregularities that may be present as a result of a large follicle or corpus luteum. There is no ovulation fossa similar to that seen in mares.

The ovary is enclosed within a peritoneal sac called the **ovarian bursa** (Figure 4.15). The ovarian bursa is

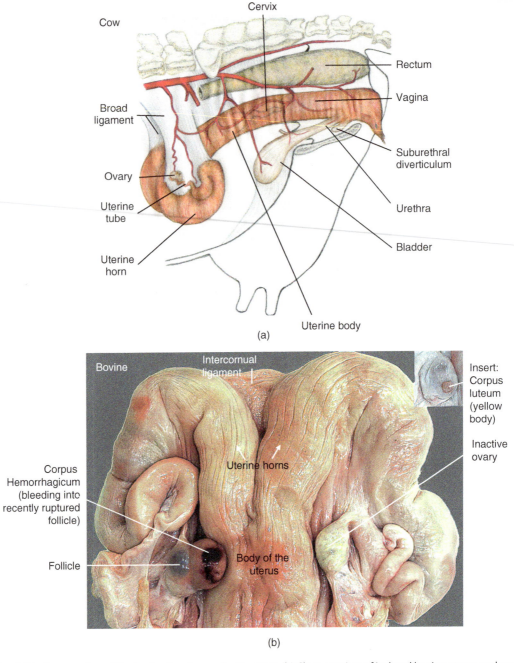

Figure 4.14 (a) In situ overview of the bovine (cow) reproductive tract. (b) Close-up view of isolated bovine uterus and ovary of another cow in the inset (upright hand corner). *Source:* Minnesota Veterinary Anatomy, University of Minnesota. (c) Isolated dorsal view of ovine uterus. *Source:* Minnesota Veterinary Anatomy, University of Minnesota.

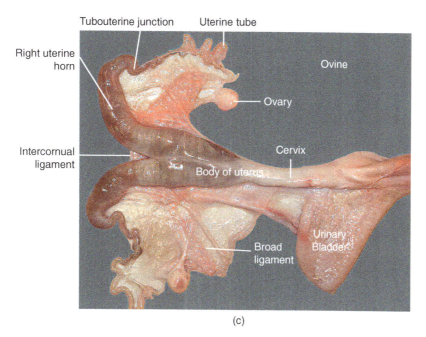

Figure 4.14 (Continued)

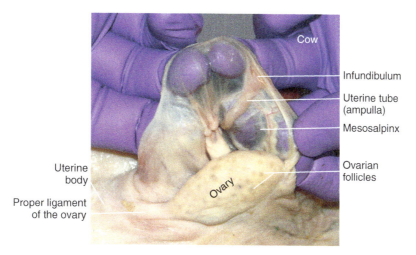

Figure 4.15 Bovine ovary (cow). Ovarian bursa opened.

formed by the **mesovarium** and **mesosalpinx.** Both are more cranial components of the broad ligament. The ovary is attached to the tip of the uterine horn by the **proper ligament of the ovary**.

Follicles released from the ovary pass into a thin-walled **infundibulum,** which is the funnel-shaped proximal, or free end, of the **uterine tube** (Figure 4.15). Finger-like projections, fimbriae, are located on the free edge of the infundibulum. Oscillations of the fimbria help attract the newly released ovum.

4.6.2 Uterine Tubes

The uterine tube (Figure 4.15) can be hard to identify on a nonpregnant tract. It is divided into proximal **ampulla** and distal, relatively thin, **isthmus** parts.

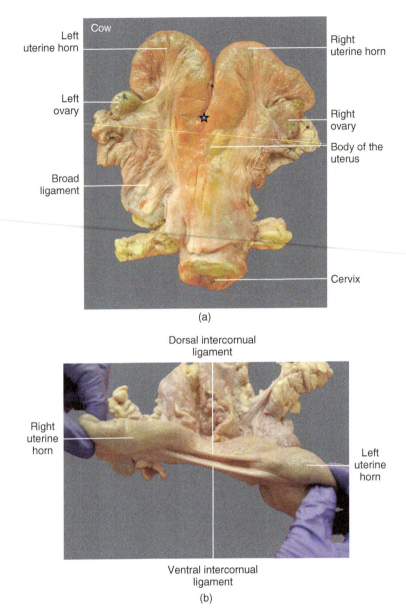

Figure 4.16 (a) Isolated bovine (cow) uterus: dorsal view. * Location of intercornual ligament. (b) Bovine (cow) dorsal and ventral intercornual ligaments: cranial view. Small ruminants have a single intercornual ligament.

Fertilization takes place in the ampulla. *There is no need to identify the ampulla and isthmus.*

4.6.3 Uterine Horns

Identify the tip of the uterine horn. This is where the uterine tube opens. Next, follow the uterine horns distally. The left and right horns are connected by the **intercornual ligament**. The cow has both dorsal and ventral **intercornual ligaments** (Figure 4.14b,c and 4.16b) compared with small ruminants that have a single ligament. Consult Box 4.12 for clinical application.

4.6.4 Uterine Body

The uterine body is relatively short. Lining the internal surface of the uterus is the endometrium that features many mushroom-shaped elevations called

Box 4.12

In rectal palpation, the examiner can insert an index finger into the space between the dorsal and ventral intercornual ligaments and pull the reproductive tract caudally toward the pelvic cavity for easier manipulation.

caruncles. During pregnancy, attached to each caruncle is a cotyledon that is part of the placenta. The unit formed by the **maternal** caruncle and **fetal** cotyledon is called a **placentome** (Figure 4.17a–c). The caruncles are dish-shaped in small ruminants (goat and sheep) and mushroom-shaped in cattle. The placenta of ruminants is classified as **cotyledonary**. In artificial

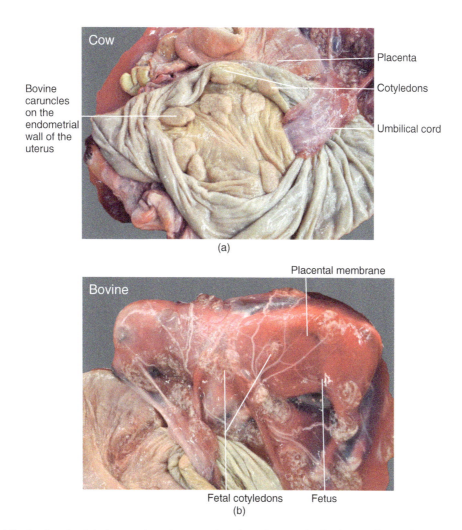

Figure 4.17 (a) Bovine (cow) cotyledonary placenta opened to show the round, raised caruncles on the internal surface of the uterus (endometrium). Union of the caruncles and cotyledons form the placentomes. The placentome is mushroom-shaped in the cow and dish-shaped in small ruminants (goat and sheep). (b) Bovine (cow) fetus surrounded by placenta. The fetus has been pulled out of the interlocking of the caruncles (maternal side of the placentome) and cotyledons (fetal side of the placentome). (c) Pregnant sheep uterus opened to show a fetal lamb connected by the umbilical cord (black asterisk) to the fetal membranes that are attached to numerous placentomes (yellow asterisks). Source: Minnesota Veterinary Anatomy, University of Minnesota.

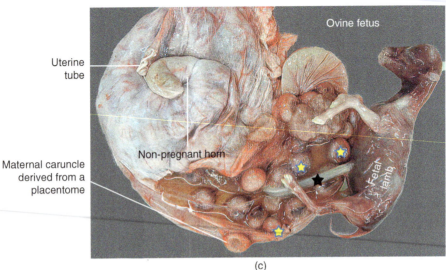

Figure 4.17 (Continued)

> **Box 4.13**
>
> In artificial insemination (AI) and embryo transfer, the uterine body is the major site for semen and embryo deposition. In AI, if the tip of the inseminating rod is inserted too far into the uterus, semen is deposited in only one of the uterine horns.

insemination (AI) semen is deposited into the uterine body (consult Box 4.13).

Failure to expel the placenta a few hours after parturition is known as retained placenta. It can be due to abortion/difficult birth or microbial infection. Untreated cows may develop metritis.

Make a longitudinal incision into the dorsal wall of an isolated female (cow) reproductive tract to open the interior as shown in Figure 4.18. *Identify the ball-shaped caruncles on the endometrium. Identify the cervix and observe its interlocking folds.*

4.6.5 Uterine Cervix

The ruminant cervix has longitudinal and transverse folds (Figures 4.18 and 4.19). The cervix remains closed most of the time by a mucous plug except in estrus or calf delivery.

The cervix projects into the vagina as the **cervix portio vaginalis** (Figure 4.21). The annular space around the portio vaginalis cervix in the cranial part of the vagina is the **vaginal fornix** (Figure 4.19). Cervical assessments are conducted during health examination (Box 4.14).

The opening of the cervix into the uterine body is the **internal uterine (or cervical) ostium** and that into the vagina is the **external uterine (or cervical) ostium** (Figure 4.19).

Pregnancy in cattle commonly involves one fetus. Twins in cattle are likely to have shared placental circulation and thus twin pregnancy is undesirable because of the likelihood that a male twin partner can inhibit the reproductive tract development of a female mate, resulting in a condition known as a **freemartin**. This condition is thought to be caused by the secretion of the antimullerian hormone by the male twin. The antimullerian hormone causes regression of the female duct system (mullerian ducts). Pregnancy in small ruminants, however, can involve more than one fetus without ill effects.

Pregnancy in cattle involves one uterine horn, resulting in significant asymmetry of the horns detectable in rectal palpation (Figure 4.20).

4.6.6 Vagina

The vagina is the chamber between the cervix and vestibule. It is three times longer than the vestibule (Figure 4.21). The vagina has circular and longitudinal mucosal folds.

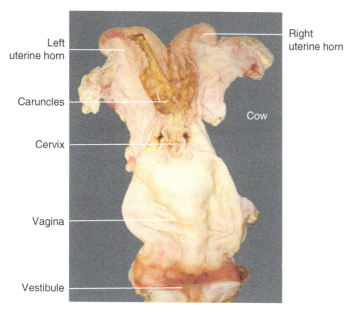

Figure 4.18 Bovine (cow) reproductive tract with uterus opened dorsally to show the caruncles on the surface of the endometrium: dorsal view.

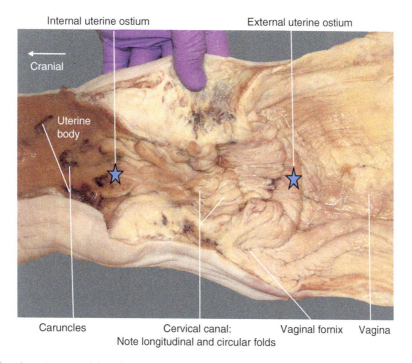

Figure 4.19 Bovine (cow) cervix opened dorsally to demonstrate the **cervical canal,** and **the internal** (toward the uterine body) and **external** (toward the vagina) **uterine orifices**.

Box 4.14

The cervix of the cow can by examined by speculum, using a vaginal speculum for discharges (blood or watery cervical discharge). A bloody vulvar discharge is commonly seen in cows during metestrum (1–2 days after estrus). A watery cervical discharge that contains whitish-yellow flakes of pus caused by a flagellated protozoan, *Trichomoniasis fetus*, can be transmitted by AI and by natural breeding.

Diagnosis of pregnancy by rectal palpation involves detection of one or more of the following (depending on the stage of pregnancy): (i) fetal membrane slip between the thumb and index fingers; (ii) amniotic vesicle (blister-like structure containing the developing conceptus and amniotic fluid; (iii) palpation of cotyledons of the fetal placenta/uterine caruncles (placentome); (iv) pulsation in the uterine artery (fremitus) on the ipsilateral side of the pregnant horn or both; (v) presence of corpus luteum on the contralateral ovary; and (vi) detection of a fetus.

If available, an ultrasound will speed up the process of pregnancy detection and is relatively more accurate than rectal palpation.

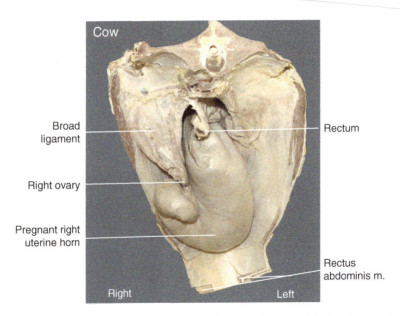

Figure 4.20 Bovine (cow) pelvic cavity showing pregnancy in the right uterine horn: cranial view. Note the significant enlargement of the right uterine horn (palpable feature of pregnancy). Gestation in cattle is about 280 days.

4.6.7 Female Pudendum

The vulva is part of the female pudendum. The pudendum consists of the vulva, clitoris, and vestibule.

4.6.7.1 Vestibule

The vestibule is the region caudal to the vagina or between the external urethral orifice and the vulva. Both urine and reproductive secretions pass through the vestibule.

4.6.7.2 Suburethral Diverticulum

The **suburethral diverticulum** is a pouch or recess below the external urethral orifice near the cranial-most extent of the floor of the vestibule (Figures 4.14a and 4.21). Identify the suburethral diverticulum and the external urethral orifice by inserting your probe in each (Box 4.15).

In the caudoventral floor of the vestibule, identify the **glans clitoris** located within the **clitoral fossa**.

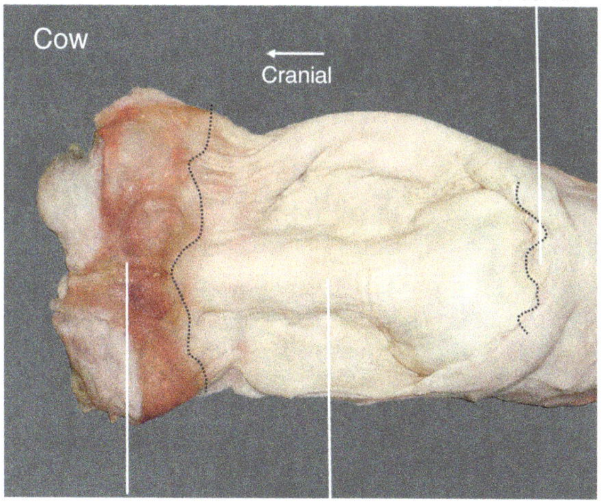

Box 4.15

The suburethral diverticulum is a depression located below the external urethral orifice. It should be avoided when performing catheterization. A useful technique is to deliberately insert the catheter into the suburethral diverticulum and then to turn the catheter 180° and draw it caudally very slowly; you can then feel the catheter entering the urethra.

Figure 4.21 Bovine (cow) reproductive tract (vagina and vestibule): dorsal view. The tract is opened ventrally looking into the roof. Note the large dorsal longitudinal fold on the roof of the vagina. For clarification of the location of the suburethral diverticulum see Figure 4.23b.

4.6.7.3 Vulva

In domestic animals, the vulva forms the only visible part of the female pudendum. It is composed of the **left** and **right labia (lips).**

The left and right labia meet dorsally to form a **dorsal commissure** and ventrally forming a **ventral commissure** (Figure 4.22).

4.6.8 Blood Supply of the Female Genital Tract

From cranial to caudal, the female reproductive tract is supplied by three main arteries: the **ovarian artery** (arises from the aorta), **uterine artery** (from the umbilical artery), and **vaginal artery** (from the internal iliac artery) (Figure 4.23a,b). Consult Box 4.16 on the clinical significance of the uterine artery.

The **uterine artery** is the largest source of blood supplying the reproductive tract. It divides into cranial and caudal parts when it courses close to the lateral sides of the uterine body. The **ovarian artery** supplies

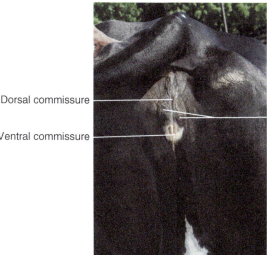

Figure 4.22 External genitalia of the cow.

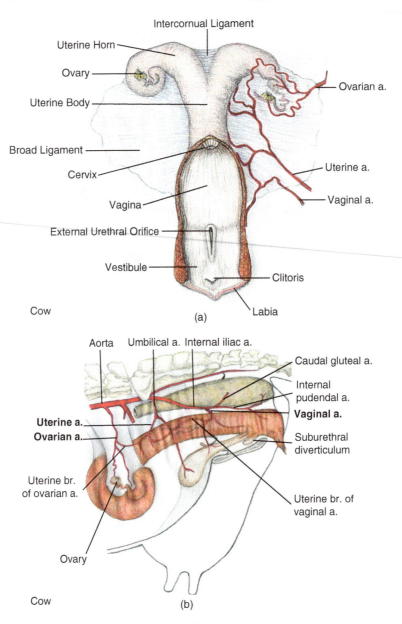

Figure 4.23 (a) Schematic illustration of arterial blood supply to the ruminant (cow) reproductive tract (isolated tract). (b) In situ schematic illustration of arterial blood supply to the bovine (cow) reproductive tract.

Box 4.16

The **uterine artery** increases in size during pregnancy. A palpable pulsation can be detected in the artery when palpated per rectum in a cow in the advanced stage of pregnancy (4–5 months). This pulsation is diagnostic of pregnancy and is referred to as whirling, thrill, or fremitus. Fremitus or thrill in the uterine artery is detected first (within about five months of pregnancy) on the ipsilateral (same) side of the pregnant horn and a month later on both the left and right sides at about the middle of the broad ligaments.

the ovary and gives rise to a uterine branch that anastomoses with the cranial branch of the uterine artery. Likewise, the **vaginal artery** supplies the vagina and also gives rise to a uterine branch that supplies the uterus (Figure 4.23a,b).

The ovarian artery is wrapped by extensive coiled branches of the ovarian vein. This arrangement is thought to help with countercurrent exchange of hormones where prostaglandins pass from the vein to the artery to be returned to the reproductive tract.

The three arteries to the female reproductive tract can be identified within the broad ligament (Figure 4.23a,b).

4.6.9 Udder

Goal: Identify the external features of the bovine and caprine udders (number of teats, intermammary groove), duct system (lactiferous ducts and lactiferous sinus), suspensory apparatus (lateral and medial laminae or ligaments), vascularization, innervation, and lymph drainage. **At the end of the female section, watch Video 20.**

The bovine udder is composed of **four mammary glands** (each is known as a **quarter**). Each gland has a single, finger-like **teat** that has one **teat orifice**. Typically, a quarter is named as right front, right hind, left front, or left hind quarter (Figure 4.24). Consult Box 4.17 for clinical application.

Small ruminants have only two glands with two teats (left and right separated by the **intermammary groove**). Supernumerary (accessory) teats may be present in some breeds of cattle.

In cows, each quarter has an independent duct system. The left and right halves of the udder are completely separated by connective tissue but the two quarters on each side appear to be merged together; however, they maintain the two separate duct systems.

In small ruminants (doe and ewe), the left and right mammary glands are also completely separated by an intermammary groove. Each gland has a single teat that carries a single teat orifice.

The udder has modified skin that has a small amount of hair.

4.6.9.1 Suspensory Apparatus and Interior Structures of the Udder

The udder is suspended from the caudal ventral body wall by **lateral** and **medial laminae** (also called ligaments). The two laminae collectively make the **suspensory apparatus** of the udder.

The **lateral laminae** (mostly fibrous) are located deep to the skin of the left and right lateral walls of

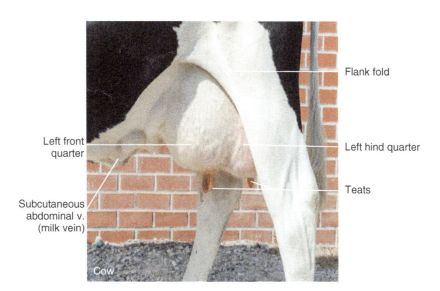

Figure 4.24 The bovine udder: left lateral view. The whole udder is composed of four quarters, two on each side.

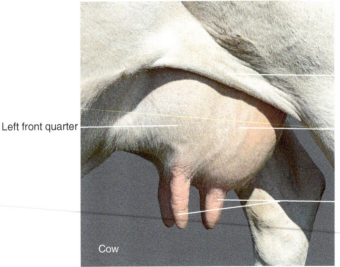

Figure 4.24 (Continued)

> **Box 4.17**
>
> Anesthesia for teat surgery is performed by several techniques including a ring block in which local anesthetic solution is injected around the base of the teat in a ring pattern.

the udder. The laminae suspend the udder from the symphysial tendon caudally, and tunica flava abdominis cranially. The lateral laminae send fibrous septa into the substance of the udder.

Dissect the skin on the lateral side of the udder and reflect it ventrally. Cut the lateral lamina at its dorsal aspect and reflect it ventrally.

Deep to the lateral lamina, find the large external pudendal artery and vein close to the mammary lymph nodes.

The paired **medial laminae** are elastic sheets. They are located between the left and right halves of the udder. These laminae are highly elastic and allow for lateral sagging of the udder when filled with milk.

*With help of Figure 4.25(a), identify the lateral and medial laminae of the suspensory apparatus of the udder. Make a sagittal section of the udder to identify the **teat canal**, **teat sinus**, and **gland sinus** (Figure 4.25a,b). A synonymous term for the sinus is **cistern**.* The combination of the gland and teat sinuses form the **lactiferous sinus**.

To understand the duct system in the udder, there follows a brief description of how milk is transported within the udder. Milk passes from milk-secreting alveoli within the substance of the udder to small excretory ducts that merge to form large lactiferous ducts. Several lactiferous ducts empty into the gland sinus at the ventral base of the udder. From the gland sinus, milk passes into the teat sinus, teat canal, and to the exterior via the teat orifice.

An annular fold and erectile venous circle (Furstenberg's venous ring) are present at the junction between the gland and teat sinuses. The teat canal has longitudinal folds that project into the teat sinus forming **Furstenberg's rosette** (Figure 4.25b,c).

4.6.9.2 Blood Supply and Venous Drainage of the Udder

Milk synthesis requires that a large amount of blood pass through the udder. This has been estimated as 600 liters of blood for each liter of milk produced. The main blood supply to the udder is from the **external pudendal artery** (also known as the **mammary artery**). In cattle, a small amount of blood comes to the udder from the mammary branches of the ventral perineal artery and dorsal labial branch from the internal pudendal artery.

Identify the **external pudendal artery** and **vein** passing out of the abdomen through the superficial inguinal ring. The external pudendal artery originates from the **pudendoepigastric trunk**. The trunk is a branch of the deep femoral artery from

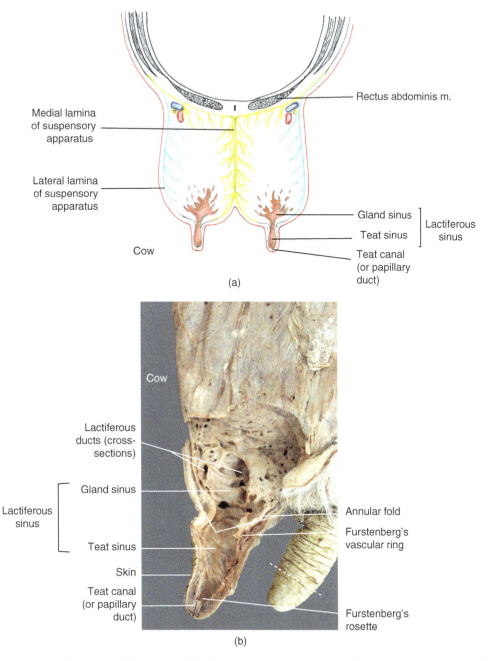

Figure 4.25 (a) Schematic illustration of the interior of the bovine (cow) udder: longitudinal section passing through left and right hind quarters of the udder. (b) Bovine (cow) teat and distal part of the udder: longitudinal section. A white dotted line shows location of the cross-section seen in Figure 4.25(c). (c) Cross-section of bovine (cow) teat to show layers and inner longitudinal folds of the teat canal: dorsal view.

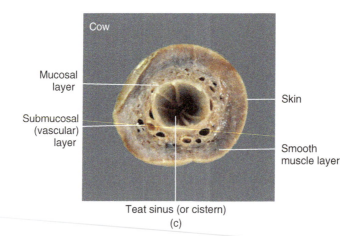

Figure 4.25 (Continued)

the external iliac artery. In large dairy cows, the external pudendal artery has a sigmoid flexure at the base of the udder to allow for stretching of the artery when the udder is laden with a large amount of milk.

Close to the proximity of the udder, the external pudendal artery divides into the cranial mammary artery (known as caudal superficial epigastric in goats) and caudal mammary artery (known as ventral labial artery in goats).

Venous drainage of the udder is through a circular venous ring around the base of the udder. This ring is formed by transverse connections between subcutaneous abdominal (milk) veins, left and right external pudendal veins, and left and right ventral labial veins (branches of ventral or dorsal perineal veins).

The **subcutaneous abdominal vein** (known by laymen as the **milk vein**) is formed by the end-to-end anastomosis of the cranial and caudal superficial epigastric veins during the first pregnancy (Figure 4.26). This vein is well developed in lactating cows. It courses cranially from the udder to enter the thorax through an opening in the ventral thoracic wall known as the **milk well**. The milk vein joins the internal thoracic vein within the thorax.

4.6.9.3 Lymphatics of the Udder

The **superficial inguinal lymph nodes** (also known as mammary lymph nodes) drain lymph from the udder and neighboring regions (vulva, clitoris, and skin of the medial thigh region). The mammary lymph nodes are two nodes on each side of the udder. They are located at the base of the udder close to the superficial inguinal ring.

In the live animal, the mammary lymph nodes can be palpated from behind between the left and right thigh regions, especially if the udder is inflamed (mastitis). Superficial lymphatic vessels can also be seen coursing caudodorsally whereas superficial veins course craniodorsally.

4.6.9.4 Innervation of the Udder

The innervation of the udder is provided by four nerves: the first and second lumbar nerves (L1 and L2), the genitofemoral nerve (from L3/L4, supplies the substance of the udder), and mammary branches of the pudendal nerve. Identify the **genitofemoral nerve** coursing with the external pudendal vein and artery through the inguinal canal to the udder and medial thigh region. Figure 4.8 shows the location of the genitofemoral nerve in the male. It runs in the same location in the female.

4.7 Live Cow

Goal: With the help of Figures 4.27 and 4.28, palpate the two important bony features of the ox pelvis: the tuber coxae and tuber ischium. They are commonly called the "hook" and "pin," respectively. Know that, unlike in horses, the hook and pin bones in dairy cows are sharply defined and angular in appearance with no discernable fat pad. Consult Box 4.18 for a random list of clinical conditions affecting the pelvic region and hindlimbs.

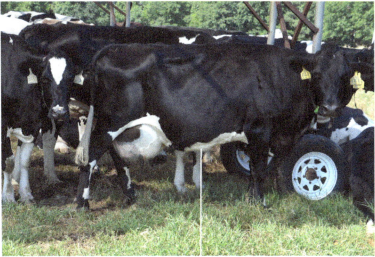
Subcutaneous abdominal (milk) vein

Figure 4.26 Milk vein in a Friesian dairy cow. The **milk vein** is formed during the first lactation period by the fusion of the **cranial** and **caudal superficial epigastric veins**.

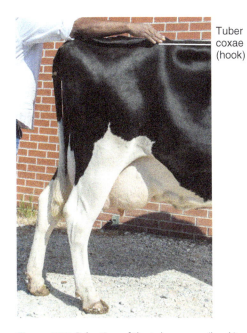

Figure 4.27 Palpation of the tuber coxae (hook).

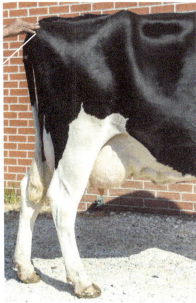

Figure 4.28 Palpation of the tuber ischium (pin).

Box 4.18
Downer Cow Syndrome: A cow that is unable to stand, which could be due to many causes, some of them relating to the reproductive system: <ul><li>Mastitis, milk fever, or metritis</li><li>Calving paralysis: obturator or sciatic nerve damage due to difficult parturition</li></ul>

- Low calcium, phosphorous, magnesium, and potassium (Ca, P, Mg, and K)
- Injury to spine or legs: sacroiliac or coxofemoral luxation
- Bacterial infections: septic metritis or acute coliform mastitis
- Compartmental syndrome: increased pressure develops in an osteofascial compartment
- Crush syndrome: release of myoglobin from muscle damage
- Pressure syndrome: ischemic necrosis if a cow is sitting in the same position for long hours (six or more)

4.8 Lab ID List for the Pelvis and Reproductive Structures

There is no need to identify items in *italics*.

A. **Bones:** Important bony landmarks of the pelvis (know some of the lay terms such as hooks and pins):
 1. Coxal tuber (hook)
 2. Ischial tuber (pin)
 3. Sacral tuber
 4. Pecten
 5. Ischiatic spine
 6. Promontory of the sacrum
 7. Know the obstetric term *conjugate* (the line connecting the promontory with the pecten) – vertical diameter larger than horizontal – pelvimeter (measuring device for pelvic dimensions)

B. **Arteries and veins**
 8. Internal iliac a.
    a. Umbilical a →gives the uterine a.
    b. *Vaginal (uterine branch)/prostatic*
    c. Internal pudendal a. (know the following branches but do not identify them)
       i. *Deep artery of the penis*
       ii. *Artery of bulb*
       iii. *Dorsal artery of the penis*
    d. Caudal gluteal a. (passes out of the pelvis through the lesser sciatic or ischiatic foramen)
 9. Testicular a. and v. (vein forms pampiniform plexus)
 10. Ovarian a.
 11. External pudendal a. and v.
    a. Cranial and caudal mammary aa.
 12. Milk v. (subcutaneous abdominal vein)

C. **Pelvic fossa and pouches**
 13. Pararectal fossa
 14. Rectogenital pouch
 15. Vesicogenital pouch
 16. Pubovesical pouch

D. **Accessory sex glands**
 17. Ampullary glands
 18. Prostate gland (know the difference between small and large male ruminants)
 19. Vesicular glands
 20. Bulbourethral glands

E. **Pelvic viscera**
 21. Urinary bladder
 22. Ureter
 23. Genital fold
 24. Median ligament of the bladder
 25. Left and right lateral ligaments of the bladder
 26. Rectum
 27. Anal canal → *anus*

F. **Male penis (fibroblastic type)**
 28. Urethral process (identify in small ruminants [buck or ram])
 29. Apical ligament (bull)
 30. Retractor penis m.
 31. Sigmoid flexure
 32. Corpus cavernosum (CCP) and corpus spongiosum (CSP) on a cross section of the penis
 33. Tunica albuginea penis
 34. Dorsal nerve of the penis
 35. Bulbospongiosus m.
 36. Ischiocavernosus m.

G. **Others**
 37. Sacrosciatic ligament (or broad sacrotuberous ligament)
    a. Major ischiatic (or sciatic) foramen
    b. Minor ischiatic foramen
 38. Urethral recess (dorsal urethral diverticulum in male)
 39. Subiliac lymph nodes

H. **Testis**
  40. Cremaster m.
  41. Tunica dartos
  42. Pampiniform plexus (testicular v.)
  43. *Scrotal ligament*
  44. Ligament of the tail of the epididymis
  45. Proper ligament of the testis
  46. Parietal and visceral vaginal tunics
  47. Ductus deferens
  48. Mesorchium and mesoductus deferens

I. **Female reproductive tract**
  49. Ovary and ovarian bursa
  50. *Uterine tube*
  51. Uterine horn
  52. Intercornual ligament (dorsal and ventral parts in cow)
  53. Uterine body
  54. Cervix
  55. Vagina
  56. Vestibule
  57. Suburethral diverticulum (know clinical significance)
  58. External urethral opening
  59. Glans of the clitoris
  60. Broad ligament (know names of three regions)
  61. Round ligament of the uterus
  62. Know type of placenta in ruminants
     a. Caruncle (mother)
     b. *Cotyledons (fetus)*

J. **Udder**
  63. Lateral lamina of suspensory apparatus
  64. Medial lamina of suspensory apparatus
  65. *Lactiferous ducts*
  66. Lactiferous sinus
     a. Gland sinus
     b. Teat sinus
  67. Teat orifice
  68. Mammary (superficial inguinal) lymph node

K. **Nerves**
  69. Obturator n.
  70. Sciatic n.
  71. Genitofemoral n.
  72. Pudendal n. → *caudal rectal n.*

5

The Forelimb

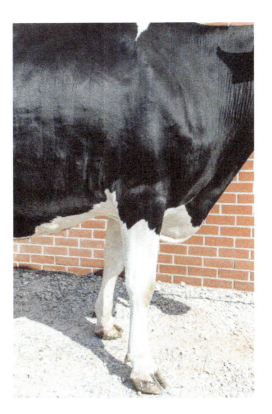

Learning Objectives
• Identify the major bones of the forelimb and understand that some bones and their features are palpable in the live animal. • Identify the major muscles, tendons, synovial structures such as bursae (e.g., infraspinatus), and tendon sheaths.

Guide to Ruminant Anatomy: Dissection and Clinical Aspects, Second Edition. Mahmoud Mansour, Ray Wilhite, Joe Rowe, and Saly Hafiz.
© 2023 John Wiley & Sons, Inc. Published 2023 by John Wiley & Sons, Inc.
Companion website: www.wiley.com/go/mansour/dissection2

- Identify and know the major nerves and blood vessels of the forelimb, especially the blood vessels and nerves in the distal limb (i.e., the median nerve and median artery on the palmar aspect, and the radial nerve on the dorsal aspects of the large metacarpal bone and digits).
- Know the nomenclature for vessels and nerves on the dorsal and palmar aspects of the large metacarpal bone and digits.
- Understand the clinical signs associated with nerve damage (e.g., damage to radial and suprascapular nerves).
- Identify and know the clinical importance of superficial veins (i.e., cephalic, accessory cephalic, and dorsal common digital vein III). The superficial veins of the forelimb are used for injection of antibiotics and for retrograde anesthesia.
- Know some of the clinical aspects (e.g., corkscrew, interdigital dermatitis, interdigital phlegmon, and interdigital hyperplasia) associated with damage to the hoof and its contents (digital cushion, superficial and deep digital flexor tendons, navicular bursa, navicular bone), and the proximal and distal interdigital ligaments that join the weight-bearing digits together.
- At the end of the thoracic limb section, watch Videos 21 and 22.

5.1 Introduction

One of the most important clinical problems in cattle is lameness. Lameness can be caused by several factors, including infections of soft tissue in the foot (e.g., interdigital fat pad) and by structural and bone malformations. Most clinical work on ruminant limbs involves the distal limb (carpus and below). You should focus most of your attention on the study of forelimb structures from the elbow distally. Some of the most common conditions causing lameness include:

- Slipper foot (laminitis)
- Inflammatory processes (foot rot, sole abscess)
- Wound in the skin around heels
- Coronary band inflammatory process
- Fissures and/or cracks in hoof wall
- Splayed toes
- Wounds in the interdigital space
- Interdigital fibroma
- Sole ulcer
- White line disease
- Hematoma under the sole
- Heel erosion
- Lesions of the dewclaws
- Bone fractures/ malformations.

Consult a textbook on bovine medicine to learn more about these conditions (a list of clinical and anatomical books is provided in Appendix C). You will learn more about these conditions in your clinical years.

5.2 Bones of the Thoracic Limb

Goal: Identify the major bones of the thoracic limb and their features. Compare with bones of the thoracic limb of the horse and other small animals (e.g., dog).

Use the bovine skeleton and the figures provided here to study the bones of the thoracic limb (Figure 5.1). The bones of the goat and sheep thoracic limb are like those of the bovine.

5.2.1 Scapula

The scapula is a flat, roughly triangular bone of the shoulder region. It is very similar to that of the horse except for one feature. The **acromion** is present in the scapula of ruminants but is absent in the scapula of the horse and pig. The lateral surface of the scapula has a large **infraspinous fossa** and relatively small **supraspinous fossa** (Figure 5.2).

The "shoulder blade" is a common name for the scapula that you may hear in the clinic.

The scapula has three borders (dorsal, cranial, and caudal), three angles (cranial, caudal, and ventral), and two surfaces (medial and lateral). The lateral surface has the **spine of the scapula** that separates the supra- and infraspinous fossae. A prominence in the middle of the spine is the tuber of the spine of the scapula: the tuber spinae scapulae.

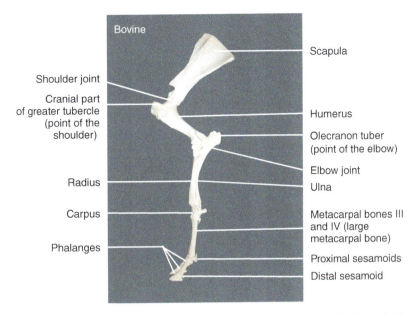

Figure 5.1 Bones of the bovine thoracic limb: left lateral view. Forelimb regions are the shoulder (scapula), brachium (humerus), antebrachium (radius and ulna), and manus (carpus, metacarpals, and digits).

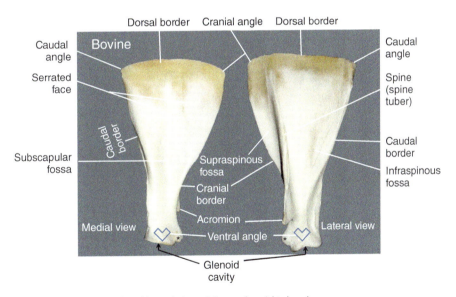

Figure 5.2 The left bovine scapula: medial and lateral views * Supraglenoid tubercle.

The depression on the distal end (ventral angle) of the scapula is the **glenoid cavity**. The glenoid cavity articulates with the head of the humerus to form the **shoulder joint**. Use Figure 5.2 to study the main features of the scapula.

On the medial surface of the scapula, identify the **subscapular fossa** and the **serrated face**.

The supra- and infraspinous fossae are for attachment of the supra- and infraspinatus muscles, respectively. The subscapular fossa is for attachment of the subscapularis muscle, and the serrated face is for attachment of the serratus ventralis muscle.

In the live animal or fresh specimen, the dorsal border of the scapula has a large **scapular cartilage** that extends its length dorsally.

5.2.2 Humerus

The humerus forms the bone of the arm or **brachium**. It is a very strong and robust bone in both cattle and horses. There are minor differences in the shape of the humerus between small and large ruminants that will not be discussed.

In the proximal part of the humerus, note that the **greater tubercle** (point of the shoulder) is well-developed and deviates toward the medial side (Figure 5.3). It is larger than the **lesser tubercle** located on the medial side. The greater tubercle is located at a higher level than the head of the humerus (see Box 5.1). The round **head** of the humerus articulates with the **glenoid cavity** to form the shoulder joint. Both the greater and lesser tubercles are divided into cranial and caudal parts.

In the horse, the greater and lesser tubercles are mostly equal in size. In addition, the horse has an intermediate tubercle. No intermediate tubercle is present in ruminants.

The **deltoid tuberosity** on the lateral surface of the humerus is well developed in both the cow and horse. It is the site for attachment of the deltoideus muscle.

Use Figure 5.3 to study the major bony prominences on the proximal and distal parts of the humerus. On the proximal humerus, identify the greater and lesser tubercles and **intertubercular groove**. The tendon of biceps brachii muscle passes in this groove.

Identify the **brachialis groove**, the attachment site for the brachialis muscle. The **humeral crest** forms the cranial border of this groove. The **body** (shaft) of the humerus is the part between the proximal head and distal humeral condyle.

On the distal humerus, identify the palpable **medial** and **lateral epicondyles**. The **radial fossa** is the shallow depression on the cranial surface of the humeral condyle. The relatively deep depression on the opposite caudal side of the humeral condyle is the **olecranon fossa**.

The condyle of the humerus articulates distally with the radius and ulna to form the **elbow joint**.

> **Box 5.1**
>
> The greater tubercle of the humerus is palpable in the live animal and forms the point of the shoulder.

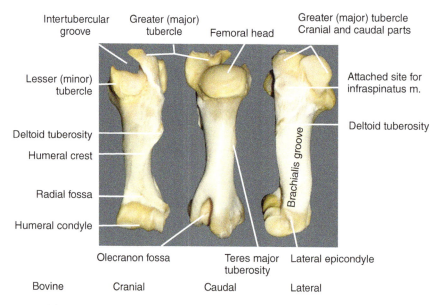

Figure 5.3 Left humerus of the ox: cranial, caudal, and lateral views.

5.2.3 Radius and Ulna

The radius and ulna are the bones of the **antebrachium** or forearm. Note that the ulna is complete in ruminants compared with that of the horse. The ulna in the bovine is fused to the radius except for proximal and distal interosseous spaces (Figure 5.4). In the horse, the ulna ends in the middle of the antebrachium.

On the proximal ulna, and with the help of Figure 5.4, identify the **olecranon tuber** or **(tuberosity)**, the palpable point of the elbow in the live animal, the **trochlear notch,** and the **anconeal process.** The olecranon tuberosity and anconeal process form the olecranon. The olecranon tuberosity is the attachment site for the extensor muscles of the elbow (e.g., triceps brachii and tensor fasciae antebrachii). See Box 5.2 for clinical application.

The distal extremity of the ulna is called the lateral styloid process or **styloid process of the ulna**. In the horse, the styloid process of the ulna is developmentally fused to the radius.

The radius is shorter and thicker than the ulna. Near the proximal extremity (head), identify the **radial tuberosity** on the medial side. The head of the radius and the trochlear notch of the ulna articulate with the humeral condyle to form the **elbow joint**.

> **Box 5.2**
>
> The olecranon tuber is palpable in the live animal and forms the point of the elbow. The point of the elbow approximates the distal part of the fifth intercostal space in the live animal.

The distal medial end of the radius is the **styloid process of the radius** (Figure 5.4).

The distal articular ends of the radius (trochlea) and ulna articulate with the proximal row of carpal bones to form the **radiocarpal joint**.

5.2.4 Carpus (Proximal and Distal Rows)

The bones of the carpus, metacarpus, and phalanges are known as the **manus**. At the end of this unit, watch **Video 21.**

As in the horse, the carpus in ruminants is composed of **two** rows (Figure 5.5a). The proximal row is like that of the horse and contains four bones. From lateral to medial, these are the **accessory carpal, ulnar, intermediate**, and **radial** carpal bones (Figure 5.5a). The accessory carpal is a palpable

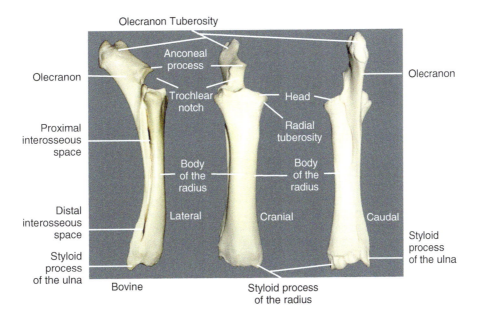

Figure 5.4 Left bovine radius and ulna: lateral, cranial, and caudal views.

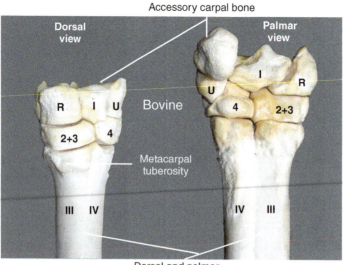

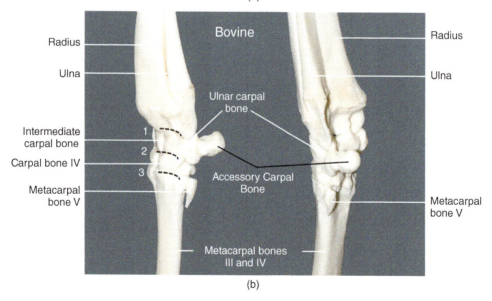

Figure 5.5 (a) The left bovine carpus and proximal metacarpal region: dorsal and palmar views. The carpus has two rows. The **proximal row** contains four carpal bones: accessory carpal (**AC**), ulnar (**U**), intermediate (**I**), and radial (**R**), from lateral (L) to medial (M). On the dorsal view, the AC bone is obscured but can be seen on the palmar view palmar to the ulnar carpal bone. The **distal row** contains two bones, the fourth carpal and fused second and third carpal bones. The distal row articulates with fused metacarpals III and IV (large metacarpal bone). Rudimentary metacarpal V is shown in (b). (b) Lateral (left) and laterocaudal (right) views of bovine left carpus showing metacarpal V bone. 1, radiocarpal joint; 2, midcarpal joint; 3, carpometacarpal joint.

landmark on the lateral surface of the carpus. It provides an attachment point for the ulnaris lateralis and flexor carpi ulnaris muscles.

The distal row is composed of two bones in ruminants. From lateral to medial, these are the **fourth carpal** and fused **second** and **third carpal bones** (Figure 5.5a). Carpal one is not present.

The horse has three or four bones in the distal row including the fourth, third, second, and first carpal bones from lateral to medial, respectively. The first carpal bone in the horse may be absent, as in ruminants.

Articulation between the proximal and distal rows of carpal bones forms the **midcarpal joint**. The articulation between the distal row of carpal bones and the large metacarpal bone (fused III and IV metacarpals) forms the **carpometacarpal joint**.

5.2.5 Metacarpal Bones (Large Metacarpal or Cannon Bone)

Metacarpals 3, 4, and 5 (**Mc III, Mc IV**, and **Mc V**) are present in ruminants. Mc III and Mc IV are fused forming a single **large metacarpal bone** (Figures 5.5 and 5.6). Identify the **metacarpal tuberosity** on the proximal dorsomedial surface of the large metacarpal bone. This is the attachment site for the tendon of the extensor carpi radialis muscle.

In the horse, only the Mc III (cannon bone) is present. Because of the presence of two weight-bearing digits in ruminants, the distal end of the large metacarpal bone has two parts with an articulating trochlea at each end. The space formed by this separation is the **intertrochlear notch**. Each trochlea articulates with the proximal phalanx (P1) of the corresponding digit.

The term **cannon bone** is a common name used for the **third metacarpal** (Mc III) bone in horses but also for the large metacarpal or fused Mc III and Mc IV bone in ruminants.

In ruminants, a small metacarpal 5 (**Mc V**) is present as a rudimentary bone on the proximolateral aspect of fused Mc III and Mc IV (Figure 5.5b). You should not confuse Mc V with a fracture or bone growth when examining an X-ray of ruminant carpal–metacarpal regions.

The axial line of fusion of Mc III and Mc IV forms the **dorsal** and **palmar axial longitudinal grooves** (Figure 5.6). In the live animal, blood vessels occupy the dorsal and palmar metacarpal longitudinal grooves. The dorsal longitudinal groove is more distinct than the palmar groove.

Note the **proximal** and **distal metacarpal canals** (openings) at the proximal and distal ends of the longitudinal grooves (Figure 5.6). These canals allow for the passage of blood vessels between the dorsal and palmar sides of the large metacarpal bone. See Box 5.3 for the clinical relevance of the axial dorsal and palmar longitudinal grooves.

> **Box 5.3**
>
> The axial dorsal and palmar longitudinal grooves on the large metacarpal bone (fused Mc III and IV bones) can be seen as an opaque fusion in the midline on X-ray films. This should not be confused with a fracture.

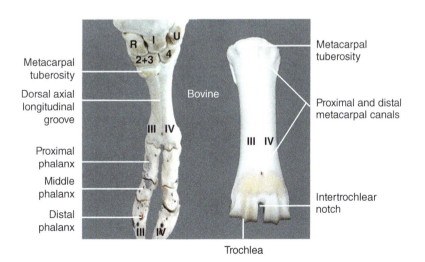

Figure 5.6 Bovine left manus (carpus, metacarpals, and digits): dorsal view. The image on the left shows the articulation of the large metacarpal bone with the carpus proximally, and digits III and IV distally. The image on the right shows an isolated bovine large metacarpal bone. Each digit has a proximal (P1), middle (P2), and distal phalanx (P3).

5.2.6 Digits

Limbs of domestic ruminants have two digits. The medial digit (**digit III**) and lateral digit (**digit IV**) are weight-bearing (Figure 5.6). The medial and lateral **dewclaws** form **digit II** and **digit V**, respectively. They are non-weight-bearing in cattle and may not have any bony skeleton. Skeletal elements of these digits are present in some ruminants.

The weight-bearing **third** and **fourth digits** have three phalanges each. From proximal to distal, these are **proximal (P1), middle (P2),** and **distal (P3) phalanges** (Figure 5.6). Each phalanx is divided into base, body, and head, from proximal to distal.

The P1 and P2 are similar in shape but the length of P1 is twice as long as P2. The shape of P3 (coffin bone) is different from P1 and P2 (Figure 5.7).

Identify the **extensor process** on the proximodorsal surface of P3. This is the site for attachment of the axial extensor tendons from the common digital extensor muscle. A similar arrangement occurs with the axial extensor tendons of the long digital extensor tendons in the hind limb.

The common name for the distal phalanx (P3) is the **coffin bone** because it is embedded inside the hoof capsule, analogous to a coffin.

Each digit has two **proximal sesamoid bones** (at the palmar surface of the fetlock joint) and a single **distal sesamoid bone** (at the palmar surface of the coffin joint). Overall, a total of four proximal sesamoid bones and two distal sesamoid bones are present in the two weight-bearing digits of each limb (Figure 5.7). The **navicular bone** (analogous to a boat) is a common name for the distal sesamoid bone.

The nomenclature and general shape of the bones in the single digit of the horse is generally like a single digit (III or IV) in ruminants.

Bones of the hind limb digits are like those of the forelimb.

The articulation between fused Mc III and Mc IV and P1 on each digit forms the metacarpophalangeal joint (**MCP**) or the **fetlock joint**. Distal to the fetlock joint is the proximal interphalangeal joint (**PIP**) or **pastern joint** formed by the articulation of P1 with P2. More distally, articulation of P2 and P3 forms the distal interphalangeal (**DIP**) or the **coffin joint**. See Box 5.4 for clinical application.

> **Box 5.4**
>
> The medial digit (digit III) of the forelimb is larger and carries more weight than the lateral digit (digit IV). This is thought to subject the medial digit to more stress. Consequently, amputation of the medial digit has a poorer prognosis than the mostly good long-term prognosis for amputation of the lateral digit.

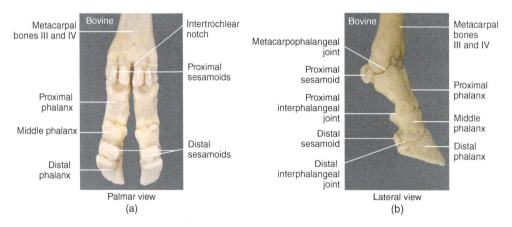

Figure 5.7 The left bovine digits: (a) palmar and (b) lateral views. In the live animal, digit IV (lateral) and digit III (medial) are interconnected by proximal and distal interdigital ligaments.

5.3 Muscles and Tendons of the Thoracic Limb

Goal: Identify the extrinsic and intrinsic muscles of the thoracic limb and know the general area of origin and insertion for each muscle. Emphasis will be placed on the musculoskeletal structures of the distal limb. Use a goat or cow thoracic limb skeleton to help you visualize the location of each muscle by identifying points of origin and insertion.

Use a bovine or caprine limb to dissect muscles of the thoracic limb depending on what is available to you (there are no differences between the two). In this guide, the extrinsic muscles of the thoracic limb, which attach the limb to the axial skeleton, are dissected on a goat cadaver while the intrinsic muscles (attached to appendicular bones of the thoracic limb) are dissected on both goat and cow limbs. Use the text description below and any prosections prepared by your instructor to help you identify muscles and tendons.

Follow the dissection plan in Appendix A to remove goat forelimbs. Alternatively, your instructor may provide you with isolated bovine or caprine limbs. It will be convenient to study the cutaneous and extrinsic muscles on a goat cadaver with the limbs attached (Figure 5.8).

Use a new scalpel blade to carefully skin the entire limb. Clean the fat and connective tissue off the regions of the limb and identify the muscles. Ask your instructor if you should preserve the blood vessels and nerves. We recommend that you use one limb (left) for dissection of muscles and a second limb (right) for dissection of blood vessels and nerves, but you can always have a mixture of both.

Pay attention to the carpal fascia (carpal extensor retinaculum) and deep antebrachial fascia when skinning the limb. When dissecting the blood vessels and nerves of the forelimb, preserve the superficial vessels (dorsal common digital vein III, cephalic, and accessory cephalic veins) and nerves (branches of the superficial branch of the radial nerve) on the antebrachium and the dorsal surface of the large metacarpal bone.

If you started your work with the whole cadaver and opted to preserve the cutaneous muscles, identify the **cutaneus omobrachialis muscle** on the lateral surface of the shoulder and caudal scapula (Figure 5.8). Identify the **cutaneus trunci muscle** located further caudally from the cutaneus omobrachialis (Figure 5.8). The cutaneus trunci does not cover the dorsal part of the flank region. It is thicker in two places: the area cranial to the stifle forming the **fold of the flank**, and close to the axilla. **In small animals (dogs and cats), the cutaneous trunci reflex (twitching of the muscle**

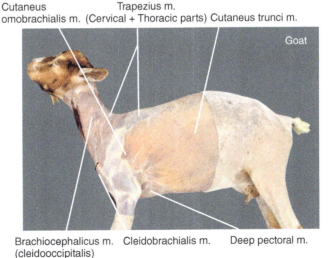

Figure 5.8 The cutaneous trunci and cutaneous omobrachialis muscles in the goat: left lateral view. The dotted line denotes the location of the clavicular intersection.

upon pinching the skin) is used for localization of thoracolumbar spinal cord injuries.

We will focus on the anatomy of the distal limb, but we will also attempt to give some information on the proximal muscles. Ask your instructor which muscles you need to identify. Your laboratory identification (ID) list for the forelimb (combined with the lab ID list for the hind limb in Chapter 6) has a few of the extrinsic muscles listed. However, all the distal intrinsic muscles (from the elbow and below) warrant your attention and are part of your ID list.

5.3.1 Extrinsic Muscles of the Forelimb

Goal: Identify the major extrinsic muscles of the thoracic limb. Make sure you identify the brachiocephalicus (an extrinsic muscle of the thoracic limb) and sternocephalicus (sternomandibularis and sternomastoideus) muscles that form the dorsal and ventral boundaries for the external jugular groove, respectively.

The muscles of the thoracic limb are divided into two groups: **extrinsic** and **intrinsic muscles**. Extrinsic muscles attach the limb to the axial skeleton. The axial skeleton comprises the skull, vertebrae, ribs, and the sternum. The extrinsic muscles of the forelimb include nine muscles (see the following list).

Although the sternocephalicus muscle (specifically, the sternomandibularis part) forms the ventral boundary for the external jugular groove in cattle and goats, the muscle is not included with the extrinsic muscles of the forelimb. This is because it does not have an attachment on the limb. The extrinsic muscles must be severed to remove the thoracic limb.

The extrinsic muscles are generally similar in different domestic animals with minor variations. In ruminants, they include the following muscles:

1) **Trapezius muscle** (has two divisions, **thoracic** and **cervical parts**)
2) **Rhomboideus muscle** (has two divisions, **cervical** and **thoracic parts**)
3) **Brachiocephalicus muscle** (has two divisions, **cleidocephalicus** and **cleidobrachialis muscles**, with the cleidocephalicus muscle further divided into two parts, **cleidooccipitalis** and **cleidomastoideus**)
4) **Omotransversarius muscle**
5) **Latissimus dorsi muscle**
6) **Superficial pectoral muscle** (has two divisions, **transverse** and **ascending parts**)
7) **Deep pectoral muscle**
8) **Subclavius muscle**
9) **Serratus ventralis muscle** (has two divisions, **cervical** and **thoracic parts**).

There follows a detailed description of the extrinsic muscles. Some of these muscles are described in Chapter 1 (head and neck). Ask your instructor which muscles you need to identify. Stumps of several extrinsic muscles can be identified on an isolated limb.

5.3.1.1 Trapezius Muscle (Cervical and Thoracic Parts)

The trapezius muscle is a thin triangular muscle. The base of the triangle lies toward the vertebral column along the dorsal border of the scapula and caudal cervical region. The apex courses distally on the lateral surface of the scapula and inserts by an aponeurosis (flat shiny connective tissue sheet) on the spine of the scapula. The trapezius muscle has **cervical** and **thoracic parts** (Figures 5.8 and 5.9).

Origin: Funicular part of the nuchal ligament on the cervical and thoracic region.

Insertion: Spine of the scapula by a flat aponeurosis.

Action: Contraction of the trapezius elevates the scapula.

5.3.1.2 Rhomboideus Muscle (Cervical and Thoracic Parts)

The rhomboideus muscle is located deep to the trapezius muscle. As in the horse, the rhomboideus in ruminants has two parts: **cervical** and **thoracic**. In the dog, a third part, called the rhomboideus capitis, is present.

Reflect the cervical and thoracic parts of the trapezius dorsally to identify the two parts of the rhomboideus muscle.

Origin:

- Rhomboideus cervicis: funicular part of the nuchal ligament that spans the distance between C2 and T2.
- Rhomboideus thoracis: thoracic spines.

Insertion: Dorsal and medial borders of the scapular cartilage.

Action: Draw the scapula dorsally.

The **hump** present in some breeds of cattle is an enlargement of the rhomboideus muscle. A hump is present in zebu cattle (*Bos indicus*) in Africa, and in Brahman (*Bos taurus indicus*) or Brahman crosses from *Bos indicus* cattle. *Bos taurus* cattle (European breeds) do not have a hump.

5.3.1.3 Brachiocephalicus Muscle (Cleidocephalicus and Cleidobrachialis)

The brachiocephalicus muscle is a compound muscle that extends craniodorsally from the distal cranial surface of the humerus to the dorsal lateral surface of the skull.

In ruminants, it has three parts: the **cleidobrachialis, cleidooccipitalis,** and **cleidomastoideus** muscles. The cleidooccipitalis and cleidomastoideus form the **cleidocephalicus** muscle.

The prefix **cleido-** in the names of the divisions of the brachiocephalicus means clavicle. No bony clavicle is present in ruminants.

The divisions of the brachiocephalicus originate from the clavicular intersection cranial to the shoulder region and course to the brachium (cleidobrachialis division) or to the head (cleidocephalicus division that itself has cleido-occipitalis and cleidomastoideus parts) (Figure 5.9). Consult Box 5.5 for clinical application.

The cleidooccipitalis is absent in the horse.

The cleidooccipitalis and cleidobrachialis, the respective cranial and caudal divisions of the brachiocephalicus muscle, are immediately visible when you remove the skin and clean the superficial fascia from the neck and brachium regions (Figure 5.9). The cleidomastoideus forms the ventral part of cleidocephalicus and is not readily visible. It directly forms the dorsal boundary of the external jugular groove and is located ventral and medial to the cleido-occipitalis muscle.

Identify the clavicular intersection, cleido-occipitalis, cleidomastoideus, and cleidobrachialis divisions. Note that the cleido-occipitalis division is much larger and broader than the cleidomastoideus division and covers most of the dorsal neck region (Figure 5.9).

Origin: Clavicular intersection cranial to the shoulder joint.

Insertion: Brachium or crest of the humerus (cleidobrachialis), nuchal crest and funicular nuchae (cleidooccipitalis), and the mastoid process of the petrous division of the temporal bone (cleidomastoideus).

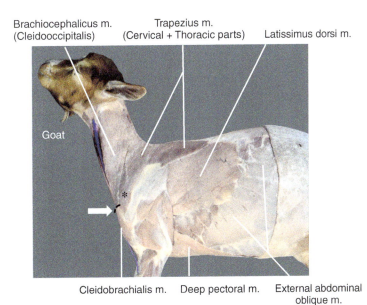

Figure 5.9 Superficial muscles of the goat showing several of the superficially located extrinsic muscles of the thoracic limb: left lateral view. Dotted line (white arrow) denotes the location of the clavicular intersection. * Omotransversarius muscle.

> **Box 5.5**
>
> As previously discussed in the neck region, the cleidomastoideus muscle (the ventral division of the cleidocephalicus) forms the dorsal border of the jugular groove in cattle, goats, and sheep. The ventral border is formed by the sternomandibularis muscle in cattle (sternozygomaticus in goats). The stermandibularis muscle represents the ventral division of the sternocephalicus muscle. Sheep lack the sternozygomaticus muscle.

> **Box 5.6**
>
> The superficial cervical lymph nodes (commonly known as prescapular lymph nodes in the clinic) drain the skin around the neck and proximal limb and are routinely examined in meat inspection. They become enlarged in infections involving the neck region.

Actions: The brachiocephalicus muscle has complex actions that depend on several factors such as whether the limb is weight-bearing or free to swing. During motion, it extends the shoulder joint and advances the whole limb. Contraction of ipsilateral muscle moves the neck and head laterally. When both left and right brachiocephalicus muscles contract, they pull the head ventrally.

5.3.1.4 Omotransversarius Muscle

The omotransversarius muscle extends between the spine of the scapula (acromion) and the atlas, the first cervical vertebra (C1). It is a flat, strap-like muscle.

The caudal portion of the omotransversarius muscle can be viewed close to the cranial border of the scapula between the cervical part of the trapezius and the cleido-occipitalis muscles (Figures 5.8 and 5.9). The cranial part of the omotransversarius is covered by the cleido-occipitalis muscle (Figure 5.9).

Transect the cleido-occipitalis muscle in the middle and reflect the two ends to uncover the cranial part of the omotransversarius muscle coursing toward the wing of the atlas.

Origin: Acromion of the scapula.

Insertion: Part of the axis and wing of the atlas (C1, the first cervical vertebra).

Action: It bends the neck laterally.

*Transect the omotransversarius in the middle of the neck and reflect both ends. Preserve the **superficial cervical lymph nodes** that are located deep to the omotransversarius and directly cranial to the cranial border of the scapula. Consult Box 5.6 for clinical application related to superficial cervical lymph nodes.*

5.3.1.5 Latissimus Dorsi Muscle

The latissimus dorsi (L. dorsi) is a large triangular muscle that lies dorsally caudal to the scapula and courses cranially medial to the proximal part of the humerus. The broad part of the muscle courses from the thoracolumbar region caudally, to the axilla (armpit) cranially (Figure 5.9). It inserts on the proximal medial surface of the humerus in conjunction with the teres major muscle (Figure 5.9). Depending on whether the forelimb is free or fixed (weight-bearing), the L. dorsi flexes the shoulder joint and draws the trunk forward, respectively.

Origin: Thoracolumbar fascia on the dorsal midline of the thorax and lumbar regions.

Insertion: Teres major tuberosity, on the medial–proximal side of the humerus.

Action: The action depends of the limb position. The L. dorsi draws the limb caudally when the limb is free (non-weight-bearing). It draws the trunk cranially when the limb is fixed (weight-bearing).

5.3.1.6 Superficial Pectoral Muscle (Descending and Transverse Parts)

The superficial pectoral muscle is located ventrally between the forelimbs and courses between the cranial part of the sternum and the proximomedial aspects of the humerus and the antebrachium region (radius and ulna) (Figure 5.10). The superficial pectoral muscle has two parts: **descending** and **transverse** pectoral muscles.

The actions of the superficial pectoral muscles include limb adduction when not bearing weight or prevention of limb abduction when weight is placed on the body.

The horse has well-developed superficial pectoral muscles when compared with cattle.

Origin: Manubrium (descending pectoral), and 2–6 sternebrae (transverse pectoral).

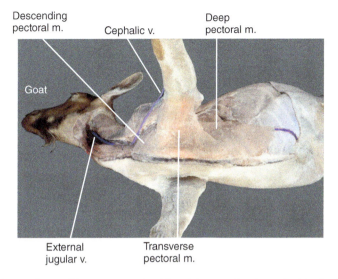

Figure 5.10 The superficial (descending and transverse pectorals) and deep pectoral muscles (goat): ventral view.

Insertion: Crest of the humerus (descending pectoral), proximal one-third of the medial forearm (transverse pectoral).

Action: To prevent abduction of the forelimbs when bearing weight. To adduct the forelimbs when not bearing weight. One of the most important functions of the pectoral muscles is to suspend and support the weight of the body between the limbs (sling system analogous to the role of the serratus ventralis muscle discussed later).

5.3.1.7 Deep (Ascending) Pectoral Muscle

The deep pectoral muscle is located ventrally behind the transverse pectoral muscle. It is thicker than the superficial pectoral muscle (Figure 5.10).

Origin: Median raphe along the entire ventral surface of the sternum.

Insertion: Lesser and greater tubercles on the proximal humerus.

Action: Adducts and draws limb caudally when the limb is free to swing. The deep pectoral advances the trunk when the limb is advanced and fixed.

5.3.1.8 Serratus Ventralis Muscle

The serratus ventralis muscle is a fan-shaped muscle located deep (medial) to the scapula. It has a critical role, along with other extrinsic muscles, in attaching the forelimb to the axial skeleton (ribs and cervical vertebrae). This type of attachment (bone–muscle–bone) is different from a conventional joint and is called **synsarcosis**. The left and right muscles act as a sling system to carry the weight of the body between the limbs as do the pectoral muscles mentioned earlier.

The thoracic limb covers much of the serratus ventralis muscle except for the cranial and caudal parts. The muscle fibers of the serratus ventralis muscle extend from the middle parts of the ribs and transverse cervical vertebrae to attach on the medial (deep) surface of the scapula along the **serrated face**.

Remove the thoracic limb to uncover the full extent of the serratus ventralis muscle (Figure 5.11). Detach the insertion from the serrated face of the scapula. To completely remove the limb, transect the remaining extrinsic muscles at the cranial, dorsal, and caudal borders.

Following removal of the thoracic limb, note the fan-shaped appearance of the serratus ventralis (Figure 5.11). On the ribs, note that the fibers of the serratus ventralis interdigitate in a serrated manner with those of the external abdominal oblique muscle, hence the name serratus.

Identify the **cervical** and **thoracic** parts of the muscle.

Origin: Last 4–5 cervical vertebrae (cervical part) and first 7–8 ribs (thoracic part).

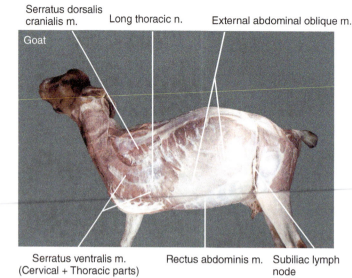

Figure 5.11 Dissection of serratus ventralis muscle (goat: left lateral view; the left forelimb has been removed). Note the fan-shaped cervical and thoracic parts of the serratus ventralis muscle (insertion of the muscle cut along the dotted line). The long thoracic nerve (from the brachial plexus) supplies the serratus ventralis muscle.

Insertion: Serrated surface of the scapula.

Action: The cervical part draws the scapula cranially when the limb swings caudally. The thoracic part does the opposite (moves the scapula caudally) when the limb is advanced cranially. The left and right muscles act as a "sling system" to support the trunk.

5.3.1.9 Subclavius Muscle

The subclavius muscle courses along the cranial border of the scapula and supraspinatus muscle. It is well developed in goats, pigs, and horses but is absent in dogs. *Do not look for it.*

Origin: First rib cartilage.

Insertion: Clavicular intersection of the brachiocephalicus muscle.

Action: No action that deserves attention.

5.3.2 Intrinsic Muscles of the Thoracic Limb

Goal: Identify the major intrinsic muscles from proximal to distal. Emphasis will be placed on muscles and tendons in the distal limb (elbow and below). Study muscle actions on the joints.

Skin the entire limb and clean the superficial fascia and fat. To keep your specimen looking fresh between labs, make sure that you keep it moistened by regularly spraying it as needed with water or InfuTrace solution (neutralizes and reduces formaldehyde in embalmed specimens). We suggest dissecting muscles and vessels on separate limbs.

Muscles in proximal limb (shoulder and brachium):

- Supraspinatus muscle
- Infraspinatus muscle
- Deltoideus muscle
- Teres minor muscle
- Teres major muscle
- Subscapularis muscle
- Triceps brachii muscle (long, lateral, accessory, and medial heads)
- Anconeus muscle
- Tensor fasciae antebrachii muscle
- Coracobrachialis muscle
- Biceps brachii muscle
- Brachialis muscle.

Muscles and structures of the distal limb (antebrachium, and manus [carpus, metacarpus and digits]). Depending on their location, the muscles of the antebrachium are broadly divided into two groups: caudolateral and caudomedial (Figures 5.12 and 5.13).

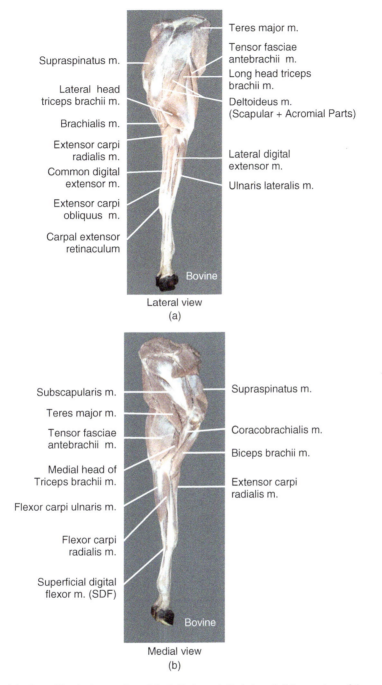

Figure 5.12 (a) Overview of the lateral intrinsic muscles of the **left** thoracic limb (goat); (b) overview of the medial intrinsic muscles of the **left** thoracic limb (goat).

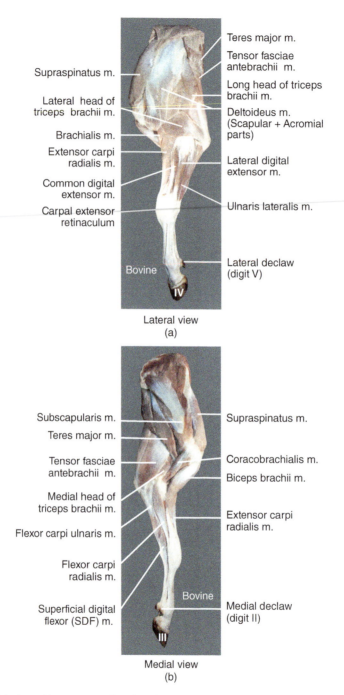

Figure 5.13 (a) Overview of the lateral intrinsic muscles of the **left** bovine thoracic limb. The bovine intrinsic thoracic limb muscles are like those of the goat (Figure 5.12a). IV, lateral digit; (b) overview of the medial intrinsic muscles of the **left** bovine thoracic limb. The bovine intrinsic thoracic limb muscles are like those of the goat (Figure 5.12b). III, medial digit.

Craniolateral group: Use the acronym "**ECLU**" to remember the first four of the following extensor muscles.

- Extensor carpi radialis muscle
- Common digital extensor muscle (has two bellies and three tendons coursing to digits III and IV)
- Lateral digital extensor muscle (has one tendon inserting on the lateral digit)
- Ulnaris lateralis muscle (has long and short tendons)
- Extensor carpi obliquus muscle.

Caudomedial group:

- Flexor carpi ulnaris muscle
- Flexor carpi radialis muscle
- Superficial digital flexor (SDF) muscle-flexor manica
- Deep digital flexor (DDF) muscle
- Interosseus muscle (suspensory ligament) axial and abaxial extensor branches.

Retinacula:

- Extensor retinaculum (deep fascia-dorsal carpus)
- Flexor retinaculum (deep fascia-palmar carpus).

Ligaments of the digits:

- Annular ligaments (fetlock, proximal, and distal digital annular ligaments)
- Interdigital ligaments (proximal and distal).

Hoof:

- Wall
- Sole
- Bulb
- White line.

5.3.2.1 Muscles of the Proximal Limb (Shoulder and Brachium)

5.3.2.1.1 Supraspinatus Muscle

The supraspinatus muscle is a lateral shoulder muscle that occupies the supraspinous fossa of the scapula (Figures 5.13a and 5.14). Note that the supraspinatus muscle wraps around the cranial border of the scapula and is visible on the medial cranial side of the scapula (Figure 5.14). The main function of the supraspinatus muscle is to stabilize the shoulder joint. Other actions of the muscle are of minor significance. It inserts on the cranial surface of the greater and lesser tubercle.

Origin: Supraspinous fossa.
Insertion: Split insertion on the greater and lesser tubercles.
Action: Stabilizes and extends the shoulder joint.

5.3.2.1.2 Infraspinatus Muscle

The infraspinatus muscle is a lateral shoulder muscle that occupies the infraspinous fossa on the lateral surface of the scapula. It is partly covered by the deltoideus muscle (Figures 5.13a and 5.14).

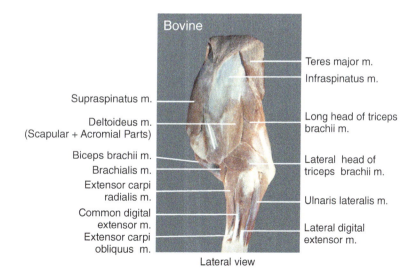

Figure 5.14 Bovine proximal muscles of the shoulder, brachium, and antebrachium: close-up left lateral view.

The infraspinatus muscle has two insertion tendons: long **superficial tendon** and relatively short **deep tendon**. Like the supraspinatus, the infraspinatus muscle stabilizes the shoulder joint.

An **infraspinatus subtendinous bursa** is present deep to the superficial tendon in ruminants and other most domestic animals (dog and horse). The bursa may, however, be absent in small ruminants.

Reflect the scapular and acromial parts of the deltoideus muscle to uncover the distal part of the infraspinatus muscle on a cow forelimb. Transect the infraspinatus belly midway between its proximal and distal ends. Reflect the distal half from the infraspinous fossa to its insertion on the humerus. Verify the presence of the subtendinous bursa.

Origin: Supraspinous fossa.

Insertion: Proximal caudal border of the greater tubercle (deep tendon) and distal to the greater tubercle (superficial tendon).

Action: Stabilizes the shoulder joint (acts like a collateral ligament). Other actions are of minor significance.

5.3.2.1.3 Deltoideus Muscle

The deltoideus muscle covers the lateral surface of the infraspinatus muscle (Figure 5.14). In ruminants, it has **scapular** and **acromial** parts. It originates from the spine of the scapula and acromion and inserts on the deltoideus tuberosity on the lateral surface of the humerus.

In the horse, the deltoideus muscle lacks the acromial part. The dog, like ruminants, has both the scapular and acromial parts.

Origin: Spine of the scapula proximal to the acromion (scapular part), and the acromion in the distal end of the scapular spine (acromial part).

Insertion: Deltoid tuberosity on the proximal lateral surface of the humerus.

Action: Flexes the shoulder joint.

5.3.2.1.4 Teres Minor Muscle

The teres minor muscle is a relatively small muscle located deep to the distal end of the scapular part of the deltoideus muscle. It lies directly over the lateral surface of the shoulder joint.

Reflect the scapular part of the deltoideus muscle to uncover the teres minor muscle.

Origin: Distal third of the caudal border of the scapula.

Insertion: Teres minor tuberosity proximal to the lateral deltoid tuberosity.

Action: Flexes the shoulder joint.

5.3.2.1.5 Teres Major Muscle

The teres major muscle is located along the caudomedial border of the scapula caudal to the subscapularis muscle. The teres major muscle flexes the shoulder joint. Look for the teres major on the medial surface of the shoulder region (Figure 5.15).

Origin: Proximal caudal border (caudal angle) of the scapula.

Insertion: Teres major tuberosity on the proximal medial surface of the humerus along with the insertion tendon of the latissimus dorsi muscle.

Action: Flexes the shoulder joint.

Note that the deltoideus, teres major, and teres minor all flex the shoulder joint. The names of these muscles can be memorized by the acronym "**DTT**," which stands for **d**eltoideus, **t**eres major, and **t**eres minor.

5.3.2.1.6 Subscapularis Muscle

The subscapularis muscle occupies the subscapular fossa on the medial surface of the scapula (Figure 5.15). The muscle has several parallel parts covered by strong white deep fascia (multipennate type muscle). Ask your instructor for explanation of the terms pennate, bipennate, and multipennate muscles.

The subscapularis muscle stabilizes the shoulder joint on the medial side in concert with the stabilizing actions of the supra and infraspinatus muscles on the lateral side of the shoulder joint. The subscapularis muscle inserts on the lesser tubercle of the humerus.

Origin: Subscapular fossa.

Insertion: Lesser tubercle.

Action: Stabilizes the shoulder joint. Other minor action includes adduction of the brachium.

5.3.2.1.7 Triceps Brachii Muscle (Long, Lateral, Accessory, and Medial Heads)

The triceps brachii muscle occupies the triangular space cranial to an imaginary line from the caudal border of the scapula to the olecranon tuber of the ulna (Figure 5.14).

The triceps brachii muscle has four heads in ruminants and dogs: **long, lateral, accessory,** and **medial**. The accessory head is small in ruminants and may sometimes be absent.

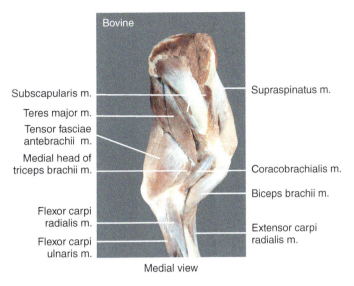

Figure 5.15 Medial bovine intrinsic muscles of the thoracic limb in the shoulder, brachium, and proximal antebrachium regions: close-up view.

In the horse, the triceps brachii muscle fits its descriptive name as it has only three heads: long, lateral, and medial. The accessory head is absent.

In all domestic animals, the heads of the triceps brachii join distally to insert on the olecranon tuber. A subtendinous bursa (**subtendinous bursa of the triceps brachii**) is located between the olecranon tuber and the combined tendon of the triceps brachii muscle.

Keep in mind that the long head is the only division of the triceps brachii that originates from the caudal border of the scapula with actions on two joints: the shoulder and elbow joints. The remaining heads originate from the proximal humerus. The triceps brachii is a major extensor of the elbow joint. Other minor extensors of the elbow (anconeus and tensor fasciae antebrachii) are of negligible significance.

Origin: Caudal border of the scapula (long head); proximal lateral humerus and tricipital line (lateral, accessory, and medial heads).

Insertion: Olecranon tuber (point of the elbow).

Action: Extend the elbow. The long head flexes the shoulder joint.

5.3.2.1.8 Anconeus Muscle

The anconeus muscle is located on the lateral surface of the elbow joint deep to the lateral head of the triceps brachii muscle. Injections through the anconeus muscles reach the elbow joint capsule.

Origin: Caudodorsal part of the humerus (olecranon tuber).

Insertion: Lateral surface of the olecranon.

Action: Extends the elbow joint. It tenses the elbow joint capsule during extension

5.3.2.1.9 Tensor Fasciae Antebrachii Muscle

The tensor fasciae antebrachii muscle is located on the caudal and part of the medial side of the antebrachium (Figure 5.15). In ruminants, the muscle covers the caudal border of the long head of the triceps brachii.

In the horse and dog, it covers a more substantial area of the medial surface of the long head of the triceps brachii muscle.

Origin: Caudal border of the scapula.

Insertion: Olecranon tuber (point of the elbow) and deep antebrachial fascia.

Action: Extends the elbow.

5.3.2.1.10 Coracobrachialis Muscle

The coracobrachialis muscle is located on the medial side of the shoulder joint and proximal brachium region. The tendon of origin obliquely crosses the shoulder joint. The muscle belly lies behind the biceps brachii superficial to the distal insertion of the teres major (Figure 5.15). It has several functions, including stabilization of the shoulder joint, adduction of the brachium, and flexion of the shoulder joint.

Origin: Coracoid process of the scapula.
Insertion: Teres major tuberosity (in the horse) and distal medial surface of the humerus distal to the teres major tuberosity (in ruminants).
Action: Flexes, adducts, and stabilizes the shoulder joint.

5.3.2.1.11 Biceps Brachii Muscle

The biceps brachii muscle is located on the cranial and medial surfaces of the humerus (Figure 5.15). It originates from the supraglenoid tubercle of the scapula and inserts on the medial–proximal surface of the radius. It is a major flexor of the elbow joint. The following two features are associated with the biceps brachii:

1) A **transverse humeral retinaculum** (a flat connective tissue structure) wraps around the tendon of origin of the biceps brachii. It prevents eversion of the tendon from the intertubercular groove.
2) An **intertubercular bursa** is present under the tendon of origin of the biceps brachii. This bursa is an independent synovial sac in bovine and equine species but is an extension of the shoulder joint capsule in dogs.

Origin: Supraglenoid tubercle.
Insertion: Radial tuberosity and medial elbow region.
Action: Flexes the elbow and extends the shoulder joint.

5.3.2.1.12 Brachialis Muscle

The brachialis muscle is located on the lateral surface of the humerus (in the brachialis groove) and is partially covered by the lateral head of the triceps brachii muscle (Figures 5.14 and 5.15). It flexes the elbow joint.

Origin: Proximal part of the caudal surface of the humerus and brachialis groove.
Insertion: Medial elbow and proximal part of the medial surface of the radius (cattle) and the medial coronoid process of the ulna (goats).
Action: Flexes the elbow joint.

5.3.2.2 Muscles and Tendons of the Distal Limb (Antebrachium and Manus [Carpus, Metacarpus, and Digits])

The muscles located on the antebrachium are divided into craniolateral and caudomedial groups. The craniolateral group are general extensors of the carpus and digits and the caudomedial group have the opposite effect (flexors of the carpus and digits).

5.3.2.2.1 Craniolateral Group (Located on the Cranial and Lateral Forearm)

To identify the extensor group of carpus and digits, turn the limb so the lateral side is facing up. From cranial to caudal, these muscles include extensor carpi radialis, extensor carpi obliquus, common digital extensor, lateral digital extensor, and ulanris lateralis muscles (Figure 5.16).

The muscles on the craniolateral group of the antebrachium muscles share common characteristics that help you memorize several of their characteristics:

1) Common origin from the lateral epicondyle of the humerus, with the exception of the extensor carpi radialis (originates from lateral supracondylar crest) and extensor carpi obliquus (originates from body of the radius).
2) All the muscles in this group are innervated by the radial nerve.
3) They collectively extend the carpus with some muscles (common and lateral digital extensor) extending the digital joints as well (muscles with the word "digit" in their name).
4) They are located on the craniolateral aspect of the antebrachium.

Remove the superficial and **deep antebrachial fascia** to uncover the muscles of the crus or antebrachium. There follows a summary of the antebrachium muscles on craniolateral aspect of the leg (crus).

5.3.2.2.2 Extensor Carpi Radialis Muscle

The extensor carpi radialis is the most cranial muscle of the craniolateral group of the antebrachium region (Figure 5.16). It originates from the lateral supracondylar crest and radial fossa and inserts on the metacarpal tuberosity of the large metacarpal bone (fused Mc III and Mc IV). It extends the carpus.

Origin: Lateral supracondylar crest and radial fossa.
Insertion: Metacarpal tuberosity at the base of Mc III and Mc IV.
Action: Extends the carpus.

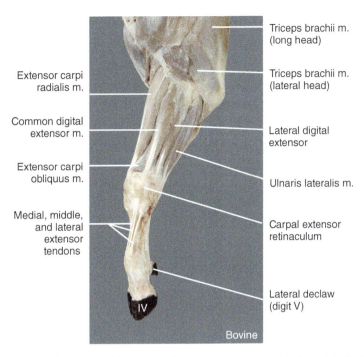

Figure 5.16 Craniolateral muscles of the antebrachium and digits (left bovine forelimb). IV-lateral digit. The superficial and deep antebrachial fascia have been removed except for the carpal extensor retinaculum.

5.3.2.2.3 Common Digital Extensor Muscle (Medial and Lateral Heads and Three Tendons)

The common digital extensor in ruminants has two bellies or heads (**medial** and **lateral**) and three insertion tendons. It is located caudal to the extensor carpi radialis muscle and cranial to the lateral digital extensor muscle (Figure 5.16). The lateral head of the common digital extensor also has superficial and deep heads. It is not necessary to dissect these heads but follow their tendons to the digits.

The common digital extensor muscle has one belly in the horse.

The tendon of the medial head of the common digital extensor is sometimes called the **medial digital extensor tendon** or **proper extensor tendon of digit III**. The tendon of the lateral head is called the **common extensor tendon of digits III and IV**.

Follow the **medial** and **lateral** (middle) tendons of the common digital extensor coursing distally on the dorsal surface of the metacarpal region. The relatively large medial tendon inserts on the medial digit (digit III). The lateral (or middle) relatively thin tendon splits into two tendons that course to the interdigital space to insert on the extensor processes of P3 of digits III and IV.

Origin: Lateral epicondyle of the humerus.

Insertion: Medial tendon inserts on P2 with extension to P3 (ox) of the medial digit (digit III); the lateral tendon splits into two thin tendons that insert on the extensor processes of P3 of digits III and IV.

Action: Extends the carpus and digital joints.

5.3.2.2.4 Lateral Digital Extensor Muscle

The lateral digital extensor muscle lies caudal to the common digital extensor (Figure 5.16). Like the common digital extensor muscle, it originates from the lateral epicondyle of the humerus. The tendon of the lateral digital extensor inserts on the lateral digit (digit IV) in the same manner as the insertion of the medial (proper) tendon of the common digital extensor on the medial digit (digit III).

Origin: Lateral epicondyle of the humerus and lateral collateral ligament of the elbow.

Insertion: On P2 and P3 (in the ox) of the lateral digit (digit IV).

Action: Extends the carpus and the phalangeal joints of digit IV.

Note that the tendon of the **lateral digital extensor muscle** to the lateral (IV) digit and the **medial tendon of the common digital extensor muscle** to the medial (III) digit are wider in size than the extensor tendons that course to the interdigital space. They are known as the "**proper**" digital extensor tendons of digits IV and III, respectively (Figures 5.16 and 5.17).

5.3.2.2.5 Ulnaris Lateralis Muscle

The ulnaris lateralis muscle is the most caudal muscle of the craniolateral group (Figure 5.16). It inserts on the AC bone and on metacarpal IV and/or V by **short** and **long tendons**, respectively. The ulnaris lateralis muscle flexes carpal joints and extends the elbow joint.

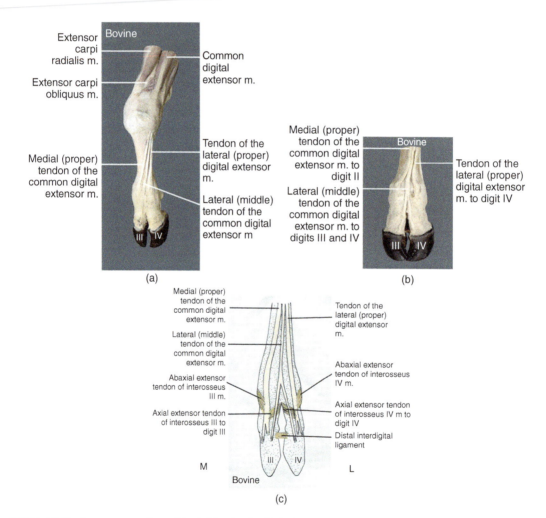

Figure 5.17 (a,b) Distal extensor tendons of the left bovine forelimb. Extensor tendons originate proximally from the common and lateral digital extensor muscles in the forearm region (a); (c) distal insertion of extensor tendons of the lateral and common digital extensor muscles, and axial and abaxial extensor branches of the interosseus III and IV muscles. Goat right forelimb: dorsal view. Source: Garrett P.D. (1988), Iowa State University Press.

Origin: Lateral epicondyle of the humerus.

Insertion: Accessory carpal bone (short tendon) and Mc IV and/or Mc V (long tendon).

Action: Flexes or extends the carpus depending on position and action of other muscles.

5.3.2.2.6 Extensor Carpi Obliquus Muscle

The belly of the extensor carpi obliquus muscle is located deep to the muscles of the craniolateral antebrachium group. It is known as the abductor pollicis longus or abductor digiti I longus in the dog. Its tendon of insertion courses obliquely over that of the extensor carpi radialis muscle to insert on the proximal medial surface of the large metacarpal bone (Figure 5.16).

Origin: Lateral distal half of the body of the radius deep to the common and lateral digital extensor muscles.

Insertion: Medial–proximal surface of large metacarpal bone (fused Mc III and Mc IV).

Action: Extends the carpus.

5.3.2.3 Caudomedial Muscle Group of the Antebrachium

Goal: Identify the flexors of the carpus and digits and know their general area of origins and insertions especially that of the distal digital flexor tendons (SDF and DDF).

To identify muscles in this group, turn the limb so the medial side is facing up (Figure 5.18). Clean the muscles and tendons by removing the overlying fascia and fat.

5.3.2.3.1 Flexor Carpi Ulnaris Muscle

The flexor carpi ulnaris muscle lies next (caudal) to the ulnaris lateralis muscle on the caudomedial side of

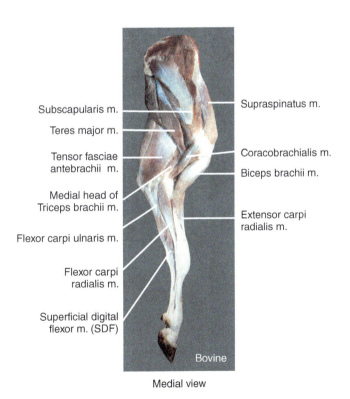

Figure 5.18 Bovine left forelimb. Caudomedial flexor muscles of the antebrachium and digits.

the antebrachium. It has a small **ulnar head** and a large **humeral head**. It is one of two muscles that insert on the **AC bone** (Figure 5.18). The other muscle is ulnaris lateralis previously discussed with extensors of the carpus. Identify the flexor carpi radialis and ulnaris lateral on a caudal view of the forelimb (Figure 5.19b).

The flexor carpi ulnaris flexes the carpus and extends the elbow.

Origin: Medial epicondyle of the humerus (humeral head) and olecranon (ulnar head).
Insertion: Accessory carpal bone.
Action: Flexes the carpus and extends the elbow.

5.3.2.3.2 Flexor Carpi Radialis Muscle

The flexor carpi radialis muscle has one belly and is located on the medial surface of the antebrachium directly caudal to the radius (Figure 5.19a). It originates

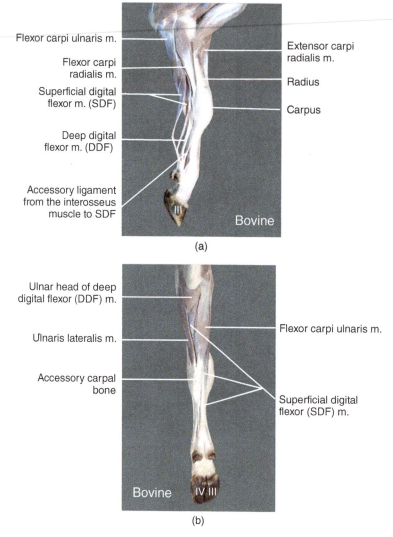

Figure 5.19 (a) Bovine left forelimb. Figure shows caudomedial flexor tendons of the distal forelimb. Tendons are separated apart to demonstrate the heads of the superficial digital flexor (SDF) and a band analogous to accessory (check) ligament coursing from the interosseus muscle to the SDF tendon. Proximally, the flexor retinaculum is incised and removed to open the carpal canal. (b) Bovine left forelimb: caudal view. The figure shows the caudal view of flexors of the carpus and digits. The flexor retinaculum is incised.

from the medial epicondyle and inserts on the lateral surface of the proximal end of the large metacarpal bone (fused Mc III and Mc IV). As you will see later, this muscle must be reflected to uncover the median artery and median nerve on the medial surface of the antebrachium region.

Note that there is no muscle covering the medial surface of the radius.

Origin: Medial epicondyle of the humerus.
Insertion: Proximomedial surface of large metacarpal bone (fused Mc III and Mc IV).
Action: Flexes the carpus.

5.3.2.3.3 Pronator Teres Muscle

In ruminants, the pronator teres muscle is a small vestigial entity of little significance (Figure 5.12b).

The muscle is fleshy in dogs and cats. There is no need to identify this muscle.

5.3.2.3.4 Superficial Digital Flexor with Superficial and Deep Parts: Flexor Manica

The SDF lies deep to the flexor carpi ulnaris muscle. It originates on the medial epicondyle of the humerus and inserts by split tendons on the palmar surface of phalanx 2 (P2) of digits III and IV.

The SDF has two bellies: **superficial** and **deep** (Figure 5.19). The tendon of the deep belly of SDF passes through the carpal canal deep to the deep layer of the flexor retinaculum while the tendon of the superficial belly of the SDF muscle passes between the superficial and deep layers of the flexor retinaculum.

The superficial and deep tendons of the SDF muscle join in the mid-metacarpal region to form a single tendon.

Above the fetlock joint, the SDF tendon receives a band from the interosseus muscle. This band is similar to the distal check ligament of the SDF in the horse except that this band connects two muscles (SDF and interosseus) instead of bone and muscle (radius and SDF) as is the case with the check ligament of the SDF in the horse. Additionally, this band is located in the metacarpus instead of the antebrachium where the check ligament of the SDF in the horse is located.

The SDF and the band from the interosseus help form the **flexor manica**, a sleeve for the passage of the DDF tendon to the palmar surface of P3.

The SDF muscle flexes the metacarpophalangeal (MCP–fetlock) and the proximal interphalangeal (PIP or pastern) joints.

Origin: Medial epicondyle of the humerus.
Insertion: Palmar surface of the middle phalanx (P2) of digits III and IV.
Action: Extends the elbow and flexes the carpal, fetlock, and pastern joints.

5.3.2.3.5 Deep Digital Flexor Muscle

In the metacarpal region, the tendon of the DDF lies cranial to that of the SDF tendon. The DDF muscle has three parts: **ulnar**, **radial**, and **humeral** heads.

Identify the tendons of the SDF and DDF muscles (Figure 5.19a). It is not necessary to identify the individual heads of the DDF muscle.

Proximal to the fetlock, each of the SDF and DDF tendons split into two tendons that pass to the lateral and medial digits (Figure 5.20).

Origin: Olecranon (ulnar head), proximal medial radius (radial head), and medial epicondyle of the humerus (humeral head).
Insertion: Flexor tubercle of the distal phalanx (P3) of digits III and IV.
Action: Extends the elbow and flexes the carpal, fetlock, pastern, and coffin joints.

5.3.2.3.6 Interosseus Muscle (Suspensory Ligament) with Axial and Abaxial Extensor Branches

The interosseus muscle (suspensory ligament) in ruminants is **fused interosseus III and IV** muscles (Figures 5.20, 5.21, and 5.22). It is located on the palmar side of the large metacarpal bone (fused Mc III and Mc IV) deep to the DDF tendon.

The horse has a single interosseus III muscle (suspensory ligament). The suspensory ligament is very tendinous in horse compared with relatively fleshy muscles in ruminants.

In the distal palmar metacarpal region, the fused interosseus muscle in ruminants gives a band that joins the SDF (discussed previously with SDF) and splits into five branches. Four of the five branches insert on the four axial and abaxial proximal sesamoid bones at the level of the fetlock joints (Figure 5.7). The fifth tendon courses in the interdigital space between the axial sesamoids and gives two axial extensor branches that join the "proper" extensor

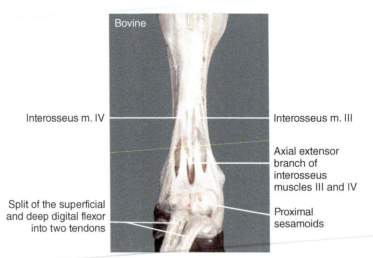

Figure 5.20 Left bovine limb: palmar view. The figure shows distal tendons of the interosseus III and IV muscles, and bifurcation of the flexor tendons (SDF and DDF) to insert on each digit. Note the attachments of four of the interosseous branches to proximal axial and abaxial sesamoid bones.

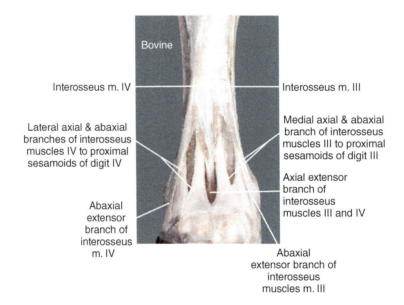

Figure 5.21 Left bovine distal metacarpal region: close-up palmar view. The SDF and DDF flexor tendons are reflected down.

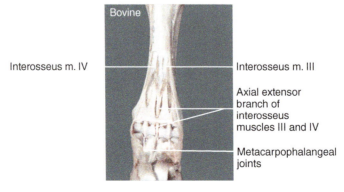

Figure 5.22 Bovine fetlock joints (left limb): palmar view. The figure shows left and right metacarpophalangeal (fetlock) joints (opened). Note the axial extensor branch from the fused interosseus muscle coursing distally between the medial and lateral distal condyles of the large metacarpal bone.

branches of the lateral and common digital extensor muscles on digits III and IV (Figures 5.17c, 5.20, 5.21, and 5.22).

The lateral and medial abaxial branches of the interosseus muscle that insert on the abaxial proximal sesamoids give rise to abaxial extensor branches that also join the "proper" digital extensor tendons on digits IV and III, respectively (Figure 5.17c). You should recall that the proper digital extensor tendons are furnished by distal continuations of the lateral digital extensor tendon and the medial tendon of the common digital extensor muscle.

Origin: Distal row of carpal bones and palmar carpal ligament.

Insertion: Proximal sesamoids bones and by continuation join the proper digital extensor tendons by axial and abaxial extensor branches.

Action: Prevents overextension of the fetlock joints produced by pressure from the weight of the animal. The interosseus muscle opposes the flexor tension of the DDF tendon on the pastern and coffin joints.

5.4 Retinacula

Goal: Know the definition of a retinaculum (a flat sheet of connective tissue that holds tendons in place over bony prominences), and give examples (e.g., extensor or flexor retinaculum).

A retinaculum is a band of flat connective tissue that wraps around and binds down muscle tendons.

In the forelimb, identify the **transverse humeral retinaculum** over the tendon of origin of biceps brachii (Figure 5.15) and the **extensor retinaculum** on the dorsum of the carpus (Figure 5.16). The carpal extensor retinaculum holds down the tendons of the extensors of the carpus and digits. A subcutaneous bursa may sometimes develop in this region. When enlarged, it is known as **carpal hygroma**. This condition results from poor management and lack of bedding.

A **flexor retinaculum** is located on the caudal aspect of the carpus. It defines the caudal boundary of the **carpal canal**. It extends from the AC bone medially, and fans over the SDF and DDF and flexor carpi radialis flexor tendons to insert on the medial surface of the carpus.

5.5 Carpal Canal

Goal: Identify the dorsal, caudal, and lateral boundaries of the carpal canal, and give examples of tendons, blood vessels, and nerves that pass through it.

The carpal canal is the space behind the carpal bones and medial to the AC bone. Flexor tendons, blood vessels, and nerves pass from proximal to distal through the carpal canal (from the medial side of the antebrachium region to the palmar side of the metacarpal region).

The thick **palmar carpal ligament** lies directly on the palmar surface of carpal bones. The palmar carpal ligament is part of the carpal fibrous joint capsule that forms the dorsal boundary for the carpal canal. Other boundaries of the carpal canal include the AC bone laterally, and the flexor retinaculum caudally. The **flexor retinaculum** has superficial and deep layers.

Vessels and flexor tendons passing through the carpal canal include the median nerve, median artery, median vein, the flexor tendons of the SDF and DDF muscle tendons, and tendon of the flexor carpi radialis muscle. The tendon of the superficial belly of the SDF passes deep to the superficial layer of the flexor retinaculum.

Identify the boundaries for the carpal canal on a cow or goat skeleton.

5.6 Ligaments of the Digits

Goal: Identify the interdigital ligaments (especially the distal interdigital ligament), annular ligaments (palmar annular ligament and proximal and distal digital annular ligaments).

There are several ligaments associated with the SDF and DDF tendons on the palmar surface of the fetlock and below. They have more clinical significance in the athletic horse than in docile ruminants. Therefore, many of these ligaments will be studied in more detail in the horse.

Ligaments unique to ruminants are the proximal and distal interdigital ligaments that prevent the lateral and medial digits from splaying (spreading apart) when they bear weight. The following discussion is an overview of the ligaments on the palmar surface of the digits. Ask your instructor which ligaments you need to identify.

5.6.1 Proximal Interdigital Ligament

This ligament courses horizontally between the proximal phalanges (P1) of digits III and IV. The proximal interdigital ligament is present in cattle and goats but is absent in sheep. Do not look for this ligament as it is difficult to identify. We recommend identifying only the **distal interdigital ligament**.

5.6.2 Distal Interdigital Ligament

This ligament courses horizontally between the proximal parts of the middle phalanges (P2) and the distal sesamoids of the opposite digits (Figure 5.23).

Identify the distal interdigital ligaments in the ox or goat. The interdigital ligaments are more developed in cattle than goats.

5.6.3 Annular Ligaments (Palmar, Proximal, and Distal Digital Annular Ligaments)

Several annular ligaments support each digit. Follow the bifurcation of the SDF and DDF tendons to digits III and IV (Figure 5.20). Identify the **palmar annular ligament** at the palmar surface of the fetlock joint. It wraps around both the SDF and DDF tendons of each digit at the level of the proximal sesamoids.

5.6.4 Digital Annular Ligaments (Proximal and Distal)

Move your probe distal to the palmar annular ligament and identify the **proximal** and **distal digital annular ligaments** on each digit. The digital annular ligaments are attached to the proximal and middle parts of the proximal phalanx (P1) on each digit.

Select one digit, transect all of the annular ligaments, and reflect the SDF and DDF tendons from the channel on the palmar side of this digit. Identify the

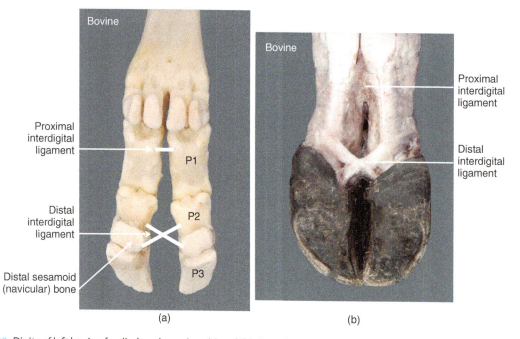

Figure 5.23 Digits of left bovine forelimb: palmar view. (a) and (b) show the proximal and distal interdigital ligaments. The proximal interdigital ligament connects the proximal parts of the proximal phalanges (P1) of digits III and IV in cattle and goats (absent in sheep). It is difficult to identify (no need to dissect it). Note that the distal interdigital ligament forms a cross (X) in the distal part of the interdigital space. Each limb of the cross courses between the distal part of the middle phalanx (P2) and the distal sesamoid (navicular bone) of the opposite digit. In sheep, the distal interdigital ligament connects the two digits transversely.

flexor manica, a sleeve from the SDF that wraps around the DDF tendon and allows for the passage of DDF tendon to its insertion on the distal phalanx (P3) (Figure 5.19a).

5.7 Hoof (Wall, Sole, Bulb, and White Line)

With the help of Figure 5.24, identify the hoof wall, sole, heel bulbs, and white line on your specimen or on a dry hoof.

The hood (or claw) structure is more clinically important in horses and so most of the details are discussed in the horse.

The hoof wall carries most of the weight of the animal. The white line is defined as the junction between the wall and the sole.

The hoof of the lateral digit (digit IV) is larger and carries more weight than the medial (digit III) hoof. This situation is reversed on the hind limb.

5.8 Arteries and Nerves of the Thoracic Limb

Goal: You should be able to identify the main arterial channels on the medial and palmar sides of the limb (axillary, brachial, and median arteries).

You should be able to use the correct nomenclature when describing the distribution and branching of the median artery and median nerve on the palmar surface, especially those nerves and vessels that course into the interdigital area. At the end of this unit, watch **Video 22. Consult Box 5.7 for clinical application.**

Box 5.7

Knowledge of blood vessels in the distal limbs of ruminants is clinically important. Intravenous regional local anesthesia (known as retrograde anesthesia or Bier block) is performed in cattle using veins in the distal limbs. Unlike in horses, extensive nerve blocks are not usually performed in ruminants (Box 5.8). Distal limb veins are also used to inject antibiotics for the treatment of hoof diseases. Typically, a tourniquet is used to compress veins so that the anesthetic or antibiotic will diffuse out to cause a localized effect. Examples of veins in the distal fore limb available for antibiotic injections or retrograde anesthesia include the dorsal common digital vein III that feeds into the accessory cephalic vein proximally.

The palmar common digital artery III represents a large source of blood coursing distally in the interdigital space. Ligation of this artery may be necessary when performing a digital amputation.

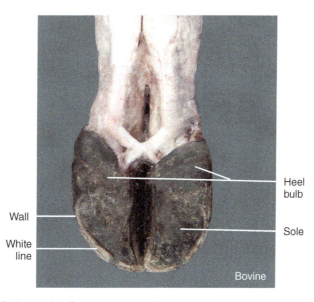

Figure 5.24 Ground surface of the bovine hoofs: palmar view. Left bovine forelimb.

5.8.1 Nomenclature of Blood Vessels and Nerves in the Distal Limb

The nomenclature of blood vessels and nerves in the distal limb needs to be understood. It is important to master some terminology such as dorsal versus palmar in the front limb, and dorsal versus plantar in the hind limb. In both limbs, you need to master the terms axial versus abaxial and common digital versus proper digital when describing the arteries, veins, and nerves of the region. Vessels and nerves lying superficially in the metacarpal region are called dorsal common digital when present on the dorsal surface, and palmar common digital when located on the palmar side of the metacarpal region.

Identify the large proximal arterial channels (axillary, subscapular, brachial, and median arteries) (Figure 5.27). The main blood supply to the distal forelimb is derived from the **median artery** that passes distally through the carpal canal in close association with the median nerve. The **palmar common digital artery III** is the largest of the distal branches of the median artery to the foot. The palmar common digital artery III enters the interdigital space between the dewclaws to provide the **axial palmar proper digital arteries to digits III and IV** (Figure 5.28). *The abaxial palmar proper digital arteries III and IV* are small and should be ignored. Dorsal common (superficial) and dorsal and palmar metacarpal (deep) arteries are also minor vessels that run on the dorsal and palmar sides of the large metacarpal bone. The deep metacarpal vessels run on the dorsal and palmar longitudinal grooves and form connections (perforating branches) between the dorsal and palmar metacarpal vessels through the proximal and distal metacarpal canals (review bones). Do not look for the dorsal common or the metacarpal vessels. Identify arteries in **red** on an embalmed cow forelimb.

Axial proper digital vessels and nerves run in the interdigital space close to the axis of the limb that runs between digits III and IV. Abaxial vessels and nerves run on the lateral sides of each digit away from the centrally located axis.

From proximal to distal, the principal arteries (main channels) of the forelimb are the **axillary, brachial,**

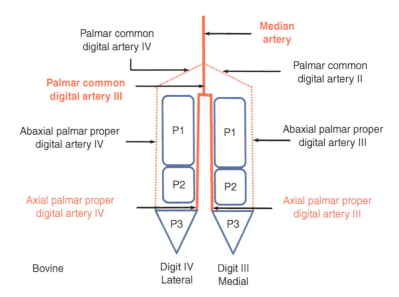

Figure 5.25 Schematic illustration for naming the branches of the **median artery** in the distal forelimb of ruminants (goat and cattle): palmar view. Identify the branches of the palmar common digital artery III in red. The remaining arteries (shown by dotted lines) are minor in size and difficult to dissect.

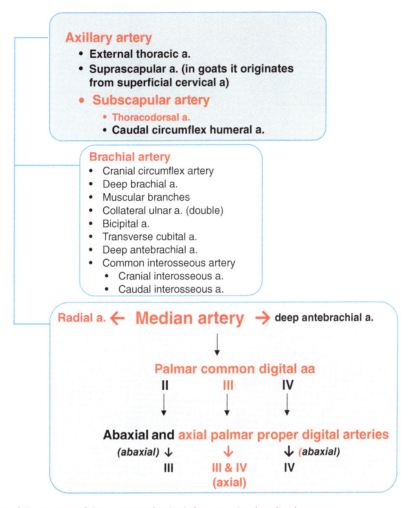

Figure 5.26 Overview of the arteries of the ruminant forelimb from proximal to distal.

median, and **palmar common digital artery III** (Figures 5.25, 5.26, and 5.27). Identify the main arterial channels in the proximal limb but focus on mastering the blood supply to the digits (clinically more important).

Locate the **median artery** in the mid-metacarpal region where it lies medial to the SDF tendon. Follow the artery distally in company with the **median nerve**. In the distal metacarpus, the median artery divides into several branches, of which the **palmar common digital artery III** is the largest (Figures 5.25 and 5.28). The palmar common digital artery III enters into the interdigital space, giving rise to the **axial palmar proper digital arteries III and IV** to the medial and lateral digits (Figure 5.28).

5.9 Veins of the Forelimb

Goal: Identify the clinically important superficial veins (cephalic and accessory cephalic) and their tributaries on the dorsal and palmar sides of the metacarpal and digital regions, especially the dorsal common digital vein III that feeds proximally into the accessory cephalic vein.

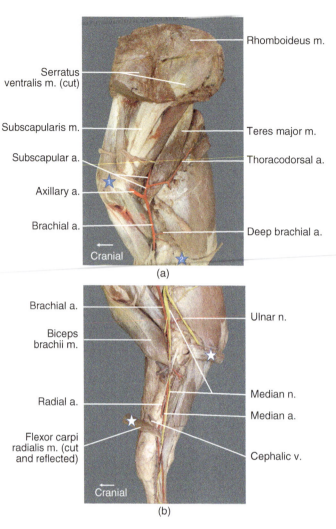

Figure 5.27 (a) Arteries of the brachium region. The figure shows the right bovine forelimb: medial view. Identify the main channels (axillary, brachial, and subscapular arteries). 1 and 2, location of shoulder and elbow joints, respectively. (b) Arteries of the antebrachium region. In the antebrachium, the brachial artery becomes the median artery. Study the distal branches of the median artery to the claws (Figure 5.28). * Flexor carpi radialis muscle transected in the middle and reflected to uncover the median artery and nerve.

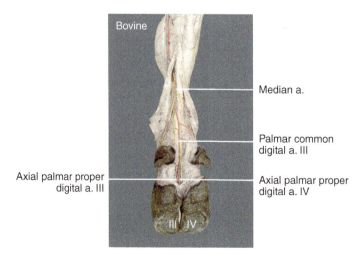

Figure 5.28 Distal branches of the median arteries and nerves to the foot. The figure shows the right bovine forelimb: palmar view. Note that the **palmar common digital III** entering the interdigital space and courses distally between the dewclaws to give axial branches (**axial palmar proper digital arteries III and IV**) to digits III and IV. There is no need to identify the small arteries to the abaxial sides of the digits.

> **Box 5.8**
>
> Conditions involving the distal foot are more commonly addressed in ruminants. The superficial veins are used for regional limb perfusion (retrograde anesthesia) of the distal limb. Injection of anesthetic in distal superficial veins in cattle is used as an alternative to the nerve block widely used in horses. It is also used for antibiotic injections for the treatment of foot infections (foot rot).
>
> A tourniquet is usually applied to either the accessory cephalic vein or, most commonly, to the **dorsal common digital vein III**. This procedure is preferable for systemic injections because it produces the maximum blood concentration of the drug in the target tissue.
>
> In surgical anesthesia, the nerve targets include dorsal (from the radial nerve) and palmar (from the median nerve) sensory nerves of the foot.

Large satellite veins (axillary, brachial, and median) follow the similarly named arteries. Some of these veins may be present as duplicate vessels (e.g., brachial and median veins). There is no need to spend time identifying deeply located satellite veins.

The superficial veins are more clinically important. Identify the **cephalic** and **accessory cephalic veins**. In the distal limb, the **dorsal common digital vein** III feeds into the accessory cephalic vein proximally. See Box 5.8 for clinical applications of the dorsal common digital vein III.

The accessory cephalic vein joins the cephalic in the distal antebrachium region. Identify the **median cubital vein** that connects the cephalic and brachial veins.

5.10 Lymphatics of the Thoracic Limb

Goal: Identify the axillary lymph nodes and know what part of the limb they drain. The axillary lymph nodes are the major lymphocenter of the thoracic limb. Identify the **axillary lymph nodes** at the medial aspect of the limb close to the shoulder joint (axilla). The axillary lymph nodes drain into the caudal deep cervical lymph nodes at the ventral end of the first rib. Next, lymph from the caudal deep cervical lymph nodes enters the major veins at the thoracic inlet.

5.11 Nerves of the Thoracic Limb

Goal: Identify the major nerves of the brachial plexus on the medial side of the shoulder and brachium regions. You should place more emphasis on understanding the distribution of the nerves to the distal part of the limb and digits. This includes the superficial branch of the **radial nerve** and the dorsal branch of the **ulnar nerve** that course on the dorsal surface of the large metacarpal bone and digits, and the **median nerve** and the palmar branch of the ulnar nerve that course on the palmar surface of the large metacarpal bone and digits. It is not necessary to identify the dorsal and palmar branches of the ulnar nerves in lab but understand their roles. For the radial and median nerves, you should focus on a relatively large nerve branch from each coursing on the dorsal and palmar metacarpal regions and interdigital spaces, respectively. These nerves are the dorsal common digital nerve III from the radial nerve, and the palmar common digital nerve III from the median nerve.

The brachial plexus (C6–T2) provides motor innervation to the intrinsic and extrinsic muscles of the thoracic limb as well as sensory innervation to the skin and joints (Figure 5.29).

Specific nerve blocks are not widely used in cattle as is the case in equine practice. The nerves in the proximal limb are similar to those of other species (horse and dog). Ask your instructor which nerves of the brachial plexus in the proximal limb you need to identify.

Nerves that supply the extrinsic muscles include *cranial pectoral nerves* (to superficial pectoral muscles), *caudal pectoral* nerves (deep or ascending pectoral muscle), *thoracodorsal nerve* (latissimus dorsi), *lateral thoracic nerve* (cutaneus trunci and cutaneus omobrachialis), and *long thoracic nerve* (serratus ventralis thoracis). Do not look for these nerves on your specimen as some of them may be torn with the removal of extrinsic muscles.

With the help of Figure 5.29a, identify the following nerves of the brachial plexus that innervate intrinsic muscles of the forelimb.

5.11.1 Suprascapular Nerve

The suprascapular nerve innervates the supra- and infraspinatus muscles. Look for the nerve on the medial side of the limb. The nerve passes laterally

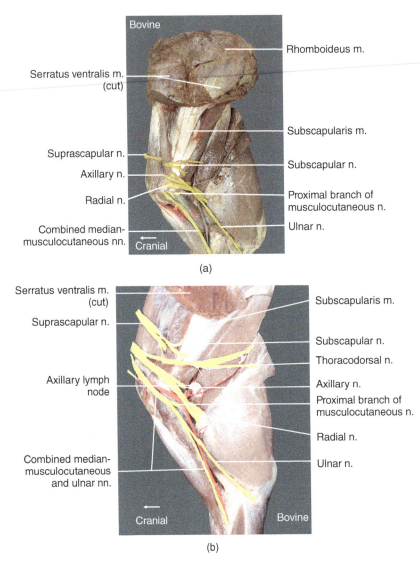

Figure 5.29 (a) Nerves of the brachial plexus (bovine). The figure shows the right shoulder and brachial regions: medial view. (b) Nerves of the brachial plexus (goat). The figure shows the right shoulder and brachial regions: medial view.

> **Box 5.9**
>
> Suprascapular nerve damage is more common in horses. The condition is known as "sweeny." Damage could be caused by physical trauma if a horse hits a metal post (jumper horses) or is kicked by other horses. Lack of an acromion in the scapula of the horse is thought to contribute to increased susceptibility but no direct evidence is present to support this claim.
>
> Atrophy of the supra- and infraspinatus muscles can occur in chronic cases of nerve damage.

between the subscapularis and supraspinatus muscles (Figure 5.29). See Box 5.9 for the clinical relevance of the suprascapular nerve.

The suprascapular nerve can be demonstrated on the lateral side of the shoulder joint by carefully scraping the distal part of the supraspinatus muscle from around the neck of the scapula and distal part of the acromion. Notice the branches to the supra- and infraspinatus muscles.

5.11.2 Subscapular Nerve

The subscapular nerve innervates the subscapularis muscle. Find the subscapular nerve diving into the subscapularis muscle on the medial side of the limb (Figures 5.29). More than one nerve could be present. No clinical significance is associated with damage to this nerve.

5.11.3 Axillary Nerve

The axillary nerve innervates the deltoideus, teres major, and teres minor muscles, and the skin on craniolateral brachium (*cranial cutaneous brachial nerve branch of the axillary*) and proximal antebrachium region (*cranial cutaneous antebrachial nerve branch of the axillary*). Look for the main stump of the axillary nerve directly behind the shoulder joint. Here, the nerve gives muscular branches to the teres major muscle and caudal part of the subscapularis muscle (Figures 5.29).

The axillary nerve passes laterally to supply the deltoideus and teres minor muscles where muscular breaches can be identified under the deltoideus coursing with the caudal circumflex humeral artery. There is no need to trace these branches or the cutaneous branches of the axillary nerve.

The muscles innervated by the axillary nerve can be memorized by the acronym "**DTT**" which stands for **d**eltoideus, **t**eres major, and **t**eres minor muscles.

5.11.4 Musculocutaneous Nerve

The **musculocutaneous** and **median nerves** are fused in ruminants as is the case in the horse. In goats, three nerves (musculocutaneous, median, and ulnar) may join in the proximal brachium region. Look for the combined trunk of the musculocutaneous, median, and ulnar nerves on the medial side of the proximal brachium region (Figure 5.29b).

At the medial shoulder region, note that the **median** and **musculocutaneous nerves** form a loop (**ansa axillaris**) around the axillary artery. The *ansa axillaris* may not be present on your specimen.

The musculocutaneous nerve remains fused to the median nerve as it courses along the cranial–medial aspect of the brachium cranial to the brachial artery. It gives a **proximal muscular branch** to the coracobrachialis and biceps brachii muscles close to the shoulder region (Figure 5.29). Proximal to the elbow, it gives a **distal muscular branch** to the brachialis muscle. Beyond the distal muscular branch, the musculocutaneous separates from the median nerve and continues as the *medial cutaneous antebrachial nerve*. There is no need to identify the *medial cutaneous antebrachial nerve.*

The muscles innervated by the musculocutaneous nerve can be memorized by the acronym "**BBC**" which stands for **b**iceps brachii, **b**rachialis, and **c**oracobrachialis muscles.

5.11.5 Radial Nerve

The radial nerve is the largest nerve of the brachial plexus. It innervates several muscles, including extensors of the elbow, carpus, and digits. It also provides sensory branches to the skin on the dorsum of the large metacarpal bone and to the structures on the dorsal surface of the front digits. It has **deep (muscular)** and **superficial (sensory) branches.**

Identify the radial nerve on medial, lateral, and dorsal sides of the limb.

On the lateral side of the distal brachium and deep to the lateral head of the triceps brachii, the radial nerve divides into **deep** and **superficial branches** (Figures 5.30 and 5.31). The deep branch supplies muscular branches to the extensor muscles of the carpus and digits.

The **superficial branch of the radial nerve** gives the **dorsal common digital nerves II and III** that run on the dorsum of the large metacarpal bone. Identify the **dorsal common nerve III** which is relatively large and courses to the interdigital space to give **axial dorsal proper digital nerves III and IV** (Figures 5.30 and 5.32b).

The dorsal common digital nerves II and IV are very small nerves that need not be dissected. Understand that the dorsal common digital nerves II courses to the abaxial side of the medial digit (digit III) to form the *abaxial dorsal proper digital nerve III*. On the other hand, the dorsal common digital nerve IV and the *abaxial dorsal proper digital nerve IV* are the continuation of the dorsal branch of the ulnar nerve (do not look for them).

5.11.5.1 Branching of the Radial and Ulnar Nerves in the Distal Limb

Reflect the lateral head of the triceps and identify the muscular branches to the triceps and the deep branch to the extensors of the carpus and digits and the superficial branch of the radial nerve on the dorsal aspect of the metacarpal region. The superficial branch of the radial nerve courses distally with the accessory cephalic vein. It gives dorsal common digital nerves II and III of which the dorsal common digital nerve III is the largest. The dorsal common digital nerve IV is from the dorsal branch of the ulnar nerve. With the help of Figure 5.32, identify the **superficial branch of the radial nerve,** *the* **dorsal common digital nerve III,** *and its* **dorsal axial proper digital nerves III and IV.** *The superficial branch of the radial nerve is located medial to the medial tendon of the common digital extensor muscle. Identify nerves in bold font in Figure 5.30.*

5.11.6 Median and Ulnar Nerves

The median, ulnar, and musculocutaneous nerves are fused on the proximal medial side of the brachium in goats (Figure 5.29b).

The **median** and **ulnar nerves** share innervation of several carpal and digital flexor muscles in the proximal region of the antebrachium (Figure 5.33).

In the metacarpal region, the median nerve divides into **medial** and **lateral branches** (this pattern could be variable) (Figure 5.34). The **medial branch of the median nerve** gives rise to **palmar common digital nerves III and II** that course to the medial digit as **axial palmar proper digital nerve III** (in the interdigital space) and **abaxial palmar proper digital nerve III,** respectively (Figure 5.34).

The **lateral branch of the median nerve** gives rise to the **axial palmar proper digital nerve IV** that courses to the lateral digit (in the interdigital space) (Figure 5.34). It also communicates with the palmar branch of the ulnar nerve to give rise to the **abaxial palmar digital nerve IV** to the abaxial side of the lateral digit (digit IV).

Identify the **palmar common digital nerves,** especially the **palmar common digital nerve III** and its **axial palmar proper digital nerves III and IV** branches in the interdigital space (Figure 5.34).

There is no need to dissect the palmar and dorsal branches of the ulnar nerve.

Note that the nomenclature for the branches of the median nerve and median artery to the digits are identical and all you need to do is replace the word "artery" with word "nerve" and vice versa (compare Figure 5.35 with Figure 5.28).

5.12 Joints of the Forelimbs

Goal: Know the bones that control each joint articulation, starting proximally from the shoulder joint working your way down to the digital joints.

Study the forelimb joint articulations on cow or goat skeleton. From proximal to distal, the forelimb joints include the shoulder, elbow, carpal, metacarpophalangeal (fetlock), proximal interphalangeal (pastern), and distal interphalangeal (coffin) joints.

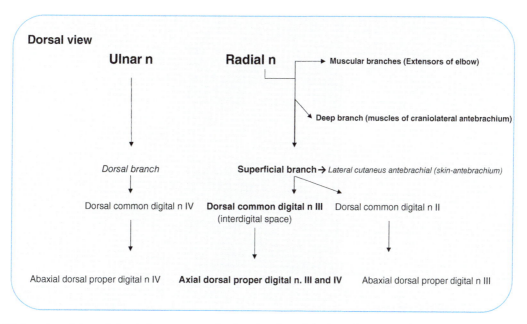

Figure 5.30 Branches of the radial and ulnar nerves to the dorsal surface of the front digits. Identify the branches of the radial nerve to the dorsal foot (Figure 5.32). In the brachial region, the ulnar nerve gives rise to a cutaneous branch, the caudal cutaneous antebrachial nerve, before it gives muscular branches to the flexor muscles of the carpus and digits (not depicted). The ulnar nerve contributes to the innervation of the dorsal and palmar sides of the lateral digit (digit IV) by the dorsal and palmar branches, respectively. The palmar and dorsal branches are depicted in Figure 5.35.

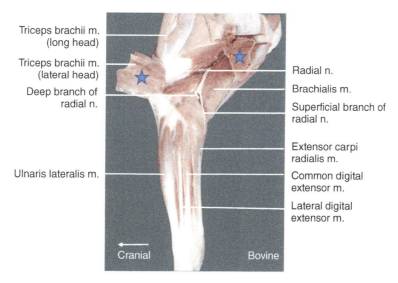

Figure 5.31 Superficial and deep branches of the radial nerve, right caprine forelimb: lateral view. * The lateral head of the triceps brachii muscle is transected in the middle and both ends are reflected to uncover the radial nerve and its deep and superficial branches.

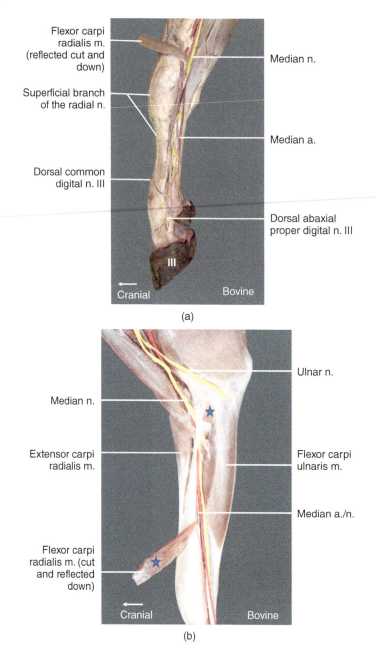

Figure 5.32 (a) The right bovine forelimb showing the course of the superficial branch of the radial nerve and median nerve: dorsomedial view. Note the superficial branch of the radial nerve coursing distally on the dorsal surface of the large metacarpal bone. It gives the dorsal common digital nerves II and III (not visible). Identify the dorsal common digital nerve III coursing to the interdigital space in Figure 5.33. (b) The right bovine forelimb: dorsal view. The dorsal common digital nerve III arises from the superficial branch of the radial nerve proximally. The radial nerve passes distally to give the large **dorsal common digital nerve III** and a small dorsal common digital nerve II to lateral digit (not shown). In the interdigital space, the dorsal common digital nerve III divides into **axial dorsal proper digital nerves III and IV**. The **dorsal common digital vein III** seen on the image feeds into accessory cephalic vein proximally.

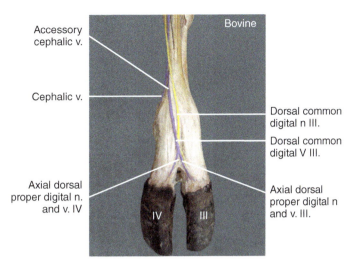

Figure 5.33 The right caprine forelimb showing the courses of the median and ulnar nerves in the distal brachium and antebrachium regions: medial view. The course of the median nerve and artery in the antebrachium region lies under (deep) to the flexor carpi radialis muscle (cut and reflected). In the antebrachium, the ulnar nerve courses distally between the flexor carpi ulnaris muscle medially, and ulnaris lateral muscle laterally. Both muscles attach to the accessory carpal bone.

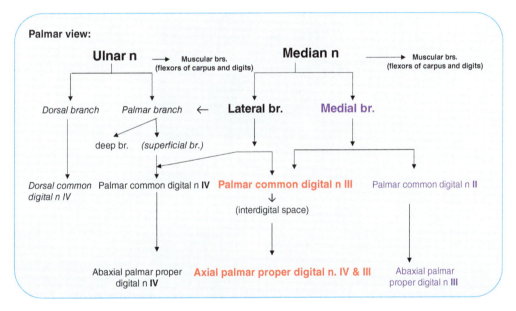

Figure 5.34 The bovine right forelimb: palmar view. Distribution of the median and ulnar nerves and the median artery in the distal foot. The branches of the median nerve and artery have the same nomenclature. Note that the median nerve divides into **medial** and **lateral branches** that course distally to innervate the digits. The medial branch gives the **axial** palmar proper digital nerve III and *abaxial palmar proper digital nerve III* (continuation of palmar common digital nerve II) to the medial digit. The lateral branch of the median nerve gives the **axial** palmar proper digital nerve IV to the lateral digit. The *abaxial palmar proper digital nerve IV* to the lateral digit is the continuation of the *palmar common digital nerve IV* formed by the union of branches from the lateral branch of the median nerve and the *palmar branch of the ulnar nerve*. Generally, the branches of the median nerves above the fetlock are called palmar common digital nerves II, III, and IV. Understand that the branching pattern can vary between specimens. Consult Box 5.10 on nerve blocks.

> **Box 5.10**
>
> Although nerve block is not widely practiced in cattle, it can be used in conditions affecting the distal limb. For complete anesthesia of the foot, three nerves should be blocked: the radial nerve (on the dorsal aspect of the limb, medial to the medial tendon of the common digital extensor muscle); branches of median nerve (on the palmar aspect of the limb, proximal to the dewclaws); and the ulnar nerve (to the lateral digit [digit IV] on both dorsal and palmar aspects). The ulnar nerve can also be blocked in the groove between the flexor carpi ulnaris and ulnaris lateralis muscles.

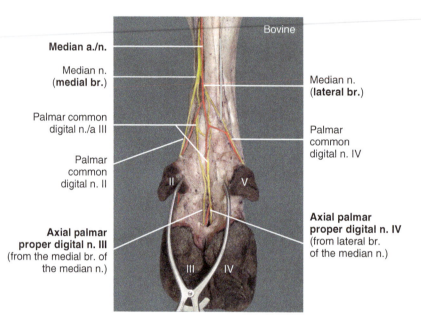

Figure 5.35 Overview of the nerves on the palmar distal forelimb of ruminants.

Joint injections are practiced widely in horses but less so in cattle. There follows a brief overview of the joints of the forelimb. Review the bones for each joint.

5.12.1 Shoulder Joint

The shoulder joint is formed by the articulation of the glenoid cavity of the scapula with the head of the humerus (Figure 5.1). The tendons of the supraspinatus, infraspinatus, subscapularis, and coracobrachialis muscles stabilize the shoulder joint by acting as collateral ligaments.

Identify the nerves in blue font. The **median nerve** gives muscular branches to the flexors of the carpus and digits in the proximal antebrachium. Distally, it passes through the carpal canal in the company of the median artery. In the mid-metacarpal region, the median nerve gives **medial** and **lateral branches** (variations may occur). The medial and lateral branches of the median nerve and the palmar branch of the ulnar nerve divide variably into **palmar common digital nerves II, III, and IV**. Typically, the **medial branch of the median nerve** gives the **axial palmar proper digital nerve III** and *abaxial palmar proper digital nerve III* to the medial digit. The lateral branch of the median nerve gives **axial palmar proper digital nerve IV** to the lateral digit. The *abaxial palmar proper digital nerve IV* to the lateral digit is formed by branches from the lateral branch of the median nerve and branches from the palmar branch of the ulnar nerve. Identify the median nerve, palmar common digital nerve III, and axial palmar proper digital nerves III and IV from the medial and lateral branches of the median nerve (Figure 5.34).

The shoulder joint capsule can be injected cranial to the tendon of the infraspinatus muscle.

5.12.2 Elbow Joint

The elbow joint is formed by articulation of several bones including the humeral condyle, proximally, the trochlear notch of the ulna and radial head, distally (Figure 5.1).

The joint is stabilized mainly by medial and lateral collateral ligaments of the elbow. The medial and lateral collateral ligaments originate from the medial and lateral epicondyles of the humerus and insert on the proximal medial and lateral borders of the radius, respectively.

5.12.3 Carpal Joints

Three joint capsules form the carpal joints (Figure 5.5a): radiocarpal or antebrachiocarpal joint (between the distal radius and the proximal row of carpal bones); midcarpal joint (between the proximal and distal rows of carpal bones); and carpometacarpal joint (between the distal row of carpal bones and fused metacarpals III and IV).

The radiocarpal and midcarpal joints do not communicate and require separate injections but the midcarpal and carpometacarpal communicate with each other.

Injections of carpal joints are best carried out on a standing animal with the carpal joints flexed.

5.12.4 Digital Joints

The digital joints include duplicate metacarpophalangeal (MCPfetlock), proximal interphalangeal (PIPpastern), and distal interphalangeal (DIPcoffin) joints (Figure 5.36a). Each of these joints is stabilized by medial and lateral collateral ligaments. Consult Box 5.11 on clinical related to joint diseases.

The metacarpophalangeal joints for digits III and IV communicate with each other but the rest of the interphalangeal joints remain as separate joint capsules.

An **interdigital fat pad** is present between the medial and lateral digits (Figure 5.36b). The interdigital fat pad can become infected under conditions involving the interdigital space such as foot rot or interdigital hyperplasia.

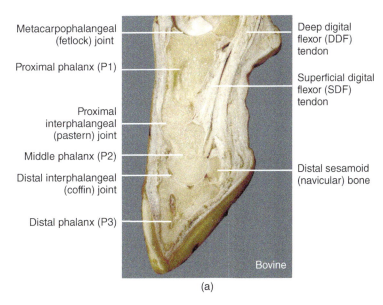

(a)

Figure 5.36 (a) Sagittal section of the bovine forelimb digits showing the digital joints and flexor tendons; (b) sagittal section of the bovine forelimb digits showing the interdigital fat pad.

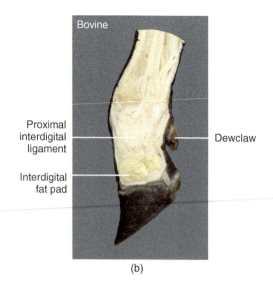

(b)

Figure 5.36 *(Continued)*

Box 5.11

Noninfectious joint diseases are common in cattle. They could be due to trauma and dietary factors. Signs include joint effusion and variable degrees of lameness. Diagnosis involves the use of one or more of several techniques that include cytology (arthrocentesis), use of radiography, ultrasonography, or computed tomography (CT). Infectious joint disease (septic joint) could result from a wide range of bacterial infections. Viruses can also infect joints, such as the arthritis of goats (big knee) is caused by caprine arthritis and encephalitis virus.

6

The Hind Limb

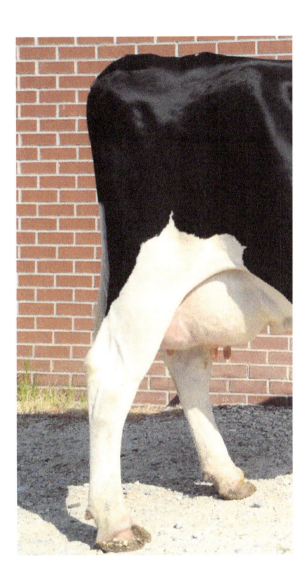

Guide to Ruminant Anatomy: Dissection and Clinical Aspects, Second Edition. Mahmoud Mansour, Ray Wilhite, Joe Rowe, and Saly Hafiz.
© 2023 John Wiley & Sons, Inc. Published 2023 by John Wiley & Sons, Inc.
Companion website: www.wiley.com/go/mansour/dissection2

Learning Objectives

- Identify the major bones of the hind limb, paying special attention to palpable features.
- Identify the major muscles, tendons, bursae (trochanteric and bicipital bursa), and tendon sheath of the superficial and deep digital flexor muscles.
- Identify and know the functions of the major nerves of the hind limb, including the femoral nerve, obturator nerve, and sciatic nerve and its major branches, tibial and common fibular (peroneal) nerves.
- Describe the clinical picture associated with damage to the common fibular, tibial, and obturator nerves.
- Know the nomenclature for the terminal branches of the common peroneal and tibial nerves on the dorsal and plantar sides of the hind limb, respectively.
- Identify the major blood supply to the foot. The dorsal metatarsal artery III carries blood to the dorsal aspect of the foot, and the plantar common digital artery III off the saphenous artery to the plantar aspect of the foot. Know the terminology for the terminal digital arteries.
- Identify and recognize the clinical importance of the superficial veins, especially the branches of the lateral saphenous vein. Superficial veins on the distal limb are used in retrograde anesthesia and for injection of antibiotics for treatment of foot infections.
- Know some of the diseases associated with damage to the hoof and its contents and structures involved (similar to those of the forelimb).
- At the end of the hind limb section, watch Video 23 Parts 1 and 2.

6.1 Bones of the Hind Limb

Goal: Study the bones of the ruminant hind limb and their palpable features. Compare and contrast with the hind limb bones of the horse.

Study the hind limb bones using a caprine or bovine skeleton (Figure 6.1). From proximal to distal, the bones of the hind limb include the os coxae (hip region), femur (thigh region), tibia and fibula (crus), tarsal bones (hock or tarsal region), fused III and IV metatarsals (cannon or large metatarsal bone) forming the (metatarsal region), and digits (each weight-bearing digit is supported by three phalanges: proximal, middle, and distal).

The term **pes** is used for the bones of the hock, metatarsals, and digits.

The bones of the metatarsal and digital regions are similar in shape to those of the front foot.

6.1.1 Os Coxae (Hip Bone)

Using Figure 6.2, take time to quickly review the bones of the os coxae and compare them with the hip bone in the horse. The bones of the os coxae are discussed in more detail in Chapter 4.

6.1.2 Femur (Thighbone)

Compare the femur in ruminants with that of the horse and note some of the major differences. The femur is the bone of the thigh region. The head of the femur articulates with the acetabulum (socket) to form the **hip joint**. Distally, the femoral condyles articulate with the tibial condyles to form the **stifle joint**.

Note the slanted or oblique orientation of the femur on the skeleton. This helps you build a mental picture of its location in the live animal.

With the help of Figure 6.3, identify the features of the femur. Proximally, identify the round **head** of the femur. The head has a small non-articular depression in the middle called the **fovea capitis femoris**. The **ligament of the head of the femur** originates here and extends from the fovea capitis to the **acetabular fossa,** the deep depression within the acetabular cavity.

The **greater trochanter** (or major trochanter) and **lesser trochanter** (also called minor trochanter) are the bony eminences on the proximal lateral and medial parts of the femur, respectively.

The greater trochanter in the horse is divided into cranial (low) and caudal (high) parts but not in ruminants.

A large third trochanter is present on the lateral proximal surface of the horse femur, but this feature is absent in ruminants.

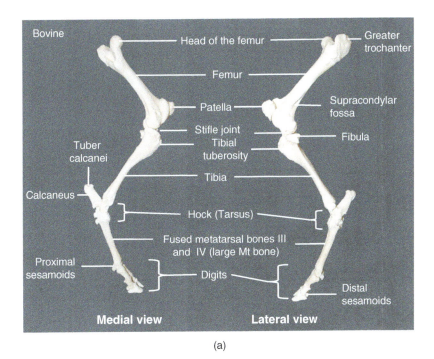

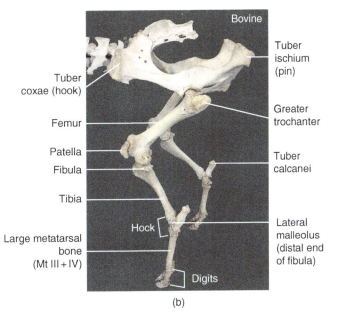

Figure 6.1 (a) Articulated bones of the left bovine pelvic limb: medial and lateral views; (b) bones of the bovine hind limb. Articulation of the femur with the hip bone (os coxae). Mt, metatarsal bone.

Identify the **trochanteric fossa** bounded laterally and caudally by the **intertrochanteric crest** (Figure 6.3).

On the distal extremity of the femur, identify the **medial and lateral femoral condyles** and the depression between them called the **intercondylar fossa**

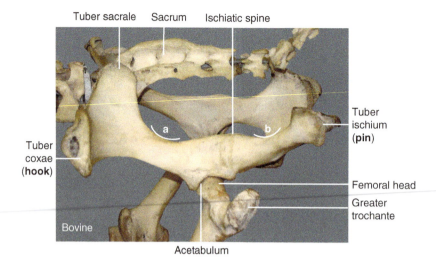

Figure 6.2 The bovine os coxae (hip bone): lateral view. (a) Greater ischiatic notch; (b) lesser ischiatic notch.

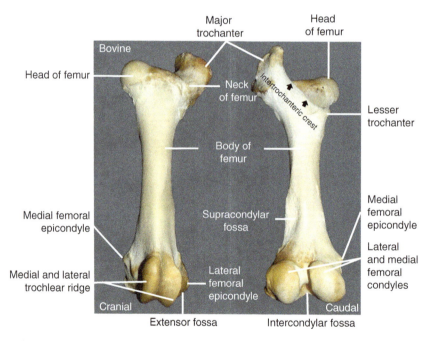

Figure 6.3 The bovine femur: cranial (left) and caudal (right) views.

(Figure 6.3). The rough surfaces on the lateral sides of the femoral condyles are the **medial and lateral epicondyles.**

The **trochlea of the femur** is the gliding surface where the patella articulates with the femur. It is situated cranial and proximal to the femoral condyles.

The depressed area between the **lateral and medial trochlear ridges** is a sliding surface for the patella. The medial ridge is generally more prominent and thicker than the lateral trochlear ridge.

The **patella** is a large diamond-shaped sesamoid bone intercalated in the tendon of insertion of the quadriceps muscle. The patella has a proximal base and distal apex.

Note the large depression on the caudolateral aspect of the distal part of the femur above the lateral condyle. This is the **supracondylar fossa.** The superficial digital flexor (SDF) muscle originates from the supracondylar fossa.

Note the small depression between the lateral trochlear ridge and lateral epicondyle of the femur. This is the **extensor fossa**. Later, you will see that the combined tendon of the long digital extensor and fibular (peroneus) tertius muscles originates from the extensor fossa.

6.1.3 Bones of the Leg (Crus)

The crus (leg) is formed by the **tibia** and **fibula** but the tibia is the only weight-bearing bone of the crus (Figure 6.4). The **fibula** is vastly reduced except for small proximal and distal parts. The proximal part is fused with the lateral tibial condyle. The distal part is a separate bone located on the most distal lateral surface of the tibia, forming what is known as the **lateral malleolus** (Figure 6.4). The lateral malleolus remains a separate bone and should be differentiated from a fracture in X-ray images of the ruminant tarsus.

Note the angulation of the tibia and how it relates to the standing animal (Figure 6.1). Identify the **medial and large condyles** on the proximal aspect of the tibia. The medial and lateral tibial condyles articulate with corresponding femoral condyles to form the **stifle joint**.

On the proximal articular surface of the tibia, observe the **intercondylar eminence** separating the medial and lateral tibial condyles. The areas cranial and caudal to the intercondylar eminence are attachment sites for the cranial and caudal cruciate ligaments, respectively. The cruciate ligaments are more clinically relevant in small animals and are not shown here.

The proximocranial eminence on the tibia is the **tibial tuberosity**. Several thigh muscles, including the quadriceps femoris, biceps femoris, and sartorius, attach on the tibial tuberosity.

Identify the **extensor groove,** the vertical notch between the lateral tibial condyle and tibial tuberosity. The combined tendon of the long digital extensor and fibularis (peroneus) tertius muscles passes from the extensor fossa of the femur through the extensor groove of the tibia.

Identify the distal depression of the tibia, called the **cochlea**. The cochlea articulates with the **proximal trochlea of the talus** to form the tibiotarsal (or tarsocrural) joint. The bony prominence on the distal medial aspect of the tibia is the **medial malleolus**. On the lateral distal part of the tibia, recall the presence of the lateral malleolus as the remnant of the fibula in the distal crus.

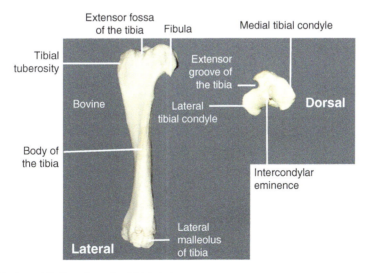

Figure 6.4 The bovine tibia: lateral (left) and proximal (right) views.

6.1.4 Tarsal Bones

The tarsus (hock) in ruminants is formed by five tarsal bones organized in three tiers (rows).

With the help of Figure 6.5, study the bones of the hock and compare them with those of the horse.

The proximal row or tier has two bones: the **calcaneus (C)** and **talus (T)**. The middle row contains one bone that represents the combined **central and fourth tarsal bones** (C+4, called the centroquartal bone). The distal row consists of two bones, fused second (T2) and third (T3) tarsal bones, and singular first (T1) tarsal bone (Figure 6.5).

The proximal enlargement of the calcaneus is the **tuber calcaneus**. The tuber calcaneus forms the **point of the hock** that serves as attachment point of the common calcanean (Achilles) tendon. By this arrangement, the calcaneus acts as a short lever arm facilitating extension of the tibiotarsal joint. The common calcanean tendon comprises several tendons that include the gastrocnemius and SDF muscles (the largest and most significant contributors).

Identify the **sustentaculum tali** on the medial surface of the calcaneus. This projection serves as a sliding surface for the deep digital flexor (DDF) muscle tendon as it passes distally past the tarsus.

Identify the **talus** bone lying medial to the calcaneus on the proximal row. The talus in ruminants has a **proximal and distal trochlea** and is more slender in shape than that of the horse.

The talus bone in the horse has only one trochlea located proximally. The distal part is flat and articulates with a similarly flat central tarsal bone. The proximal trochlea of the talus in ruminants is more slanted than that of the horse.

The distal trochlea of the talus in ruminants articulates the **centroquartal bone** (fused central and fourth tarsal bone). Its presence in ruminants is described as a characteristic for the order Artiodactyla. The proximal and distal trochleae of the ruminant talus allow for greater movements at both the **tarsocrural and proximal intertarsal joints**.

A **tarsal canal** is formed between three sets of fused tarsal bones that include fused T2+T3 tarsal bones, fused C+ 4 tarsal bones (centroquartal bone), and fused III and IV metatarsal bones. The perforating tarsal artery courses through this canal from the dorsal to the plantar aspect of the hock. A similar canal is present in the horse between the central, third, and fourth tarsal bones.

Identify the tarsal canal on articulated bovine hock.

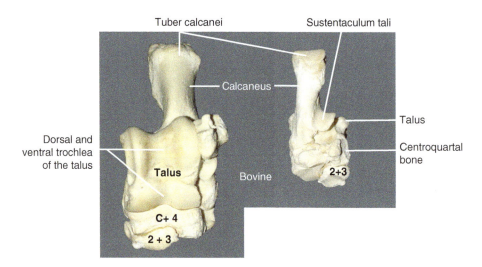

Figure 6.5 Bovine tarsus (hock): dorsal (left) and plantar (right) views. The centroquartal bone (C+4) is formed by fusion of central and fourth tarsal bones. Note the presence of proximal and distal trochleae in the talus. The small first tarsal bone is located on the plantar aspect of the distal row.

6.1.5 Fused Metatarsals III and IV (Large Metatarsal Bone)

The large metatarsal bone (Figure 6.6) is formed by fusion of the third and fourth metatarsal bones (**Mt III and Mt IV**). This bone is similar in shape to the large metacarpal bone in the forelimb except that it is slightly longer and slimmer.

The large metatarsal bone has a proximal **base** (articulates with the distal row of tarsal bones) and distal **heads** (capita) that are separated by the **intercapital notch** (Figure 6.6). The left and right heads articulate with the proximal phalanx of the corresponding digits (digits III or IV).

Identify the **axial dorsal and plantar longitudinal grooves** on the large metatarsal bone. The dorsal longitudinal groove on the dorsal surface is more distinct than the plantar longitudinal groove on the plantar surface. Note the presence of **proximal and distal metatarsal canals** that allow for blood vessels to course between the dorsal and plantar sides of the limb (Figure 6.6).

In contrast to the horse, Mt I and Mt II (splint bones) are absent in ruminants. However, a small **metatarsal sesamoid** is located at the proximal medioplantar aspect of Mt III (see discussion of the metatarsal sesamoid bone later).

Recall that the term "pes" includes the tarsal, metatarsal, and digital bones. The corresponding term in the forelimb is the "manus," which includes the carpal, metacarpal, and digital bones.

6.1.6 Metatarsal Sesamoid Bone

Identify the **metatarsal sesamoid bone** on the plantar proximal aspect of the third metatarsal bone (Mt III). The metatarsal sesamoid was once thought of as the metatarsal II bone (medial splint) found in the horse. The bone should not be mistaken for a fracture in X-ray films of the ruminant tarsus.

The digits are similar to those of the front foot. The non-weight-bearing rudimentary digits II (medial) and V (lateral) are referred to as **dewclaws**. In

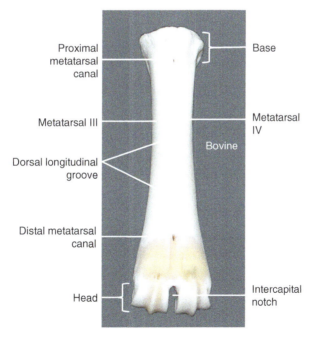

Figure 6.6 Bovine large metatarsal bone (fused third [III] and fourth [IV] metatarsal bones): dorsal view. The dorsal metatarsal artery III courses in the dorsal longitudinal groove. Proximal and distal perforating arteries course through the proximal and distal metatarsal canals from the dorsal surface to the plantar surface of the large metatarsal bone. The proximal and distal perforating branches originate from the dorsal pedal and dorsal metatarsal artery III, respectively. The bone has a proximal base and distal head regions.

ruminants, they may contain small bones that do not articulate with the other bones of the skeleton. Digits III (medial) and IV (lateral) are the weight-bearing digits. Each is formed by **proximal (P1), middle (P2),** and **distal (P3) phalanges** similar to those in the forelimb (review Figure 5.7).

A pair of proximal sesamoids and a singular distal sesamoid bone are present on each digit.

6.2 Muscles of the Pelvic Limb

Goal: Identify the major pelvic limb muscles. Have a broad understanding of their origin and insertion, especially the muscles and tendons on the distal part of the hind limb. Understand muscle actions on the joints of the pelvic limb. This is a key goal and learning objective.

Detailed descriptions of pelvic limb muscles (i.e., knowing the precise origin and insertion points) are unnecessary because they are of little clinical interest in ruminants. However, we will attempt to follow a systemic approach that would be of value for students who are studying pelvic limb muscles for the first time.

The sublumbar muscles (psoas minor, iliopsoas [psoas major plus iliacus], and quadratus lumborum) are located medially on the ventral surface of the lumbar vertebrae and may not be available for study if the pelvic limb is disarticulated from the hip joint. The sublumbar muscles possess little movement. They form the tender part of the T-bone steak cuts. Ask your instructor if these muscles should be identified. There follows a brief description of their locations and actions.

The **psoas minor** is the most medial of the sublumbar muscles. It has a long distinct tendon. In ruminants, it arises from T12–L5 vertebrae and inserts on the psoas minor tubercle on the ilium. In the horse, the psoas minor arises from T16–L5 vertebrae.

The **iliopsoas muscle** is formed by a combination of the psoas major and iliacus muscles. As a major flexor of the hip joint, it is discussed with the muscles acting on the hip joint.

The quadratus lumborum muscle has no action on the hip.

The sublumbar muscles can easily be identified on a mid-sagittal section of the caudal lumbar region, hip, and medial proximal part of the pelvic limb.

From medial to lateral, the psoas minor, psoas major, and quadratus lumborum run parallel to each other.

6.2.1 Muscles Acting on the Hip Joint

Muscles in this group include flexors of the hip joint (iliopsoas and sartorius muscles) and extensors of the hip joint (gluteal and hamstring muscles). The lateral muscles of the hip and thigh are known as "rump" muscles.

You can skin the entire limb or carry out your dissection in regions. With the help of Figure 6.7a,b, make similar skin incisions and remove the skin from the hip, thigh, and proximal leg. You may opt to keep the skin on your cadaver by reflecting it sideways or dorsally so you can use it to cover your specimen. Clean the fascia overlying the gluteal and thigh regions. Do not transect the fascia lata (insertion of the tensor fasciae latae muscle). The gluteal fascia (superficial, middle, and deep layers) covers the muscles in the hip and thigh regions. Cranially, it is continuous with the thoracolumbar fascia. Note the distinct fascial separation (intermuscular septa) of the hip and thigh muscles.

The prime flexor of the hip joint is the **iliopsoas muscle** (Figure 6.7c), a sublumbar muscle that has attachment to the ventral surface of the lumbar vertebral bodies and the ventral body of the ilium.

The iliopsoas has two parts: the **psoas major** and **iliacus muscles**. Identify the psoas major and iliacus on the medial aspect of the pelvis. The psoas major courses from the sublumbar region and proximal ends of the last few ribs to the lesser trochanter. It joins the iliacus at an area ventral to the sacrum. The iliacus is shorter and arises from L6 vertebra, ventral sacrum, and sacroiliac surface of the ilium.

Other flexors of the hip joint include the **sartorius, tensor fasciae latae, and rectus femoris muscles**. Identify these muscles on an isolated bovine or goat limb.

The major extensors of the hip joint are the lateral muscles of the hip and thigh including the **gluteal and hamstring muscles** (rump muscles) (Figures 6.7a,b and 6.8).

6.2.1.1 Gluteal Muscles

This group of hip muscles includes the **superficial, middle, and deep gluteal muscles** (Figure 6.7). The **tensor fasciae latae** (Figures 6.7a and 6.8) can be

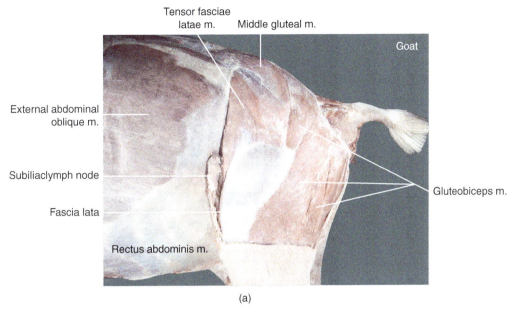

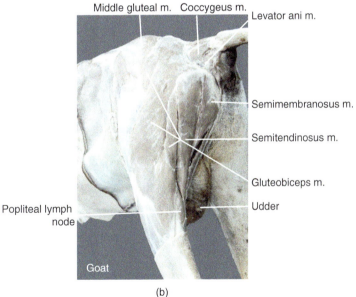

Figure 6.7 (a) Hip (gluteal) and thigh (hamstring) muscles of a goat (left pelvic limb): left lateral view. The lateral muscles of the hip and thigh are commonly known as "**rump muscles**." (b) Gluteal and hamstring muscles of a goat (left pelvic limb): left caudolateral view. (c) Hip and thigh muscles of a goat: left lateral view. Dissection of the accessory gluteal muscle by transection and reflection of the middle gluteal muscle. The gluteobiceps femoris and tensor fasciae latae muscles are removed. * Deep gluteal muscle. (d) Hip and proximal thigh of a goat: close-up left lateral view. Dissection of the deep gluteal muscle by transection and reflection of the middle and accessory gluteal muscles caudally. The gluteobiceps femoris and tensor fasciae latae muscles are removed. * Coccygeus muscle.

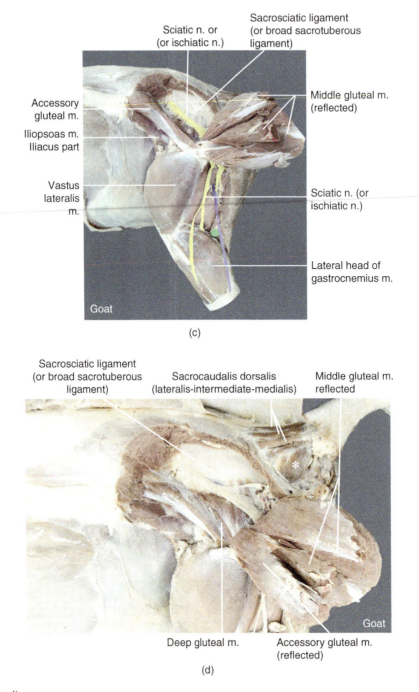

Figure 6.7 (*Continued*)

included with the gluteal group because of its position and common innervation although it has a flexor action on the hip while the gluteal muscles extend the hip.

On the lateral surface of the thigh, and with the help of Figures 6.7a and 6.8, identify the tensor fasciae latae and middle gluteal muscles.

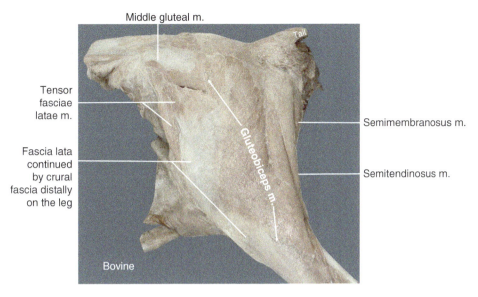

Figure 6.8 Bovine hip and thigh muscles: left lateral view. The broad gluteobiceps muscle is formed by the fusion of the biceps femoris and superficial gluteal muscles.

Understand that the gluteal fascia sends connective tissue septa that separate adjacent muscles. Clinically, these septa could hinder drainage of inflammatory exudate in an inflammatory process in the lateral hip region.

Keep in mind that the superficial gluteal muscle in ruminants fuses with the biceps femoris muscle to form the **gluteobiceps muscle**.

6.2.1.1.1 Tensor Fasciae Latae Muscle and Fascia Lata

The tensor fasciae latae is triangular. It is located laterally distal to the middle gluteal muscle and wraps around the proximal cranial thigh region (Figures 6.7a and 6.8). It inserts on the patella and cranial tibia by a broad connective tissue sheet, called the lateral femoral fascia or **fascia lata** (Figure 6.7a).

Origin: Tuber coxae and neighboring parts of the ventral surface of the ilium.
Insertion: Patella and cranial surface of the tibia by the way of fascia lata and lateral femoral fascia.
Action: Flexes the hip and tenses the lateral femoral fascia. Acts with the quadriceps femoris muscle in extending the stifle. By itself it is considered a weak extensor of the stifle joint.

6.2.1.1.2 Middle Gluteal Muscle

The middle gluteal muscle lies on the proximal lateral hip region (gluteal surface of the ilium) between the tensor fasciae latae and superficial gluteal muscles (Figures 6.7a,b and 6.8). It extends the hip joint.

Origin: Tuber coxae, wing of the ilium, and lateral surface of the sacrosciatic ligament.
Insertion: Greater trochanter.
Action: Extends the hip and abducts the limb.

Transect the middle gluteal muscle from the tuber coxae (hook) and wing of the ilium and reflect it caudally (Figure 6.7c,d). This should uncover the **accessory gluteal muscle** located on the cranioventral border of the **middle gluteal muscle** (Figure 6.7c).

The deep caudal portion of the middle gluteal muscle in dogs, the **piriformis muscle**, is thought by some to be analogous to the accessory gluteal muscle in large animals. However, this comparison raises some questions that are not answered.

The insertion of the accessory gluteal on the lateral distal part of the greater trochanter is cushioned by a subtendinous bursa called the **trochanteric bursa**. Trochanteric bursitis (inflammation) is more important in horses and can cause lameness in racehorses. Consult Box 6.1 for clinical relevance.

The trochanteric bursa can be demonstrated by transection of the middle and accessory gluteal muscles and reflection of the accessory gluteal muscle to its insertion on the distal part of the greater trochanter (Figure 6.7d).

> **Box 6.1**
>
> Trochanteric bursitis is a condition involving inflammation of the trochanteric bursa. It occurs most commonly in racehorses.

6.2.1.1.3 Deep Gluteal Muscle

The deep gluteal muscle lies deep to the middle gluteal muscle and ventral to the course of the large sciatic nerve on the lateral surface of the sacrosciatic ligament. It has a fan-shaped appearance and is covered by a glistening aponeurosis (Figure 6.7d). Study its origin and insertion on the skeleton.

Origin: Tuber coxae, ischiatic spine, and lateral and ventral surface of the body of the ilium.
Insertion: Greater trochanter.
Action: Extends the hip joint and abducts the limb.

6.2.1.2 Hamstring Muscles

The hamstring muscles include the **biceps femoris**, **semitendinosus**, and **semimembranosus muscles** (Figures 6.7b and 6.8). In ruminants, the superficial gluteal muscle fuses with the biceps femoris to form the **gluteobiceps muscle**.

The development of the hamstring muscles contributes to the shape of the pelvis (croup region). Cattle have an angular (depressed) pelvis because the hamstring muscles in ruminants have only pelvic heads (the part of the muscles that originate from the ischiatic tuberosity and run distally) but have no proximal vertebral heads covering the hip bone (i.e., no part originating from caudal vertebrae). In contrast, the hamstring muscles in the horse have both vertebral and pelvic heads. Athletic horses for example have well-developed proximal vertebral heads of the hamstring muscles. This conceals most of the bony landmarks of the pelvis. In ruminants, the bony features of the pelvis are more easily palpable than in horses.

6.2.1.2.1 Gluteobiceps Muscle

Identify the broad gluteobiceps muscle on the lateral thigh caudal to the tensor fasciae latae muscle (Figures 6.7a,b and 6.8). Study the origin and insertion of the gluteobiceps muscle on the skeleton. Note that ruminants have no separate superficial gluteal muscle. The equivalent muscle fuses with the biceps femoris muscle to form the gluteobiceps muscle (Figures 6.7a and 6.8).

Origin: Ischiatic tuberosity, gluteal fascia, and the intermuscular septum separating it from the semitendinosus muscle caudally.
Insertion: Three sites: the lateral patellar ligament, cranial tibia, and common calcanean tendon.
Action: Has multiple complex actions. In addition to extending the hip joint, this muscle can also extend or flex the stifle joint depending on whether the limb is fixed (bearing weight) or free. It also acts to extend the hock joint.

6.2.1.2.2 Semitendinosus Muscle

The semitendinosus muscle lies between the gluteobiceps muscle cranially, and semimembranosus muscle caudally (Figures 6.7b and 6.8). Its major action is to extend the hip. Additionally, it has flexor and extensor actions on the stifle and the hock joints, respectively. In ruminants, the semitendinosus has a pelvic head but the vertebral head is absent.

In horses, the semitendinosus muscle has vertebral and pelvic heads that arise from caudal vertebrae and the ischiatic tuberosity, respectively.

Origin: Ischiatic tuberosity (pelvic head).
Insertion: Medial proximal tibia, and on the tuber calcaneus via the common calcanean tendon.
Action: Extends the hip, flexes the stifle, and extends the hock.

6.2.1.2.3 Semimembranosus Muscle

The semimembranosus muscle lies between the semitendinosus cranially, and adductor muscle on the medial aspect of the thigh (Figures 6.7b and 6.8). On the medial thigh, it is covered by the gracilis muscle (Figure 6.9).

The semimembranosus muscle is shorter than the semitendinosus and its prime action is to extend the hip.

Transect the gracilis muscle on the medial aspect of the thigh to visualize the full extent of the muscle belly and its insertion on the distal medial aspect of the femur.

Origin: Ischiatic tuberosity (pelvic head).
Insertion: Medial epicondyle of the femur, caudal to the medial collateral ligament of the stifle joint.
Action: Extends the hip joint.

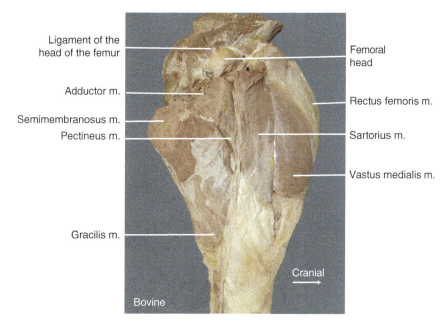

Figure 6.9 The left bovine hind limb showing adductor medial thigh muscles: medial view. The vastus medialis muscle is part of the quadriceps muscle and not the adductors. The limb is dislocated from the hip joint.

6.2.1.3 Medial Adductor Thigh Muscles

The major adductors of the hind limb can be memorized by the acronym "**PAGE**" that stands for **p**ectineus, **a**dductor, **g**racilis, and **e**xternal obturator muscles. The sartorius muscle is discussed with the medial thigh adductor group but is not a major adductor and has other actions.

6.2.1.3.1 Sartorius Muscle

The sartorius muscle is a long, relatively flat muscle in the craniomedial thigh region (Figure 6.9). It has cranial and caudal heads that are separate at their origin but are fused distally. Only at its origin does it appear to have two heads.

The sartorius muscle flexes the hip and helps to adduct the limb.

In the dog, the sartorius muscle, much like in ruminants, is divided into cranial and caudal parts, but remains undivided in the horse.

Origin: Psoas minor tendon and iliac fascia (**cranial head**) and body of the ilium (**caudal head**).
Insertion: Medial patellar ligament and fascia on the medial aspect of the stifle joint.

Action: Adducts the limb and flexes the hip joint.

6.2.1.3.2 Gracilis Muscle

The gracilis muscle is the most superficial muscle of the PAGE muscles on the medial thigh. It is a broad flat muscle that arises from the symphysial tendon (Figure 6.10).

The symphysial tendon is a condensation of connective tissue on the ventral surface of the pelvic floor (pelvic symphysis). It is a caudal extension of the prepubic tendon, the primary insertion tendon for the rectus abdominis muscle. The symphysial tendon serves as the origin for the adductor muscles and contributes to suspension of the udder in the female.

Make a note of the vessels (saphenous artery, saphenous nerve, and medial saphenous vein) obliquely crossing the superficial surface of the gracilis muscle (Figure 6.10) and note the clinical significance of the saphenous artery (Box 6.2).

Origin: Pelvis symphysis (symphysial tendon) and prepubic tendon.
Insertion: Medial patellar ligament and medial and cranial proximal border of the tibia.

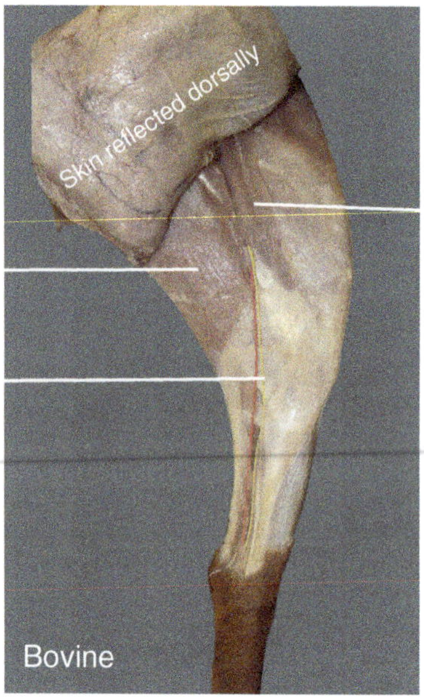

Figure 6.10 Bovine superficial medial thigh muscles. Note that the saphenous artery and saphenous nerve obliquely cross the distal part of the gracilis muscle. The medial saphenous vein (caudal branch), which accompanies the saphenous artery and nerve, is not visible (not injected).

> **Box 6.2**
>
> The femoral triangle is a site used for taking the pulse from the femoral artery in some animals. The sartorius muscle forms the cranial boundary and the pectineus forms the caudal boundary. In cattle, the pulse can be evaluated from the **saphenous artery** that lies more distally on the superficial surface of the medial thigh muscles.

Note that the tendons of the sartorius and gracilis muscles converge together distally near the medial surface of the stifle.

Action: Adducts the limb (main action).

6.2.1.3.3 Pectineus Muscle

The pectineus is a thin muscle of the PAGE group that lies between the sartorius muscle cranially, and the gracilis and adductor muscles caudally (Figure 6.9).

The pectineus muscle forms the caudal boundary of the femoral triangle.

Origin: Pectin and prepubic tendon.
Insertion: Medial epicondyle of the femur.
Action: Adducts the hind limb.

6.2.1.3.4 Adductor Muscle

The adductor muscle is the largest of the PAGE muscles and is situated on the medial aspect of the thigh (Figure 6.9). Reflection of the gracilis muscle should uncover the adductor.

Find the adductor muscle lying between the semimembranosus muscle caudally, and the pectineus muscle cranially (Figure 6.9).

The adductor muscle consists of two parts: the adductor magnus and adductor brevis. There is no need to identify these parts.

Origin: Pelvic symphysis (by the symphysial tendon).
Insertion: Medial proximal femur.
Action: Adducts the limb (major action).

6.2.1.3.5 External Obturator Muscle

In ruminants, the external obturator muscle has intrapelvic and extrapelvic parts. It lies deep to the origin of the adductor muscle and covers the ventral and dorsal surfaces of the obturator foramen. Do not look for it in your specimen but you may view its location on the skeleton.

In other domestic animals, the intrapelvic portion of the external obturator is a separate muscle called the internal obturator muscle.

6.2.2 Muscles Acting on the Stifle Joint

In this group, you should focus on the quadriceps femoris muscle (major extensor of the stifle). Identify the four parts of this muscle and their insertion on the tibial tuberosity by three patellar ligaments. Other muscles that have flexor actions on the stifle include the popliteus, gastrocnemius, and SDF muscles (Figure 6.11). The gastrocnemius and SDF are discussed with the muscles acting on the hock and digits.

6.2.2.1 Quadriceps Femoris Muscle

The quadriceps femoris muscle is the largest muscle on the cranial surface of the femur (Figures 6.11 and 6.12). It comprises four heads: the **rectus femoris, vastus lateralis, vastus medialis, and vastus intermedius.**

*Reflect the tensor fasciae latae and gluteobiceps muscles by transecting the fascia lata along the cranial border of the gluteobiceps muscle. Reflect the gluteobiceps femoris muscle distally to fully uncover the lateral head (vastus lateralis) of the quadriceps femoris muscle. Note the presence of the large **sciatic nerve** deep to the gluteobiceps femoris.*

The three vastii (vastus lateralis, vastus medialis, and vastus intermedius) muscles of the quadriceps femoris muscle originates from the proximal femur but the rectus femoris originates from a location on the body of the ilium cranial to the acetabulum. The four heads of the quadriceps femoris fuse distally and insert by three **patellar ligaments** on the **tibial tuberosity** (Figure 6.12).

The quadriceps femoris is a prime and powerful extensor of the stifle joint. The rectus femoris is the only head of the quadriceps femoris muscle that has a flexor action on the hip joint.

Origin: Proximal lateral and medial surface of the femur (vastus lateralis, vastus intermedius, and vastus medialis), and body of the ilium cranial to the acetabulum (rectus femoris).

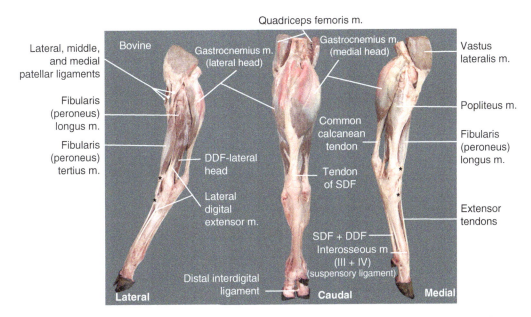

Figure 6.11 Overview of bovine pelvic limb muscles: lateral, caudal, and medial views. * Proximal (crural) and distal (metatarsal) extensor retinaculum. DDF, deep digital flexor muscle; SDF, superficial digital flexor muscle.

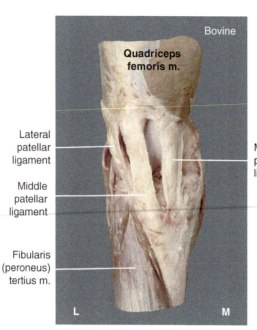

Figure 6.12 Insertion of the bovine quadriceps femoris muscle on tibial tuberosity by three patellar ligaments. The vastus intermedius (out of view) is located deep between the vastus lateralis, rectus femoris, and vastus medialis on the dorsal surface of the femur.

Insertion: Tibial tuberosity via three patellar ligaments.
Action: Extends the stifle (all four heads) and flexes the hip (rectus femoris only).

Other muscles of the hip are very small and have minor actions. These include the *internal obturator, quadratus femoris, coccygeus,* and *levator ani muscles*. The coccygeus and levator ani muscles (Figure 6.7b) originate on the pelvis and insert on the caudal vertebrae of the tail and anus. They form a **pelvic diaphragm** that supports the rectum and other pelvic viscera against herniation. These muscles are clinically more important in small animals (e.g., dogs). Their weakness is associated with incidence of perineal hernia. There is no need to dissect them.

6.2.3 Muscles Acting on the Hock and Digits

The muscles of the crus are divided broadly into two groups. The **craniolateral group** (Figures 6.11, 6.13, and 6.14) includes muscles that only flex the hock, and others that flex the hock and extend the digits.

The second group is the **caudomedial group** (Figure 6.11) that comprises muscles that extend the hock only, and others that extend the hock but also flex the digits.

The muscles in the craniolateral group are innervated by the common peroneal (fibular) nerve, the cranial division of the sciatic nerve. The muscles in the caudomedial group are innervated by the tibial nerve.

6.2.3.1 Craniolateral Muscles of the Leg (Crus)

The craniolateral muscle group comprises the **cranial tibial, fibularis (peroneus) tertius, long and (short) digital extensor, fibularis (peroneus) longus, and lateral digital extensor muscles**. The terms fibularis and peroneus are used interchangeably and both terms are acceptable.

With the help of Figure 6.13, skin your specimen down to the claws (hoofs) if you have not already done so. Keep the dewclaw in place. Isolate the extensor retinacula on the dorsal surface of the hock and proximal metatarsal region. You may also want to preserve branches of the lateral saphenous vein, especially the cranial branch.

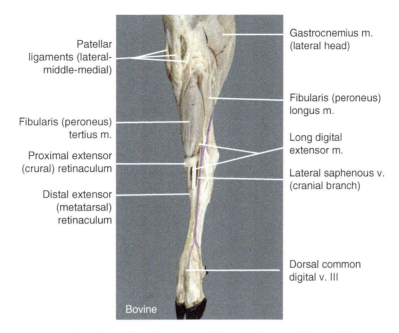

Figure 6.13 Bovine superficial craniolateral muscles of the crus on left pelvic limb: craniolateral view.

6.2.3.1.1 Fibularis (Peroneus) Tertius Muscle

The belly of the **fibularis (peroneus) tertius** muscle is the largest and most superficial and cranial of the craniolateral group (Figures 6.13 and 6.14). Unlike the horse, in which the fibularis tertius is purely tendinous, in ruminants, it is fleshy. Additionally, in the horse, the fibularis tertius lies deep to the long digital extensor muscle. This position is reversed in ruminants.

The fibularis tertius inserts on the tarsus and proximal metatarsal bones by **lateral** and **medial** tendons. It primarily flexes the hock. There is no need to dissect the tendons of insertion.

Origin: Extensor fossa of the femur, passing distally through the extensor groove on the proximal tibia by a common tendon shared with the long digital extensor muscle.

Insertion: The lateral tendon inserts on the dorsal surface of the large metatarsal bone (fused Mt III and Mt IV). The medial tendon inserts on the first tarsal and fused tarsal bones II and III, and the plantar aspect of the large metatarsal bone. Note these points of insertion on the skeleton or articulated limb but do not dissect them.

Function: Flexes the hock.

6.2.3.1.2 Long Digital Extensor Muscle

The long digital extensor muscle fuses with the fibularis tertius and is partially covered by the fibularis (peroneus) tertius muscle.

Find the belly of the long digital extensor muscle deep and lateral to the fibularis (peroneus) tertius muscle (Figure 6.14).

The long digital extensor muscle has **medial** (deep) and **lateral** (superficial) **bellies** that give **medial** and **lateral** digital extensor tendons.

Trace the tendons of insertion of the long digital extensor to the digits. Notice that the long digital extensor muscle insertion is similar to that of the common digital extensor in the forelimb.

Identify and isolate the **crural and metatarsal extensor retinacula** that hold down the tendons of the craniolateral muscles of the crus on the flexor (dorsal) surface of the hock and dorsal surface of the large metatarsal bone.

Origin: Extensor fossa of the femur.

Insertion: Medial tendon (from the medial belly) inserts on the dorsal surface of the middle (P2) and distal (P3) phalanx of the medial digit. The lateral (middle) tendon (from the lateral belly) bifurcates into two thinner tendons that insert on the extensor

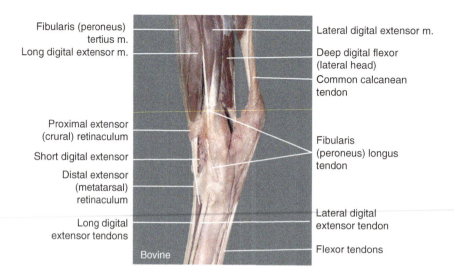

Figure 6.14 The bovine craniolateral muscles and tendons of the crus: close-up left lateral view.

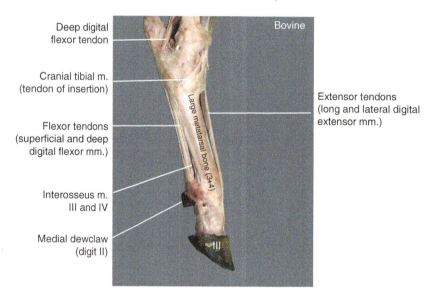

Figure 6.15 Left pelvic limb digital extensor tendons and retinacula: dorsal view. Note that three digital extensor tendons (medial, middle, and lateral) can be identified on the dorsal surface of the large metatarsal bone. Two tendons originate from the long digital extensor muscle (medial and lateral) and one (lateral) from the lateral digital extensor muscle. The lateral tendon of the long digital extensor gives two branches that insert on the extensor process of digits III and IV. The digital extensor tendons of the pelvic limb are arranged similarly to the tendons of the common and lateral digital extensor muscles in the thoracic limb.

processes of P3 on both the third (medial) and fourth (lateral) digits.

Function: Flexes the hock joints and extends the digital joints.

The **short (brevis) digital extensor muscle** is a small muscle situated on the dorsal surface of the hock. The tendon of the short digital extensor joins that of the long digital extensor (Figures 6.14 and 6.15). There is no need to dissect it.

6.2.3.1.3 Lateral Digital Extensor Muscle

The lateral digital extensor muscle lies caudal to the fibularis longus muscle (Figure 6.14). Trace the tendon of the lateral digital extensor distally to the lateral digit (digit IV). Insertion of this tendon is similar to the insertion of the medial tendon of the long digital extensor on the medial digit (digit III).

Origin: Lateral collateral ligament of the stifle and by extension from the lateral epicondyle of the femur.
Insertion: Middle (P2) and distal phalanx (P3) of lateral digit (digit IV).
Function: Flexes the hock and extends digital joints of the lateral digit.

6.2.3.1.4 Cranial Tibial Muscle
The cranial tibial muscle lies on the dorsal (cranial) surface of the tibia deep to the fibularis tertius and long digital extensor muscles.

Reflect the combined tendons of the fibularis tertius and long digital extensor muscles to uncover the belly of the cranial tibial muscle.

Origin: Proximal lateral surface of the tibia and fibula.
Insertion: First tarsal bone, fused second and third tarsal bones, and proximomedial surface of the large metatarsal bone (Figure 6.16). Identify these sites on the skeleton but do not dissect them.
Function: Flexes the hock.

6.2.3.1.5 Fibularis (Peroneus) Longus Muscle
The fibularis (peroneus) longus is a triangular muscle lying caudal to the long digital extensor muscle (Figures 6.13 and 6.14). This muscle is present in the dog but absent in the horse.

Origin: From the lateral tibial condyle, rudimentary fibula, and the lateral collateral ligament of the stifle.
Insertion: By an oblique tendon on the fourth tarsal bone and plantar aspect of the large metatarsal bone.
Function: Flexes the hock.

6.2.3.2 Extensor Retinacula

Identify the **crural (proximal) and metatarsal (distal) extensor retinacula** (Figures 6.14 and 6.15). The extensor retinacula are transverse flat bands of deep fascia that hold down the tendons of the flexor of the hock and extensor of the digits on the craniolateral aspect of the hind limb.

The **proximal (crural) extensor retinaculum** is located on the distal dorsal surface of the **crus,** hence the word "crural" in the name. It transversely crosses the tendons of three muscles on the craniolateral surface of the crus: the fibularis tertius, long digital extensor, and cranial tibial muscles.

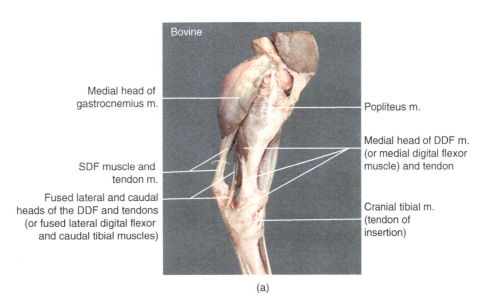

(a)

Figure 6.16 (a) Caudomedial muscles of the crus in the bovine hind limb: left medial view. Dotted line, common calcaneal tendon. (b) The metatarsal region on the left bovine hind limb showing extensor and flexor tendons on the dorsal and plantar sides, respectively: medial view.

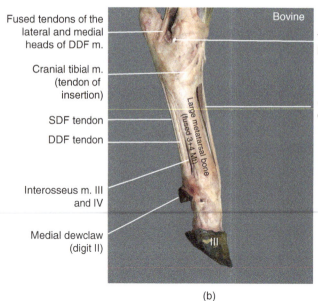

(b)

Figure 6.16 (Continued)

The **distal (metatarsal) extensor retinaculum** lies slightly distal to the hock on the proximal dorsal surface of the metatarsal region, hence the word "metatarsal" in the name. It passes over and holds down three extensor tendons: the short digital extensor, long digital extensor, and lateral digital extensor muscles (Figures 6.14 and 6.15).

6.2.3.3 Caudomedial Muscles of the Leg (Crus)

The caudomedial group includes the **soleus, gastrocnemius, SDF, DDF**, and **popliteus** muscles (Figure 6.16). Collectively, they extend the hock (except the popliteus) and some (SDF and DDF) course distally and flex the digital joints. They are innervated by the tibial nerve.

6.2.3.3.1 Soleus Muscle

This is a small muscle that originates from the rudimentary fibula. Find the soleus on the proximolateral surface of the lateral head of the gastrocnemius muscle. The tendon of the soleus muscle joins the gastrocnemius and the common calcanean tendon. No dissection is necessary.

Origin: Rudimentary fibula.
Insertion: Joins the common calcanean tendon.
Function: Helps in extending the hock.

6.2.3.3.2 Gastrocnemius Muscle (Lateral and Medial Heads)

The gastrocnemius muscle is a large muscle that lies on the caudal aspect of the stifle joint and proximal tibial. It is known as the calf muscle in humans.

The gastrocnemius has **lateral** and **medial** heads that join to form a common insertion tendon (Figure 6.16a). It originates from the **supracondylar tuberosities** and inserts on the **calcanean tuber**. It is a major component of the **common calcanean tendon** and acts to flex the stifle and extend the hock.

Find the large **tibial nerve** coursing distally between the two heads of the gastrocnemius muscle. It emerges in the space cranial to the common calcaneal tendon.

Origin: Lateral and medial supracondylar tuberosity.
Insertion: Calcanean tuber.
Function: Because the stifle and hock movement is synchronized by the reciprocal apparatus, the gastrocnemius flexes the stifle joint when the hock is flexed and extends the hock when the stifle is extended.

6.2.3.3.3 Superficial Digital Flexor Muscle

In the proximal leg, the SDF muscle lies deep to the lateral and medial heads of the gastrocnemius muscle. In the distomedial part of the leg, the SDF tendon passes medially to become superficial to that of the gastrocnemius tendon (Figure 6.16a).

Transect the medial and lateral heads of the gastrocnemius from their origins and reflect them down to uncover the SDF. At the calcanean tuber, the gastrocnemius tendon is deep to the tendon of the SDF.

The SDF in ruminants is fleshier than in the horse but has a tendinous band that courses within the muscle. It is very tendinous in the horse.

Study the origin and insertion of SDF on the skeleton. It originates from the supracondylar fossa (a depression on the caudodistal part of the femur)

Similar to the forelimb, the tendon of the SDF continues distally and separates into two components that insert on the second phalanx (P2) of the medial and lateral digits.

Origin: Supracondylar fossa (Figure 6.3).
Insertion: Calcanean tuber proximally, and middle phalanges (P2) of digits III and IV distally.
Function: Extends the hock and flexes the fetlock and pastern joints.

6.2.3.3.4 Common Calcanean (or Calcaneal) Tendon and Calcanean Bursae

The **common calcanean (Achilles) tendon** is formed principally by the tendons of the **gastrocnemius and SDF muscles** (Figures 6.14 and 6.16a). Other minor contributors include the soleus, gluteobiceps, and semitendinosus muscles.

A subtendinonus bursa (**subtendinous calcanean bursa**) is located between the SDF and gastrocnemius tendons at their point of insertion on the calcanean tuber (point of the hock). At the same location, a subcutaneous calcanean bursa (an acquired bursa by friction and/or trauma on hard surfaces) may be present under the skin over the point of the hock.

In the horse, inflammation of a subcutaneous calcanean bursa can result in an enlargement known as "capped hock."

6.2.3.3.5 Deep Digital Flexor Muscle

Proximally in the crus region, the DDF muscle has **three heads** designated as **lateral head (or lateral digital flexor muscle), medial head (or medial digital flexor muscle)**, and **caudal head (or caudal tibial muscle)** (Figure 6.16a). Distally in the metatarsal region, the combined tendons of the DDF muscle lie deep to the SDF muscle (Figure 6.16b).

The **lateral head of DDF** (the largest of the three heads) fuses with the caudal head (or tibialis caudalis muscle). The large, combined tendon of the lateral and caudal heads is surrounded by a synovial sheath as it courses on the plantar surface of the hock over the sustentaculum tali within the tarsal flexor canal (Figure 6.16). Visualize this location on the skeleton. Identify the lateral head of the DDF on the lateral side of the limb caudal to the belly of the lateral digital extensor muscle (Figure 6.14).

The relatively thin tendon of the **medial head of the DDF** passes through the medial collateral ligament of the hock (Figure 6.16). It joins the combined larger tendon of the lateral and caudal heads forming a large single tendon of the DDF muscle in the metatarsal region (Figure 6.16b).

Origin: Lateral and caudal proximal surface of the tibia.
Insertion: Distal phalanges (P3) of both digits III and IV.
Function: Flexes the digital joints of digits III and IV.

6.2.3.3.6 Popliteus Muscle

The popliteus muscle lies on the proximocaudal surface of the tibia deep to the lateral and medial heads of the gastrocnemius muscle (Figure 6.16a).

Origin: Popliteal fossa and later condyle of the femur.
Insertion: Caudomedial surface of the tibia.
Function: Flexes the stifle.

6.2.3.3.7 Interosseus Muscle (Suspensory Ligament)

Interosseus muscles III and IV in ruminants combine to form a single complex structure. The divisions and insertion of the interosseous are as described in the forelimb (see Figures 5.20–5.22). Identify the interosseus muscle deep to the DDF on the plantar surface of the large metatarsal bone (Figure 6.16b).

6.3 Blood Vessels and Nerves of the Hind Limbs

Goal: Understand the major blood channels, especially the blood supply to the distal foot. The focus in vascularization of the ruminant pelvic limb is on the arteries on both the dorsal and plantar sides of the pes (tarsus and below).

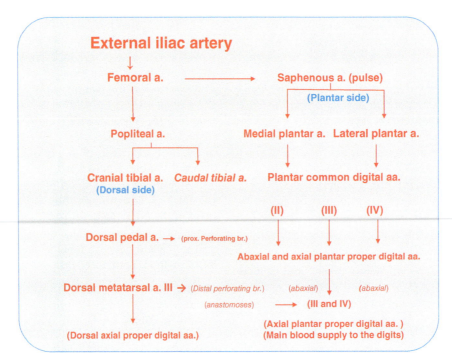

Figure 6.17 Overview of arterial **blood supply to the dorsal and plantar sides of the hind limb**. The femoral artery (main channel to the hind limb) is the continuation of the external iliac artery beyond the vascular lacuna. On the dorsal surface of the limb, blood to the digits comes from the cranial tibial, dorsal pedal, and dorsal metatarsal artery III. On the plantar side, blood comes from the saphenous and its distal branches, medial arteries, and, later, plantar arteries. The distal perforating branch from the dorsal metatarsal artery III joins with the plantar common digital artery III from the medial plantar artery. This large anastomosis runs in the interdigital space and divides into axial plantar proper digital arteries III and IV (**the main blood supply to the digits**). Do not identify arteries in *italics*.

The blood supply to the distal part of the hind limb comes from both the dorsal and plantar sides (Figure 6.17). This pattern is different from that for the forelimb where the main arterial blood supply to the front foot emanates mainly from one side, the palmar side.

6.3.1 Overview of Arterial Blood Supply to the Whole Hind Limb

In the proximal hip region, the gluteal muscles receive arterial blood from the **cranial gluteal artery**, a branch from the internal iliac artery, and from the **caudal gluteal artery**, one of two terminal branches of the **internal iliac artery** inside the pelvis.

The **cranial gluteal artery** passes out of the pelvic cavity through the **greater ischiatic foramen**. The **caudal gluteal artery** (one of the terminal branches of the internal iliac artery) courses out of the pelvic cavity via the **lesser ischiatic foramen**. The gluteal vessels are discussed with the pelvis.

Before you start your dissection of blood vessels in the hind limb, study an overview of the blood supply using Figure 6.17.

The main channel in the proximal limb that brings arterial blood to the hind limb is the **femoral artery**. This is the continuation of the **external iliac artery** out of the pelvis onto the medial surface of the thigh (Figure 6.18).

The femoral artery detaches several branches including the **saphenous artery** in the distal thigh region. The saphenous artery runs superficially on the medial thigh in association with the **saphenous nerve** and **medial saphenous vein** (Figure 6.10). Because of its superficial location on the medial thigh, the saphenous artery can be used for **pulse evaluation** in cattle.

With the help of Figure 6.18, use a fresh or embalmed bovine hind limb to dissect the major blood vessels. In the proximal medial thigh and leg, transect the gracilis muscle and medial head of the gastrocnemius muscles. Trace the femoral artery coursing from caudal thigh

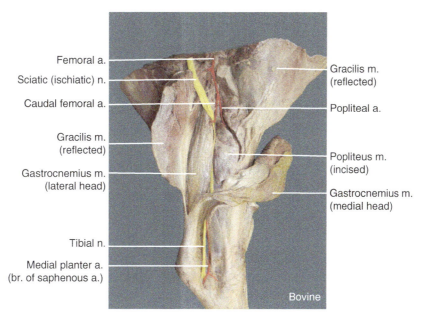

Figure 6.18 The left bovine thigh region showing the femoral artery and sciatic nerve: medial view. The medial head of the gastrocnemius and gracilis are reflected. The caudal femoral artery is the last branch off the femoral artery in the thigh region before it becomes the popliteal artery caudal to the stifle joint. Note the course of the tibial nerve between the heads of the gastrocnemius proximally, and in the space cranial to the common calcaneal tendon distally.

region distally in the popliteal notch, caudal to the stifle joint.

Here, the name of the femoral artery changes to the **popliteal artery**. The popliteal artery courses distally between the medial and lateral heads of the gastrocnemius muscle through the popliteal notch where it divides into the **cranial tibial and caudal tibial arteries.** These vessels travel to the corresponding dorsal and caudal surfaces of the tibia, respectively. Do not trace the caudal tibial artery (minor vessel). Follow the cranial tibial artery on the dorsal surface of the crus.

*On the dorsal surface of the crus, follow the **cranial tibial artery** coursing distally deep to the cranial tibial muscle in company with the **deep peroneal nerve**. With help of* Figure 6.19, *spread the muscles of the craniolateral group apart in the distal crural region.*

On the dorsal surface of the hock, the name of the **cranial tibial artery** changes to **dorsal pedal artery**. Identify both arteries. The dorsal pedal artery gives rise to a *proximal perforating tarsal artery (do not look for it)*. Distal to this branch, the dorsal pedal artery becomes the **dorsal metatarsal artery III** (Figure 6.19).

Identify the **dorsal metatarsal artery III** that courses on the axial dorsal longitudinal groove on the dorsal surface of the large metatarsal bone (Figure 6.19). This artery sends proximal and distal perforating metatarsal arteries that pass from dorsal to plantar sides of the fused third and fourth metatarsal bone through corresponding proximal and distal metatarsal canals (see groove and perforations on Figure 6.6). *Do not look for these arteries.*

In the distal third of the large metatarsal bone, the dorsal metatarsal artery III gives rise to the *distal perforating branch* and continues distally to give the small **dorsal** axial proper digital arteries III and IV. Do not look for the distal perforating or dorsal axial proper digital arteries.

On the plantar surface, the **saphenous artery** divides into **medial and lateral plantar arteries** that run with like-named nerves (divisions of the tibial nerve). The medial and lateral plantar arteries give the plantar common digital arteries, of which the **plantar common digital artery III** is the largest.

Trace the relatively large **medial plantar artery** and its largest branch, the **plantar common digital artery III**, to the interdigital space. The distal perforating artery from dorsal metatarsal artery III joins with the plantar common digital artery III from the saphenous artery. These large anastomoses are the main blood supply to the digit and give **axial plantar proper**

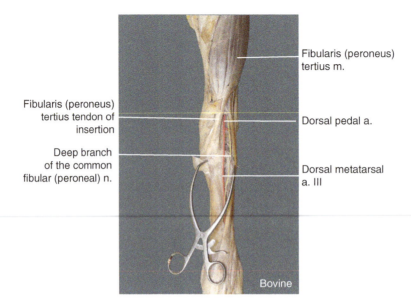

Figure 6.19 Main arteries on the dorsal surface of distal limb (cranial tibial–dorsal pedal–dorsal metatarsal artery III) to the digits. Left bovine hind limb: dorsal view.

> Box 6.3
>
> The anastomoses of the dorsal metatarsal artery III and the plantar common digital artery III are potential sources of bleeding when digital amputation is performed.

digital arteries III and IV that course to the interdigital space on the plantar surface of the foot. Consult Box 6.3 for clinical relevance.

6.3.2 Veins of the Hind Limb

Goal: Identify the superficial veins of the distal hind limb, especially branches of the lateral saphenous vein (cranial and caudal branches coursing on the lateral aspect of the hock). Identify the dorsal common digital vein III coursing on the dorsum of the metatarsal region. Know that the dorsal common digital vein III feeds into the cranial branch of the saphenous vein proximally.

Veins of the hind limb are divided into deep satellite veins that follow like-named arteries and superficial veins, some of which do not have a corresponding artery (e.g., lateral saphenous vein).

The superficial veins include the **lateral and medial saphenous veins**. The lateral saphenous vein has **cranial** and **caudal** branches. The medial saphenous vein has only a caudal branch.

In the horse, each of the lateral and medial saphenous veins has cranial and caudal branches.

The **lateral saphenous vein** is relatively large and follows an independent course on the lateral aspect of the pes with no satellite artery. In contrast, the medial saphenous vein has a satellite saphenous artery.

Identify the cranial and caudal branches of the **lateral saphenous vein** (Figure 6.20a). Trace the **dorsal common digital vein III** from the dorsal surface of the foot proximally. Note that it feeds into the cranial branch of the lateral saphenous vein (Figure 6.20a).

The lateral saphenous vein drains into the medial circumflex femoral vein deep in the medial thigh region. It courses proximally deep to the distal part of the gluteobiceps muscle (Figure 6.20b).

The medial saphenous vein, however, drains into the femoral vein in the mid-thigh region. It courses with a satellite saphenous artery and saphenous nerve (Figure 6.10).

6.3.3 Lymphatic Structures of the Hind Limb

Goal: Identify the popliteal and deep inguinal lymph nodes and know how the lymph flows from the distal limb.

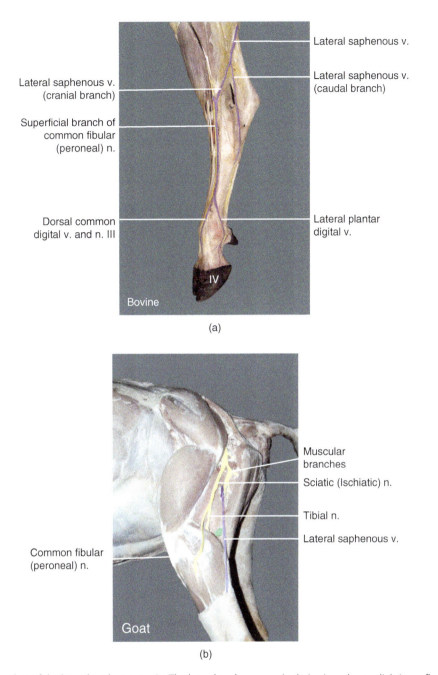

Figure 6.20 (a) Branches of the lateral saphenous vein. The lateral saphenous vein drains into the medial circumflex femoral vein on the medial thigh region. Note that the dorsal common digital vein III and the lateral plantar vein drain into the cranial branch of lateral saphenous vein. Bovine left hind limb: lateral view. These veins are used for injection of antibiotics and retrograde anesthesia (Box 6.4). (b) The lateral saphenous vein coursing deep to the distal part of the gluteobiceps muscle (removed) to join the medial circumflex femoral vein on the medial side of the thigh region.

Box 6.4

Like in the forelimb, the superficial veins are of clinical importance in the injection of antibiotics or anesthetics (retrograde anesthesia) intended to act on the distal foot. The cranial branch of the lateral saphenous vein or its branches (e.g., the dorsal common digital vein III or lateral plantar digital vein) are frequently used for these procedures. Anesthetic injected in the veins diffuses out and anesthetizes digital nerves to allow surgical procedures on the digits. Consult Box 5.8.

Lymph from the lower limb collects into the **popliteal lymph node**. The popliteal lymph node is located in a depression between the biceps femoris and semitendinosus muscles at the caudal level of the stifle joint (Figure 6.7b).

Lymph from the distal limb passes proximally to the popliteal lymph node. Efferent (outflow) lymph vessels from the popliteal lymph nodes eventually drain to medial iliac lymph nodes along the caudal segments of the aorta near the branching of the external iliac arteries. Other lymph centers that drain the pelvis and hind limbs in ruminants (lumbar, external iliac, sacral, ischial, and anorectal nodes) are discussed with the pelvis.

6.3.4 Nerves of the Hind Limb

Goal: Identify the major nerves (sciatic, obturator, and femoral) and their branches. Identify the location and know the major functions of hind limb nerves so you can diagnose nerve damage and avoid causing nerve-associated damage. Describe the nomenclature for branching of the tibial and common peroneal nerves in the distal limb (Figures 6.21 and 6.22). Understand that nerve block for diagnosis of lameness, such as that widely

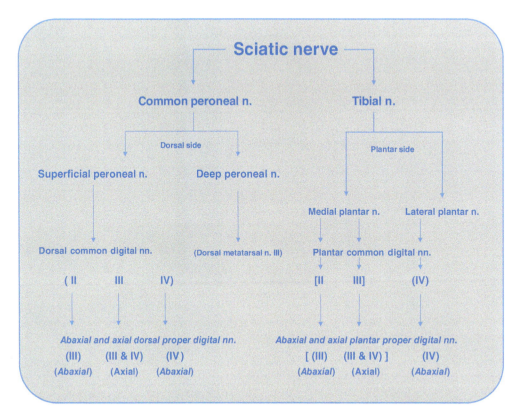

Figure 6.21 Overview of the innervation of the ruminant hind limb.

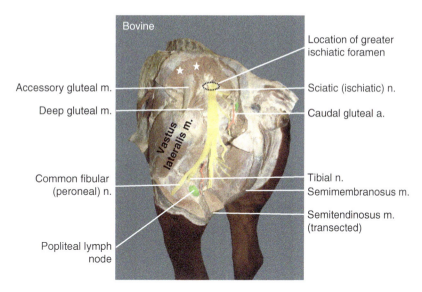

Figure 6.22 The structures deep to middle gluteal and gluteobiceps muscles (bovine): caudolateral view. * Middle gluteal muscle transected.

performed in equine medicine, is limited in bovine clinical practice.

The motor and sensory nerve supply of the hind limb structures originates from the **lumbosacral plexus** that extends from L6 to S5 lumbar and sacral spinal cord segments.

On the lateral surface of the sacrosciatic ligament find the **cranial gluteal nerve** emerging from the greater ischiatic foramen with the large **sciatic nerve**. The cranial gluteal nerve innervates the middle and deep gluteal muscles, and tensor fasciae latae muscles.

The **caudal gluteal nerve** innervates the gluteobiceps muscle along with the muscular branches from the main trunk of the sciatic nerve.

The major nerves of the hind limb are the **femoral nerve, obturator nerve, sciatic nerve**, and its two major tributaries, the **common fibular (peroneal)** and **tibial nerves** (Figures 6.21 and 6.22).

Study the branching pattern of the sciatic nerve, especially in the distal limb (Figure 6.21).

Akin to arterial blood supply, the distal foot is supplied from nerves that run on the dorsal surface of the foot (from the common peroneal or fibular nerve and its branches) and from nerves on the plantar surface (medial and lateral plantar nerves from the tibial nerve).

The **common peroneal** (fibular) and **tibial** nerves are the two major divisions of the sciatic nerve deep to the biceps femoris muscle. At the level of the lateral surface of the stifle joint, the common peroneal nerve divides into **superficial and deep peroneal (fibular) nerves** that can be traced between the fibularis (peroneus) longus and lateral digital extensor muscles. The superficial peroneal runs distally on the dorsal surface of the large metatarsal bone and gives the **dorsal common digital nerves** II, III, and IV, of which the **dorsal common digital nerve III** is the largest. The dorsal common digital nerves course on the dorsal surface of the foot to form **axial dorsal proper digital nerves III and IV** in the interdigital space, and *abaxial dorsal proper digital nerves III and IV* to the medial and lateral digits, respectively. **The deep peroneal** nerve gives a small and minor *dorsal metatarsal nerve III* that joins the **dorsal common digital nerve III** above the fetlock. On the medial side of the crus and just proximal to the hock, the tibial nerve divides into **medial and lateral plantar nerves**. These branches run in the metatarsal region on each side of the flexor tendons. The **medial plantar nerve** gives **plantar common nerves** II and III above the fetlock. These nerves course distally to form the **axial plantar proper digital nerves** III and IV in the interdigital space, and *abaxial plantar proper digital nerve III* to the abaxial surface of the medial digit. The **lateral**

plantar nerve gives *plantar common digital nerve IV*, which in turns gives the *abaxial plantar proper digital nerve IV* to the lateral digit. Identify the nerves in bold.

6.3.4.1 Femoral Nerve

The **femoral nerve** (Figure 6.23) supplies the quadriceps femoris muscle and gives a cutaneus branch, the **saphenous nerve**. The saphenous nerve runs on the medial thigh in company with the saphenous artery and medial saphenous vein (Figure 6.10). The saphenous nerve is sensory to the skin on the medial side of the leg as far distally as to the mid-metatarsal region. Consult Box 6.5 for clinical relevance of the femoral nerve.

6.3.4.2 Obturator Nerve

The **obturator nerve** supplies the adductor (PAGE) muscles. This nerve is studied with the pelvis. Find the nerve coursing along the medial shaft of the ilium and passing distally through the obturator foramen to the medial thigh or on lateral view of the pelvis where the hind limb is removed (see Figure 4.12). Consult Box 6.6 for clinical relevance of the obturator nerve.

Box 6.5

Femoral nerve damage is reported in calves that have a difficult birth when forcible traction of the fetus damages the nerve. A calf with femoral nerve damage will not be able to carry weight on the affected limb. Loss of skin sensation will be localized to the medial thigh, medial crus, and medial pes as the result of damage to the saphenous nerve, a branch of the femoral nerve.

Box 6.6

Obturator nerve damage can occur by compression of the nerve by a large fetus during difficult parturition. The condition is characterized by failure to adduct the limb, especially on a slippery floor.

6.3.4.3 Sciatic Nerve

Now let us study the branches of the sciatic nerve in the distal limb in more detail (Figures 6.21, 6.22, 6.23, 6.24, 6.25, 6.26 and 6.27). **The sciatic nerve** leaves the pelvis via the **greater ischiatic foramen** (Figure 6.22). It enters the lateral thigh deep to the gluteobiceps by

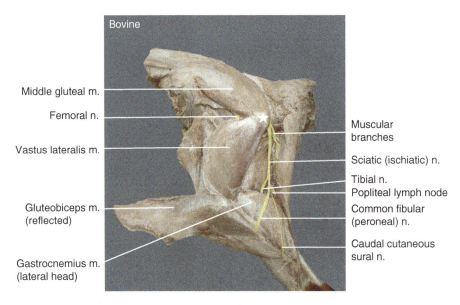

Figure 6.23 Proximal branches of the sciatic nerve (ox). The tensor fasciae latae muscle was removed and the gluteobiceps transected and reflected down.* Greater trochanter of the femur.

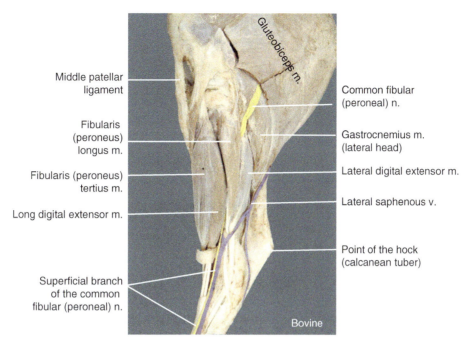

Figure 6.24 The bovine pelvic limb showing the **common peroneal nerve** and branches of the lateral saphenous vein: left lateral view.

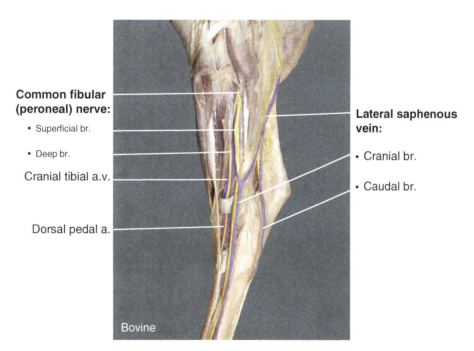

Figure 6.25 Superficial and deep branches of the common fibular (peroneal) nerve on the lateral crus and proximal metatarsal regions. The left bovine pelvic limb: lateral view.

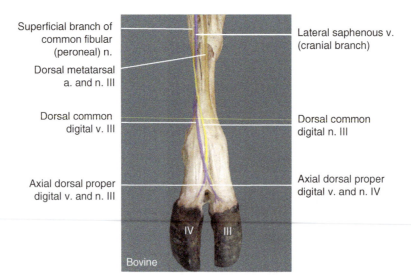

Figure 6.26 The right bovine pelvic limb: dorsal view. Distribution of the superficial and deep branches of the common fibular (peroneal) nerve on the dorsal aspect of the metatarsal and digital regions. Identify the superficial branch of the peroneal nerve and the dorsal common digital nerve III (coursing with the dorsal common digital vein III) in the metatarsal region above the fetlock joint. The dorsal common digital nerve III gives the axial dorsal proper digital nerves III and IV in the interdigital space. The deep peroneal course in the metatarsal region is the dorsal metatarsal nerve III.

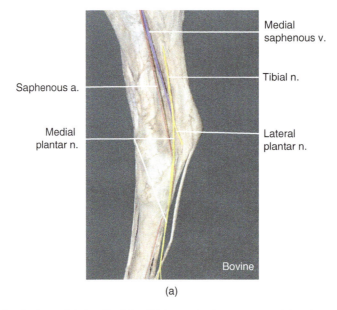

(a)

Figure 6.27 (a) The bovine hind limb: medial view. Find the tibial nerve in the groove cranial to the common calcaneal tendon on the medial side of the leg. It is accompanied by the medial saphenous vein. (b) The bovine left hind limb: plantar view. The figure shows the tibial nerve above the hock and its medial and lateral plantar branches below the hock on each side of the flexor tendons. (c) The medial and lateral plantar nerves course distally forming plantar common digital nerves II, III, and IV in the distal plantar metatarsal region, and axial and abaxial plantar proper digital nerves in the foot region. Identify the **plantar common digital nerve III** and its **axial plantar proper digital nerves III and IV** coursing distally in the interdigital space.

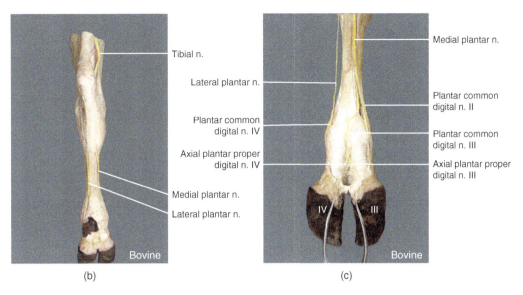

Figure 6.27 (Continued)

passing medial to the greater trochanter and caudal to the hip joint.

Reflect the gluteobiceps ventrally and find the two major branches of the sciatic nerve: the common fibular (peroneal) and tibial nerves (Figure 6.22).

6.3.4.4 Common Fibular (Peroneal) Nerve

The terms "fibular" or "peroneal" are used interchangeably and both are acceptable. The **common fibular nerve** innervates the muscles on the craniolateral aspect of the crus (flexors of the hock and extensors of the digit). It also carries sensory impulses from the dorsal aspect of the hind foot. The common peroneal nerve divides at the level of the proximal fibula into **deep and superficial peroneal nerves.**

Look for the common peroneal nerve as it emerges from under the distal part of the gluteobiceps muscle in the proximal lateral crural region (Figure 6.24). Here it divides into deep and superficial peroneal nerves.

Trace the superficial and deep peroneal nerves in the groove between the fibularis (peroneus) longus and lateral digital extensor muscles (Figures 6.24 and 6.25).

In the proximal leg, the **deep peroneal nerve** gives muscular branches to the craniolateral muscles of the leg: the fibularis (peroneus) tertius, long digital extensor, cranial tibial, and fibularis (peroneus) longus muscles. Collectively, these muscles flex the hock and extend the digits.

More distally on the dorsal surface of the metatarsal region, the deep peroneal gives the **dorsal metatarsal nerve III**. Trace this relatively small nerve coursing close to the dorsal metatarsal artery III (continuation of the dorsal pedal artery) (Figures 6.19 and 6.26). The dorsal metatarsal nerve III joins the dorsal common digital nerve III from the superficial peroneal nerve. Do not look for this union.

The **superficial peroneal nerve** innervates the lateral digital extensor muscle in the proximal crural region. It courses distally along the lateral side of the crus. At the distal end of the metatarsal region, it gives the **dorsal common digital nerves II, III, and IV**, of which the **dorsal common digital nerve III** is the largest (Figure 6.26). The dorsal common nerves course to the dorsal aspect of the digits and give rise to the **axial and abaxial dorsal proper digital nerves** as they pass distal to the dewclaws.

Identify the **dorsal common digital nerve III** that passes distally in the interdigital space and gives the **axial dorsal proper digital nerves III and IV** to the medial and lateral digits, respectively (Figure 6.26).

6.3.4.5 Tibial Nerve

On the medial aspect of the crus, locate the tibial nerve in the depression between the common

> **Box 6.7**
>
> Although retrograde anesthesia in the distal veins of the foot is widely used in cattle, a four-point nerve block of the dorsal common digital nerves, dorsal metatarsal nerve III, and medial and lateral plantar nerves can be performed.

calcanean tendon and the DDF muscle (Figures 6.18 and 6.27a). Identify the branching of the tibial nerve using Figure 6.21. Proximally, the tibial nerve gives a cutaneous branch and runs between the medial and lateral heads of the gastrocnemius muscle where it gives muscular branches to the muscles caudal to the tibia (extensors of the hock and flexor of the digits).

Medially above the hock, the tibial nerve divides into a larger **medial** and a relatively thinner **lateral plantar nerves**. The plantar nerves run in the metatarsal region on each side of the flexor tendons (Figure 6.27b,c).

Trace the larger **medial plantar nerve** through the metatarsal region where it is situated medial to the flexor tendons (Figure 6.27b,c). Proximal to the dewclaws, the medial plantar nerve gives rise to the **plantar common digital nerves II and III.** Of these, the **plantar common digital nerve III** is the largest (Figure 6.27c). The lateral plantar nerve forms the **plantar common digital nerve IV** (Figure 6.27c) and abaxial plantar proper digital nerve IV.

Trace only the **plantar common digital nerve III** to the interdigital space where it forms the **axial plantar proper digital nerves III and IV** (Figure 6.27c). Do not look for the abaxial plantar proper digital nerves but you should know the nomenclature. Consult Box 6.7 for nerve block on the distal hindlimb.

In some texts, the term "proper" is omitted when the digital nerves and arteries are described.

6.4 Joints of the Hind Limb

Goal: Identify the bones that form each joint of the hind limb.

From proximal to distal, the major joints of the hind limb are the **hip (or coxofemoral) joint, stifle joint, hock joints (tarsocrural or tibiotarsal, proximal intertarsal, distal intertarsal, tarsometatarsal)**, and **digital joints (fetlock, pastern, and coffin)**. Identify these joints on a cow or goat skeleton and on your dissection specimen. To save time, your instructor may prepare prosected specimens of selected joints (e.g., stifle) for demonstrating the ligamentous structures. Joint injections and aspirations of synovia "arthrocentesis" are more widely used in equine practice than in cattle or goats. This makes detailed anatomy of ruminant joints unnecessary.

6.4.1 Hip Joint

The hip or coxofemoral joint is the articulation between the head of the femur and the acetabulum. The **ligament of the head of the femur** stabilizes the joint. There is no accessory ligament similar to that in the horse.

6.4.2 Stifle Joint

Like in the horse, the stifle joint of large ruminants (cattle) has three patellar ligaments (Figure 6.12) compared with a **single** patellar ligament in small ruminants and dogs.

Other ligaments of the stifle (medial and lateral collateral, medial and lateral femoropatellar, cranial and caudal cruciate, and meniscofemoral ligaments) are similar among domestic animals. They can be demonstrated on prosected specimens.

The stifle joint capsule consists of femoropatellar and femorotibial joints. The femorotibial joint has medial and lateral compartments. The femoropatellar joint always communicates with the medial compartment of the femorotibial joint and occasionally with the lateral femorotibial joint.

The lateral and medial femorotibial joints usually communicate with each other. In contrast, no communication exists between these two compartments in the horse or dog. Consult Box 6.8 for clinical relevance of the stifle joint.

> **Box 6.8**
>
> Inflammation of the stifle joint is known as **gonitis**. It is caused by inflammatory or structural damage in the joint. This condition can cause severe pain in bulls and failure to breed. Other conditions that affect the stifle include patellar luxation and torn cruciate ligaments.

6.4.3 Hock (or Tarsus) Joint

The hock joint is a complex joint formed by four articulations. From proximal to distal, they are the **tibiotarsal** (or tarsocrural), **proximal intertarsal**, **distal intertarsal**, and **tarsometatarsal** joints. Review the bones that make up each joint. Consult Box 6.9 for clinical relevance.

Know that the tarsocrural joint communicates with the proximal intertarsal joint. Likewise, the distal intertarsal joint communicates with the tarsometatarsal joint.

> **Box 6.9**
>
> Several conditions affect the hock joints. Examples include formation of subcutaneous hygroma, inflammation of the tarsocrural joint (bog spavin), and arthritic changes affecting various tarsal bones.
>
> Joint infection of goats with caprine arthritis and encephalitis virus can lead to progressive arthritis and lameness in dairy goats raised under intensive farming management.

The digital joints are similar to the digital joints of the forelimb.

6.5 Live Cow

Several bony prominences and soft structures can be palpated on the pelvic limb. Examples include the tuber calcanei (point of the hock joint), medial and lateral malleoli, extensor tendons of the long and lateral digital extensor muscles, and the cranial and caudal branches of the saphenous vein (Figure 6.28). The lateral saphenous vein and the dorsal common digital vein III are frequently used for intravenous injection of anesthetic drugs to obtain anesthesia of the foot in cattle (Box 6.4).

6.6 Lab ID List for Forelimb and Hind Limb

You should be able to identify differences and similarities between the appendicular bones of ruminants and equine as outlined in the relevant chapters. There is no need to identify items in *italics*.

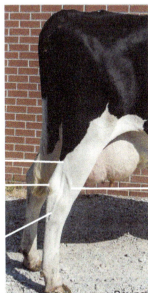

Figure 6.28 Right hind limb showing the cranial and caudal branches of the lateral saphenous vein: lateral view.

A. **Bones of Forelimb and Hind limb**
   1. Scapula (compare with horse and dog)
   2. Humerus (compare with horse and dog)
   3. Fused radius and ulna
   4. Carpus (collective term)
      a. Proximal row – radial, intermediate, ulnar, and accessory (landmark) carpal bone.
         iv. No first carpal
      b. Distal row – fused second and third carpal bones, fourth carpal bone
   5. Metacarpus (collective term): (compare with horse)
   6. Metacarpal or metatarsal 3+4 (cannon or large metacarpal or metatarsal bone)
   7. Intertrochlear notch
   8. Fifth metacarpal bone is present (metacarpal 5)
   9. Digits III and IV (P1, P2, and P3)
   10. Proximal sesamoids
   11. Distal sesamoids
   12. Dewclaws (digits II and V)
   13. Tuber coxae = hook bone (common name)
   14. Tuber ischia = pin bone (common name)
   15. Femur
   16. Medial trochlear ridge in cattle (compare with small ruminants)
   17. Fibula
   18. Lateral malleolus (compare with horse)
   19. Tarsus (hock)
      a. Proximal tier:
         i. Talus (compare with horse)
         ii. Calcaneus – calcanean tuber
      b. Middle tier:
         i. Centroquartal bone (fused T4 and central tarsal bone) – compare these bones with horse
      c. Distal tier:
         i. T1, combined T2/T3 (compare with horse)

B. **Joints**
   1. Shoulder joint: know puncture location
   2. Elbow joint: know puncture location
   3. Carpus: know joint communication between:
      a. Antebrachiocarpal
      b. Middle carpal
      c. Carpometacarpal
   4. Fetlock joint
      a. Dorsal and palmar pouches
   5. Pastern joint capsule: know that it has *dorsal and palmar pouches*
   6. Coffin joint
   7. *Proximal interdigital ligament*
   8. Distal interdigital ligament (P2): know function
   9. Stifle joint:
      a. Patellar ligaments (lateral, intermediate, and medial): know clinical significance of medial patellar ligament – compare the patellar ligaments in cattle with small ruminants
      b. Know joint capsule communication and puncture sites
   10. Hock joint: know joint communication
      a. Tarsocrural joint
      b. Proximal intertarsal joint
      c. Distal intertarsal joint
      d. Tarsometatarsal joint

C. **Muscles of the forelimb**
   1. Brachiocephalicus m.
   2. Omotransversarius m.
   3. *Subclavius m.* (rudimentary)
   4. Rhomboideus m. (hump in Zebu cattle)
   5. Serratus ventralis m.
   6. Infraspinatus m. (subtendinous infraspinatus bursa)
   7. Biceps brachii m.
      a. Independent intertubercular bursa in the ox (compare with small ruminants)
   8. Triceps brachii
      a. Subtendinous bursa
      b. Inconstant subcutaneous bursa at the olecranon

D. **Tendons and muscles in the forearm:** only the digital **extensors and flexors** among the muscles of the forearm merit notification. Three extensor tendons (**medial, middle, and lateral**) can be palpated side by side on the dorsal surface of the large metacarpal bone.
   1. Common digital extensor m.
      a. Medial tendon
      b. Lateral (middle) tendon

2. Lateral digital extensor m. Note: the medial tendon of the common digital extensor and the lateral digital extensor tendon are sometimes called the proper digital extensor tendons.
3. Superficial digital flexor (SDF)
4. Deep digital flexor (DDF)
5. Interosseus m. (study the branching pattern: axial and abaxial extensor branches)

E. **Muscles of the hindlimb**
   1. Hip region
      a. Quadriceps femoris m.
      b. Middle gluteal m.
      c. Hamstring m. (biceps femoris, semitendinosus, and semimembranosus muscles)
      d. Gluteobiceps m. (biceps + superficial gluteal mm.)
   2. Muscles of the leg (craniolateral and caudomedial groups)
   2a. Craniolateral group
      a. Tibialis cranialis m.
      b. Peroneus tertius m. (compare with horse)
      c. Long digital extensor m.
      d. Lateral digital extensor m.
   2b. Caudomedial group:
      a. Gastrocnemius m.
      b. SDF m.
      c. DDF m.
      d. Popliteus m.
      e. Soleus m.

F. **Nerves of the forelimb (from the brachial plexus)**
   1. Suprascapular n.
   2. Median n.
   3. Palmar common digital n. *II*, III, *IV* (identify palmar common digital n. III only)
      a. Axial and abaxial palmar proper digital nn. III and IV
   4. Ulnar n.
   5. Radial n.
      a. Superficial branch
      b. Deep branch
   6. Dorsal common digital n. III
      a. Axial dorsal proper digital nn. III and IV

G. **Nerves of the hind limb (from lumbosacral plexus)**
   1. Obturator n. (know clinical significance)
   2. Femoral n. (know clinical significance)
   3. Sciatic n.
      a. Tibial n. (medial and lateral plantar n.)
      b. Common peroneal or fibular (superficial and deep peroneal nn.)
   4. Superficial peroneal (fibular) n.
      a. Dorsal common digital n. III
      b. Axial dorsal proper digital nn. III and IV
   5. Deep peroneal (fibular) n.
      a. *Dorsal metatarsal n. III*
   6. Plantar common digital n. III (from medial plantar n.)
      a. Axial plantar proper digital nn. III and IV

H. **Main arterial blood supply of the forelimb (mainly from the palmar side)**
   1. Axillary a.
   2. Brachial a
   3. Median a. *(radial a.)*
      a. **Palmar common digital a. III (largest) → axial** palmar proper digital arteries III and IV (follow them in the interdigital space of forelimb)

I. **Main arterial blood supply of the hind limb**
   1. Dorsal aspect of the hind limb
   2. Cranial tibial a.
   3. Dorsal pedal a.
   4. Dorsal metatarsal a. III (travels from dorsal to plantar aspect through intertrochlear notch and anastomoses with the plantar common digital a. III from the saphenous a.)
   5. Plantar aspect of the hind limb
      a. Saphenous a. (medial *and lateral plantar branches*)
      b. Medial plantar a. (largest) plantar common digital a. III (joins with the dorsal metatarsal a. III)
      c. Axial plantar proper digital arteries III and IV (follow them in the interdigital space of hind limb)

J. **Veins (forelimb)**
   1. Cephalic v.
   2. Accessory cephalic v.
      a. Dorsal common digital v. III: know clinical significance

K. **Veins (hind limb)**
   1. Lateral saphenous v.
      a. Cranial branch of lateral saphenous v.
         i. Dorsal common digital v. III: know clinical significance

L. **Digits (sagittal section)**
   1. Navicular bone
   2. Digital cushion
   3. Interdigital insertion of SDF and DDF
   4. *Proximal interdigital ligament*
   5. Distal interdigital ligament
   6. Interdigital fat pad
   7. Hoof wall and sole (hoof)
   8. White line (junction of the wall and sole)

Appendix A

Dissection Instructions for a Goat Cadaver

A.1 Dissection Labs

The time frame for dissection of a goat cadaver will be determined by your instructor based on your course contents and schedule. The dissection plan described requires a minimum of nine labs. The head can be demoed as a stand-alone lab. The bovine and caprine heads are compared for musculoskeletal structures, blood vessels, and nerves (watch Videos 4, 5, and 6).

Suggested setup for the head lab is as follows: mid-sagittal and lateral views of the bovine and caprine heads could be discussed on one side of the lab while teeth (aging), horn structures, and paranasal sinuses could be discussed on the other side. Specimen/station numbers needed for this lab depend on the student numbers.

When dissecting the limbs, the first lab covers the musculoskeletal system while the second lab covers the blood vessels and nerves. Dissection of the neck and body cavities (thorax, abdomen, and pelvis) are completed as one unit in four sequential labs. Organs and structures in the thorax, abdomen, and pelvis should be studied first in situ (for topography) and later as isolated viscera (for a more detailed study of the heart, abdominal viscera, and isolated male and female reproductive tracts).

A.2 Dissection of Goat Neck and Body Cavities (Labs, 1, 2, and 3)

- Each group of six students should have one goat or sheep. From here on, we refer to the goat, but the sheep is very similar. We would like the **even numbered groups** to **open the right side** of the animal and the **odd numbered groups** to **open the left side**.
- You may use a large knife for some of the skinning, but we suggest using no. 20 or 22 scalpel blades and handle no. 4 for most of the dissection (see **Video 24**).
- It is very important for you to follow each step of these directions and see *all* the structures listed on your lab ID before moving on. We move quickly through the ruminant anatomy so get as much as you can out of each lab.

A.2.1 Removal of the Thoracic Limb

- Lay the goat on its side on the table and have someone pull the thoracic limb you will be removing away from the body.
- Using a sharp knife or scalpel, cut through the skin and muscles just behind the thoracic limb. You will feel the blade against the ribs when you are deep enough.
- Extend the cut behind the thoracic limb from the dorsal midline down close to the sternum.
- Turn the blade so that it lies flat against the body wall and cut the deep and superficial pectorals from caudal to cranial as close to the sternum as possible (Figure A.1).
- When you reach the level of the thoracic inlet, turn the blade and cut dorsally in front of the limb.
- Return to your ventral cut and sever any remaining brachial plexus or axillary blood vessels on the medial side of the limb. Finally, cut through

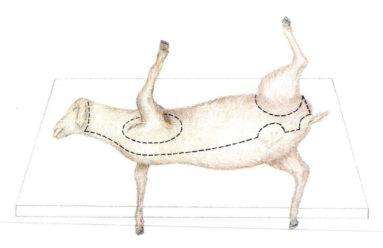

Figure A.1 Outline of skin incisions for removal of forelimb and hind limb and reflection of the skin off the neck and flank.

the attachments of the **serratus ventralis** muscle on the deep surface of the scapula and the remaining **rhomboideus** muscle attachment at the dorsal border of the scapula. Now you will be able to remove the thoracic limb.
- *The instructor will provide you with a plastic bag to place the limb for further dissection later.*

A.2.2 Removal of the Pelvic (Hind) Limb

- Have someone elevate the pelvic limb that is to be removed to allow the dissector good access to the inguinal area with his or her blade (Figure A.1). A knife would be the best tool to use here.
- The purpose of the first cut is to sever the adductor muscles where they attach to the pelvic symphysis. Incise the skin between the legs just lateral to the midline on the side you will be removing (Figure A.1).
- If you have a male, be careful not to cut the penis. The penis should remain with the pelvis when the limb is removed.
- Make a deep cut dorsally through the adductor muscles with the person elevating the limb lifting as the cut is made to open the space between the limb and the pelvis.
- If the initial cut is made correctly, you should feel the knife hit the bottom of the pelvis or possibly the acetabulum (review this area on a skeleton). Use your blade tip to find the bottom of the hip joint and cut into it. When you find the joint, you will probably see synovial fluid. Also, as you cut the **ligament of the head of the femur**, you will find the leg much easier to elevate.
- At this point, the hard work is done. Cut the lateral thigh muscles from the pelvis, leaving some muscles covering the **sacrosciatic ligament**.
- *Once the hind limb is free, put it in the plastic bag with the thoracic limb or in a separate bag for later dissection.*

A.2.3 Skinning of the Neck and Flank on the Side Where the Limbs Are Removed

- Now it is time to skin your specimen. Because of the rapid pace, we will be moving at, we are going to skin the entire left/right side.
- Make a skin incision just behind the ear from the dorsal midline to the ventral surface of the neck (Figure A.1).
- Make another skin incision along the ventral midline connecting your first cut on the ventral neck and extending all the way back to the inguinal area. There will be big holes in your skin where the thoracic and hind limbs used to be.
- As you continue the skin incision back toward the inguinal area, cut lateral to the penis if you have a male or lateral to the udder if you have a female.
- Join the ventral incision in the inguinal region with the cut you made to remove the pelvic limb (Figure A.1).
- Now you should remove the skin, folding it dorsally and exposing the neck, thorax, and abdomen.

Do not worry about the cutaneus trunci that should remain with the skin.
- Reflect the skin to just a little beyond the dorsal midline, and leave it attached to the body. The skin will help hold in moisture when you put the cadaver away. Now it is time to see some anatomy!

A.2.3.1 Neck

- Clean the superficial neck fascia. The **external jugular vein** lies in the **jugular groove.** Identify the muscular boundaries for the jugular groove. In the goat, the jugular groove is bounded by the **sternomandibularis (sternozygomaticus) muscle** ventrally, and the **cleidomastoideus muscle** (distal part of the brachiocephalicus muscle) dorsally.
- The **sternomandibularis** muscle is commonly referred to as the **sternozygomaticus** muscle in the goat as it attaches to the zygomatic arch (see Figure 1.20 in Chapter 1).
- The sternomandibularis muscle is absent in the sheep, making the jugular groove less distinct in this species.
- You should see another muscle lying deep to the external jugular vein in the cranial part of the neck. This muscle is the **sternomastoideus.** Find the sternomastoideus muscle where it divides from the **sternomandibularis** muscle in the middle of the neck. The sternomandibularis and sternomastoideus form the **sternocephalicus muscle**.
- Cut the **sternomastoideus** muscle just beyond its origin and reflect it dorsally to reveal the **carotid sheath**. By now, you should know what is in the carotid sheath. Identify its main contents (the **common carotid artery** and **vagosympathetic nerve trunk**) and move on.

A.2.4 Opening the Thorax and Abdomen for Studying the Topography on the Left and Right Sides

Now you are ready to open the thorax and abdomen. Remember we said we were moving fast! (See **Video 10** if you have not already done so.)

- Identify the following nerves on the thoracic wall:
  - **Long thoracic nerve** (see Figure 2.7 in Chapter 2). This is a motor nerve that supplies the serratus ventralis muscle.

> **Box A.1**
>
> Surgical incision into the thorax should be made in the middle of the ribs away from the caudal border to avoid damaging the intercostal neurovascular bundle.

  - **Intercostal nerves, arteries, and veins**. The intercostal vessels and nerves follow the caudal border of the ribs. You may see them better from the interior of the ribs when you reflect the rib cage dorsally. See Box A.1 for clinical relevance.
- Using Figures 2.6 and 2.7, quickly identify the muscles on the lateral wall (some are cut with the forelimb). Because of time, your instructor may decide to skip the identification of these muscles as they have little clinical relevance. However, understand that a rupture of the **serratus ventralis muscle** in cattle could result in the displacement of the scapula dorsally above the vertebral column. This condition is commonly known as "**flying scapula.**" Remove all the muscles over the ribs exposing their sternal attachments ventrally.
- Next, remove as much epaxial musculature (see Figure 2.6) as you can to expose the proximal ends of the ribs. This includes the longissimus and iliocostalis systems primarily. There is no need to identify these muscles by their individual names.
- Find the first rib by looking just caudal to the remnant of the brachial plexus.
- Using a scalpel blade, expose the cranial border of the first rib and open the thoracic inlet. There should be copious amounts of embalming fluid in the pleural cavity.
- Using the rib cutters provided, cut the distal attachment of the ribs as close to the sternum as possible. Begin at the thoracic inlet cutting the first rib and working your way backward.
- Cut any intervening tissue between each rib as you go.
- When you reach the caudal end of the sternum, use a blade to continue a ventral midline incision through the abdominal wall cutting back toward the inguinal region.
- As with the skin incision, cut lateral to the penis or mammary gland.
- Stop your incision at the level equal to the cranial surface of the hind limb still attached to the opposite

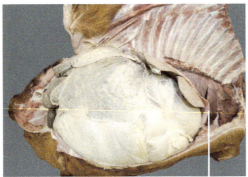
Figure A.2 Opening of the thorax and abdomen: right lateral view. Make similar incisions on the left side.

side of the animal. The goal here is to avoid cutting into the spermatic cord, mammary gland, or superficial inguinal ring.
- Next, make an incision perpendicular to your ventral incision dorsally toward the back of the animal.
- You have essentially created a giant flap now, which we will elevate to see the left or right thoracic and abdominal cavities as seen in Figure A.2 and **Video 10**.
- Now use the rib cutters to cut the proximal shaft of the ribs as close to the thoracic vertebrae as possible (Figure A.2). **Do not** cut the tissue between the ribs. The aim is to leave the ribs attached.
- With someone pulling up on the body wall flap, cut the diaphragm free from its attachment to the body wall. This part sounds much easier than it is, but take your time and you will get it right.
- As you cut the diaphragm free, you should be able to fold back the entire body wall to reveal the thoracic and abdominal organs in situ (Figure A.2).

A.2.5 Thorax

Study the surface landmarks on the thoracic wall including the **basal border of the lungs** and **diaphragmatic line of pleural reflection**.

A.2.5.1 Thoracic Landmarks
A.2.5.1.1 Basal Border of the Lungs
The basal border of the lungs is defined as the most caudal extent of the lungs. Lung sounds should be listened to cranial to this line. Review the boundaries of the basal border of the lungs in the ox, goat, and sheep as outlined in Chapter 2.

A.2.5.1.2 The Diaphragmatic Line of Pleural Reflection
This line represents the most caudal extent of the pleural cavity where the costal parietal pleura becomes the parietal diaphragmatic pleura, or vice versa. A needle inserted cranial to the line is in the pleural cavity and a needle puncture caudal to the line is in the peritoneal cavity. Review the boundaries for the diaphragmatic line of pleural reflection as outlined in Chapter 2.

- Study the ribs and thoracic vertebrae using articulated skeletons in lab. Compare the ribs of the ox with the equine. (Can you state the difference in shape between the bovine and equine ribs?)
- You will need to identify the structures within the thorax listed on the lab ID list. Use Figures 2.8, 2.11, 2.12, and 2.13 in Chapter 2 to help you.
- To see the internal structures of the thoracic cavity, you will need first to remove the lungs.
- Remove the lungs by making your cut as close as possible to the hilus. Avoid cutting the vagus and phrenic nerves by reflecting the lungs toward you as you make your cut. The aim is to remove the lungs as one unit with all the lobes attached to each other. Those working on the right side will encounter a **tracheal bronchus**, which feeds the right cranial lobe of the lung. Additionally, the accessory lobe of the right lung wraps around the caudal vena cava. To remove all the lobes of the right lung, push this lobe out using your fingers. If you opened the left thorax, make sure you see the tracheal bronchus and right lung lobes as well.
- Identify lung lobes on the left and right sides (see Figure 2.9a,b). Unlike equine lungs, ruminant lungs

are lobulated. Their lobe divisions are like those of the dog. The **left lung** has **cranial and caudal lobes,** with the cranial lobe divided into **cranial and caudal parts**. The right lung has four lobes: **cranial, middle, caudal,** and **accessory lobes**.
- Identify the **tracheal bronchus**, a unique feature in the right ruminant lung. It ventilates the cranial lobe of the right lung (see Figure 2.9c). Review the clinical significance of the tracheal bronchus (in the live animal, be cautious not to obstruct the tracheal bronchus when using an endotracheal tube with inflatable cuffs during anesthesia).
- **Note:** You will be responsible for identifying structures on both *left and right* sides because of some differences. Groups working on the opposite side should exchange tables when their dissection is complete. Using the lab ID list and appropriate figures in the book will help you move through the dissection more efficiently.

A.2.5.2 Nerves and Vessels Within the Thorax

After you have removed the lungs, use your forceps to carefully remove the parietal pleura and any fat (no scalpel).

Using the lab ID list and with the help of Figure 2.8, study the structures within the thorax. Those who are working on the left side should identify the **thoracic duct** before starting to look for other structures (ask your instructor for help). The thoracic duct is very delicate. Preserve this structure for the other group to see.

Thoracic surgery in ruminants is not common. Most of the structures in the ruminant thorax are like those you have seen in the dog and horse with fewer differences. Identify the following structures:

1) **Caudal mediastinal lymph node**. The caudal mediastinal lymph node is elongated in shape and is in the caudal mediastinum between the descending aorta and esophagus (see Figure 2.8). Review the clinical significance of this node as discussed in Chapter 2. It is not necessary to identify other nodes.
2) **Phrenic nerve**. The phrenic nerve is a motor nerve to the diaphragm. Find the nerve running across the lateral surface of the heart within the parietal mediastinal pleura (see Figure 2.8). Clean the nerve and follow the nerve to its destination on the diaphragm. The phrenic nerve originates from the ventral spinal branches of C5–C7.
3) **Vagus nerve.** Identify the ventral and dorsal vagal trunks (see Figure 2.13).
4) Left recurrent laryngeal nerve (see Figure 2.11).
5) Sympathetic trunk (see Figure 2.13).
6) Cervicothoracic ganglion (CTG) (see Figure 2.12).
7) Brachiocephalic trunk (see Figures 2.11 and 2.15a).
8) Pulmonary trunk (see Figure 2.15a).
9) Cranial vena cava (see Figure 2.15b).
10) Caudal vena cava (see Figure 2.15b).
11) Left azygos vein (see Figures 2.11 and 2.15a). This vein drains into the coronary sinus in the right atrium. The dog and horse do not have a left azygos vein but cattle, sheep, goats, and swine do. A right azygos vein is usually present in ruminants and sometimes in pigs.
12) **Right azygos vein.**
13) Thymus (young animal) – may be seen in the neck.
14) Longus colli muscle.
15) Thoracic duct (see Figures 2.8 and 2.11).
16) Trachea.
17) Esophagus.

A.2.6 Abdomen (In Situ and on Extirpated Viscera)

- Those who opened the **right** side should mark the structures on this side with words "**right side**" on their ID list.
- The abdominal discussion for the **left** will use the same approach and mark the structures on this side with the words "**left side**" in front of them.
- **Note:**
  – Your instructor may ask you to skip the abdominal wall. Study any salient points from the abdominal wall using the figures in Chapter 3 (see Figures 3.6, 3.8, and 3.9).
  – To have some intact animals for the exam, your instructor may ask some groups to leave the viscera in their animals. There is still much you can observe with the viscera in situ, but these groups will need to mingle with their neighbors in order to see cut organs.
- The main discussion of the abdominal contents can be found on the lab ID list in Chapter 3. Use the figures in Chapter 3 to study the in situ contents on your side. In this or the next lab, you will remove the abdominal organs and examine them more closely.

- Work your way through the lab ID list on the abdomen to make sure you have seen all the relevant structures on the right and left sides.
- *Now it is time to remove the head by sawing at the C3 level. Store the head in the plastic bag provided.*
- **Cleanup:** You will be provided with either a plastic bag or sheet with which to wrap your animal. Make sure you wet your specimen before you wrap it up and use the body wall flap you made to cover the exposed viscera.
- Use the time in the next lab to follow on with the ID list. Use the extirpated abdominal viscera (gastrointestinal tract–liver, spleen–kidney) and pelvic viscera (male and female reproductive tracts) for closer inspection and discussion with your group and the instructor.

A.2.7 Dissection of Male and Female Pelvis (Lab 4)

- Your goal is to dissect structures on the medial and lateral sides of the pelvis and on isolated reproductive viscera. Your instructor should provide you with isolated male and female genitalia for a more detailed study.
- After you have removed the abdominal viscera, cut the pelvis from L6 and store in a plastic bag.
- Use the sagittal section to study the **peritoneal pouches** (see Figure 4.3a). Clean the fat from the pelvis and remove the peritoneum to isolate the vessels and nerves on the medial side. Make sure that you follow the branches of the **internal iliac artery** and identify the **obturator and pudendal nerves**. The internal iliac artery is very long in ruminants compared with the equine species. It courses caudally most of the length of the pelvis before it divides into the **caudal gluteal** and **internal pudendal** arteries (Figure 4.10a–b). Identify these terminal branches of the internal iliac artery. In the middle of the pelvic cavity, the internal iliac artery gives the prostatic artery in the male and vaginal artery in the female. Do not attempt to dissect other minor branches.
- Transect the gluteal muscles off the lateral side of the pelvis to demonstrate the **sacrosciatic ligament** and some of the structures passing through the **greater and lesser ischiatic (or sciatic) foreman** (go back to Chapter 4 to review this part).
- Those who worked on the male should exchange cadavers with those working on the female cadaver.
- Use the lab ID instructions and the figures in Chapter 4 to study male and female genital tracts. On an isolated male tract, make sure you identify the bends of the **sigmoid flexure, retractor penis muscle, dorsal nerve of the penis,** and the **urethral process**. On the female tract, identify the **ovaries, uterine horns, cervix, vagina,** and **vestibule**. Identify the clinically important **suburethral diverticulum** in the cranial vestibule.

A.3 Head Dissection (Lab 5)

- You will be provided with goat and bovine heads cut into two equal halves. Use half for muscles and the other half for blood vessels, nerves, salivary glands, and lymph nodes. For sake of time, your instructor may opt to prepare prosections of the head and demonstrate this lab.
- Skin the head carefully. Leave a small zone of the skin around the eyes, mouth, ears, nose, and horns. You may be asked to preserve or remove the cutaneous muscles of the head.
- With the help of Figures 1.10, 1.17, and 1.18, identify the structures listed on the lab ID list on lateral and medial views.

A.4 Forelimb Dissection (Labs 6 and 7)

Use time in lab 6 for the study of the musculoskeletal system and lab 7 for the study of blood vessels and nerves.

- Skin the entire limb from the scapula to the digits.
- Try to preserve the **cephalic and accessory cephalic veins**, and the **superficial branch of the radial nerve**. The **dorsal common digital nerve III** is the distal continuation of the superficial branch of the radial nerve.
- Refer to figures and instructions *(in italics)* in Chapter 5. Use the lab ID list for the forelimb and hind limb.

A.5 Hind Limb Dissection (Labs 8 and 9)

Follow the same scheme as for dissection of the forelimb (lab 8 for the musculoskeletal system and lab 9 for blood vessels and nerves).

- Skin the entire limb from proximal femur to the digits.
- Try to preserve the **medial saphenous vein, saphenous nerve**, and **saphenous artery** on the superficial surface of the gracilis muscle (see Figure 6.10). On the lateral side, preserve the **cranial and caudal branches of the lateral saphenous vein** (see Figure 6.20). Preserve the **superficial branch of the common peroneal nerve** and its continuation as the **dorsal common digital nerve III**, and **dorsal common digital vein III** (see Figure 6.20).
- Study the major muscles, nerves, and blood vessels using the lab ID list, figures, and instructions in Chapter 6.

Videos Captions

Video note: with audio are available at www.wiley.com/go/mansour/dissection2

#1 Chapter 1
Video 1 part 1: Important features of the bovine skull.

#2 Chapter 1
Video1 part 2: Features of the bovine skull and detailed description of the paranasal sinuses.

#3 Chapter 1
Video 2 part 1: Features of bovine teeth and steps for aging ruminants.

#4 Chapter 1
Video 2 part 2: Features of bovine teeth and steps for aging ruminants.

#5 Chapter 1
Video 3 part 1: Features of bovine teeth and steps for aging ruminants.

#6 Chapter 1
Video 3 part 2: Features of bovine teeth and steps for aging ruminants.

#7 Chapter 1
Video 4 Selected anatomical features of the bovine and caprine lateral head.

#8 Chapter 1
Video 5 Selected anatomical features of the bovine and caprine lateral and sagittal head.

#9 Chapter 1
Video 6 Selected anatomical features of the bovine and caprine lateral and sagittal head.

#10 Chapter 1
Video 7 Selected anatomical features of the bovine neck.

#11 Chapter 1
Video 8 Selected anatomical features of the goat neck.

#12 Chapter 2
Video 9 Selected anatomical features of the bovine left thorax.

#13 Chapter 2
Video 10 Selected anatomical features of the bovine right thorax.

#14 Chapter 2
Video 11 Selected anatomical features of the caprine thorax.

#15 Chapter 3
Video 12 Features of the bovine abdominal wall.

#16 Chapter 3
Video 13 Features and topography of the bovine left abdominal organs.

#17 Chapter 3
Video 14 Features and topography of the bovine right abdominal organs.

#18 Chapter 3
Video 15 Features of the caprine left and right abdominal organs in situ.

#19 Chapter 3
Video 16 Features of the caprine left and right isolated abdominal organs.

#20 Chapter 3
Video 17 Features of the bovine left and right isolated abdominal organs.

#21 Chapter 4
Video 18 Features of the bovine male reproductive organs.

#22 Chapter 4
Video 19 Features of the bovine pelvis and female reproductive organs.

#23 Chapter 4
Video 20 Features of the bovine udder.

#24 Chapter 5
Video 21 Bovine thoracic limb musculoskeletal structures.

#25 Chapter 5
Video 22 Bovine thoracic limb blood vessels and nerves.

#26 Chapter 6
Video 23 part 1: Bovine pelvic limb musculoskeletal structures.

#27 Chapter 6
Video 23 part 2: Bovine pelvic limb musculoskeletal structures, blood vessels, and nerves.

#28 Appendix A
Video 24 Opening of the thoracic and abdominal cavities.

Appendix B

Terminology: Common Terminology and Names

A

Animal Welfare: The well-being of an animal.
Antlers: Head gears found in the deer family. The bone is covered by skin (velvet). Antlers are found in members of the deer family and are shed annually.
Artificial Insemination (AI): The act of inseminating a cow using fresh or frozen semen.
Average Daily Feed Intake: The average amount of feed consumed by an animal each day.
Average Daily Gain: The amount of weight gained by an animal during its growing cycle.

B

Bull: Sexually mature and an uncastrated male bovine (specifically cattle).
Buck (Billy): A male goat used for breeding. The term buck is also used for male deer.
Buckling: A young sexually immature male goat.
Beef: The culinary name for meat from beef cattle.
Bovid: Any of various hoofed, horned ruminant mammals of the family Bovidae. This family includes cattle, sheep, goats, buffaloes, bisons, antelopes, and yaks.
Bovine: Relating to cows or cattle.
Breeding Stock: Sexually mature male and female livestock that are retained to produce offspring.

C

Calves (calf, singular): The young of domestic cattle under one year of age. The term is used for cattle of either sex from birth to weaning. Meat from a calf is called **veal**. Calf can also refer to young from animals like camels, dolphins, elephants, giraffes, and hippopotamuses.
Camelid: Any two-toed ruminant of the family Camelidae, including the camels, llamas, and vicunas.
Caprine: Relating to goats. (The scientific name of goats is *Capra hircus*.)
Cow: A fully grown female animal of a domesticated breed of bovine, used as a source of milk or beef.
Crossbreeding: The mating of animals of different breeds. For example, breeding a Hereford cow with an Angus bull.
Calving: The act of giving birth to a calf.
Cull: To sell inferior animals for meat.
Cud: Food that has been partly digested and brought up from the rumen to the mouth for further chewing by ruminants, such as cattle or sheep.

D

Doe: A female goat.

Guide to Ruminant Anatomy: Dissection and Clinical Aspects, Second Edition. Mahmoud Mansour, Ray Wilhite, Joe Rowe, and Saly Hafiz.
© 2023 John Wiley & Sons, Inc. Published 2023 by John Wiley & Sons, Inc.
Companion website: www.wiley.com/go/mansour/dissection2

E

Ewe: A female sheep of any age.

F

Feeder Cattle: Cattle past the calf stage that have weight increased making them salable as feedlot replacements.

Feedlot: A confinement facility where cattle are fed to produce beef for the commercial trade. May be under a roof or outdoors.

G

Goat/chevon: the meat of goats.

Gestation: Carrying an unborn animal during the pregnancy.

Greenhouse Gas: An atmospheric gas that contributes to the greenhouse effect by absorbing infrared radiation produced by solar warming of the Earth's surface.

H

Heifer: A young female cow that has not given birth (typically under two years of age).

Heiferette (plural heiferettes): A heifer (less than two years in age) that gave birth to one calf and then fed for slaughter.

Horns: Two-parth eadgear. Bones covered by keratinized epithelium (horn sheath). Horns never shed. Horns are found in cattle, sheep, and goats as examples.

I

Implantation: To become attached to and embedded in the maternal uterine lining. Used for a fertilized egg.

Inbreeding: The breeding or mating of related individuals within an isolated or closed group of organisms or people. Inbreeding can sometimes result in a loss of vigor or health in offspring. However, in agriculture and animal husbandry, the continued breeding of closely related individuals can help to preserve desirable traits in a stock.

L

Lamb: A young sheep, less than one year old.
Lactation: The process of making milk.

M

Manure: Organic matter used as organic fertilizer in agriculture.

Marbling: The pattern created by intramuscular fat in meat, especially red meat. The quality of marbling in meat can be influenced by selective breeding and feeding practices. In the United States, "prime" cuts of meat have the highest marbling content.

Mastitis: An infection and inflammation of the udder in cows.

Monogastric: An animal with a stomach consisting of one compartment for digestion. Includes humans and pigs.

Mutton: name for meat from older sheep (over one year).

N

Neonatal: Relating to newborn animals.

O

Ossicones (translation bone cones): Ossified cartilage covered with skin. Ossicones never shed. Found in giraffes and male okapi.

Ovine: Relating to sheep.

Ovulation: The release of an egg cell (ovum) from the ovary in female animals, regulated in mammals by hormones produced in the pituitary glands during the menstrual cycle.

P

Parturition: The act of giving birth to offspring. In cows, parturition is called **calving**, and in pigs, parturition is called **farrowing**.

Polled: Hornless ruminant (naturally or genetically bred).

Pronghorns: Two-parth eadgear. Bones covered by a branched keratinized sheath. The sheath is shed but the bone is not. Found in animals with deer-like bodies. The pronghorn (*Antilocapra americana*) is a member of the Antilocapridae family found in North America.

Puberty: The stage in which an animal reaches sexual maturity.

R

Ram: A male sheep of any age.

Red Meat: Meat that is red when raw and not white when cooked. In the nutritional sciences, red meat includes all mammal meat. Red meat includes the meat of most adult mammals and some fowl (e.g., ducks).

Roughage: Coarse, less digestible food or fodder. It provides bulk to the food intake and promotes normal gut function.

Ruminant: Any of various even-toed hoofed mammals of the suborder Ruminantia. Ruminants usually have a stomach divided into four compartments and chew a cud consisting of regurgitated, partially digested food. Includes cattle, sheep, goats, deer, and others.

S

Sheep: Any of the various usually horned ruminant mammals of the genus Ovis in the family Bovidae, especially the domesticated species Ovis, raised in many breeds for wool, edible flesh, or skin.

Sire: The male parent. To father or become the sire of.

Sorghum: A cereal grass used mainly for feed grain or silage.

Stockers: Weaned grazing calves to enhance growth prior to finishing and slaughter. Usually of lower condition than "feeders."

U

Uterine: adjective meaning relating to the uterus.

V

Veal: The meat of young cattle (calves), as opposed to meat from older cattle. Though veal can be produced from a calf of either sex or any breed, most veal comes from male calves of dairy cattle breeds.

W

Wether: castrated male goat and/or sheep.

Z

Zoonotic: Relating to a disease communicable from animals to humans under natural conditions. Example: rabies.

References

1. *Glossary of Small Ruminants* – Angela McKenzie-Jakes, Extension Animal Science Specialist. Florida A&M University.
2. *Knowing the Livestock Lingo* – Nebraska 4-H- g2175.pdf (unl.edu).
3. *Useful Livestock Terms*, https://www.agric.wa.gov.au/sites/gateway/files/Useful%20livestock%20definitions%20for%20primary%20schools%20-%20AgLinkEd%20header%20for%20printing%20-%20final2.pdf

Appendix C

Further Reading

Andrews, A.H. (1991) *Outline of Clinical Diagnosis in Cattle*, Wiley.

Aspinall, V. and Cappello, M. (2015) *Introduction to Veterinary Anatomy and Physiology Textbook*, 3rd edn. Butterworth-Heinemann.

Ball, P.J.H. and Peters, A.R. (2004) *Reproduction in Cattle*, 3rd edn. Wiley-Blackwell.

Blowey, R.W. and Weaver, A.D. (2011) *Color Atlas of Diseases and Disorders of Cattle*, 3rd edn. Mosby Elsevier.

Burdas, K.D., Habel, R.E., Wunsche, A., Mulling, C.K., and Greenough, P.R. (2011) *Bovine Anatomy*, 2nd edn. Schlutersche.

Clark, T.L., Abbott, L.C., and Ruoff, L.M. (2016) *Guide to Dissection of the Horse and Ruminants*, 2nd edn. Bluedoor.

Cockcroft, P. (ed.) (2015) *Bovine Medicine*, 3rd edn. Wiley-Blackwell.

Constantinescu, G.M. (2001) *Guide to Regional Ruminant Anatomy Based on the Dissection of the Goat*, Iowa State University Press.

Duncanson, G.R. (2013) *Farm Animal Medicine and Surgery: For Small Animal Veterinarians*, CABI Publishing.

Dyce, K.M., Sack W.O., and Wensing C.J. (2010) *Textbook of Veterinary Anatomy*, 4th edn. Saunders.

Dyce, K.M. and Wensing, C.J.G. (1971) *Essentials of Bovine Anatomy*, Lea and Febiger.

Evans, H.E. and de Lahunta, A. (2016) *Guide to Dissection of the Dog*, 8th edn. Saunders.

Garrett P.D. (1988) *Guide to Ruminant Anatomy Based on the Dissection of the Goat*, Iowa State University Press.

Getty, R. (1975) *Sisson and Grossman's Anatomy of Domestic Animals*, 5th edn., vols 1 and 2, W.B. Saunders.

Holtgrew-Bohling, K. (2016) *Large Animal Clinical Procedures for Veterinary Technicians*, 3rd edn. Elsevier.

Hopper, R.M (ed.) (2014) *Bovine Reproduction*, 2nd edn. John Wiley & Sons, Inc.

König, H.E., Liebich, H., and Bragulla, H. (2014) *Veterinary Anatomy of Domestic Mammals: Textbook and Color Atlas*, 6th edn. Schattauer.

Lin, H. and Walz, P. (2014) *Farm Animal Anesthesia: Cattle, Small Ruminants, Camelids, Pigs*, John Wiley & Sons Inc.

Mansour, M., Steiss, J., and Wilhite, R. (2016) *Equine Anatomy Guide: The Head and Neck*. Blurb Books.

Melling, M. and Alder, M. (eds) (1998) *Bovine Practice 2: In Practice Handbooks Series*, 2nd edn. W.B. Saunders.

Nickel, R., Schummer, A., Seiferle, E., Wilkens, H., Wille, K. and Frewein, J. (1986) *The Anatomy of the Domestic Animals, vol. 1. The Locomotor System of the Domestic Mammals*, Verlag Paul Parey.

Reece, W.O. (2009) *Functional Anatomy and Physiology of Domestic Animals*, 4th edn. Wiley-Blackwell.

Schummer, A., Nickel, R., and Sack, W.O. (1979) *The Viscera of the Domestic Mammals*, 2nd edn. Springer-Verlag.

Index

a

abaxial dorsal proper digital nerves 249
abaxial palmar digital nerve IV 212
abaxial palmar proper digital nerve III 212
abdominal tendon 99
abdominal wall 95
abducent nerve (CN VI) 29, 36
abomasal groove 115, 123
abomasal volvulus 123
abomasum 105, 111, 121
accessory carpal bone 181, 200
accessory cephalic vein 209
accessory gluteal muscle 229
accessory lung lobe 72
accessory nerve 37, 53 54
accessory pancreatic duct 130
accessory sex glands 144
acetabular fossa 220
acromion 178
adductor muscles 232
adnexa 144
alar foramina 50
ampulla 161
ampullary glands 159
anconeal process 181
anconeus muscle 195
annulus 25
ansa axillaris 211
ansa subclavia 82
antebrachium 181
anterior chamber 48
antimesenteric vessels 126
aorta 79
aortic arch 76, 85
aortic hiatus 79
aortic semilunar valve 88
apical ligament 146
area for lung auscultation 66
artery of the bulb of the penis 154
artery of the penis 153
articular disc 24
arytenoid cartilage 42
ascending colon 105, 123
ascending duodenum 123, 125
atlantoaxial joint 50
atlantooccipital joint 50
atlas 24, 48
atria 84
atrioventricular valves 88
atrium ruminis 120
auricles 84
auricular surface (heart) 82
auriculopalpebral nerve 36
axial dorsal longitudinal groove 225
axial dorsal proper digital nerve 249
axial dorsal proper digital nerves III and IV 212, 249
axial palmar proper digital arteries III and IV 207, 212
axial plantar proper digital arteries III and IV 241–242
axial plantar proper digital nerves III and IV 249
axial skeleton 2
axillary artery 77, 78
axillary lymph nodes 209
axis 48

b

baby teeth 16
basal border of the lungs 65
basihyoid bone 43
bicarotid trunk 77
biceps brachii muscle 196
biceps femoris muscle 230
bile duct 130
body (shaft) of the ilium 140
body of the mandible 4
bony rim of the orbit 4
border of the lung 65
brachial artery 206–207
brachialis groove 180
brachialis muscle 196
brachiocephalic trunk 76, 77, 85
brachiocephalicus muscle 55, 186
brachium 180
broad ligament 159
broken mouth 22
buccal branches 36
buccinator muscle 28
bulbar conjunctiva 44
bulb of the penis 145, 151
bulbospongiosus muscle 145
bulbourethral glands 158
butcher's bible 120

Guide to Ruminant Anatomy: Dissection and Clinical Aspects, Second Edition. Mahmoud Mansour, Ray Wilhite, Joe Rowe, and Saly Hafiz.
© 2023 John Wiley & Sons, Inc. Published 2023 by John Wiley & Sons, Inc.
Companion website: www.wiley.com/go/mansour/dissection2

C

calcanean bursae 239
calcanean tuber 238
calcaneus 224
calyx 132
canines 16
cannon bone 183
cardia 112, 115
cardiac glands 122
carotid sheath 30
carpal hygroma 203
carpometacarpal joint 183
caruncles 163
caudal auricular artery 30
caudal auricular nerve 5
caudal compartment of the frontal sinus 13
caudal duodenal flexure 123, 124, 125
caudal gluteal artery 141, 155, 240
caudal gluteal nerve 141, 245
caudal groove 118
colic 136
caudal laryngeal nerve 37, 55, 81
caudal mediastinal lymph nodes 80
caudal mediastinum 74
caudal mesenteric artery 135
caudal mesenteric lymph nodes 136
caudal mesenteric vein 135
caudal pillar 118, 120
caudal superficial epigastric vein 78
caudal tibial artery 241
caudal tibial muscle 239
caudal vena cava 76–77, 86, 136
caudal vertebrae 141
caudate process of the caudate lobe of the liver 111
caudodorsal blind sac 118
caudoventral blind sac 118
caval foramen 77
cecocolic orifice 123
cecum 123, 126, 129
celiac artery 135
celiac lymphocenter 136
cement 17
central flexure 123, 126, 129
central tarsal bone 224
centrifugal coils 123, 126, 129
centripetal coils 123, 126, 129
centroquartal bone 224
cephalic vein 209
ceratohyoid bone 43
cervicothoracic ganglia 82
cervix portio vaginalis 164
cheek teeth 16
chordae tendineae 86, 87
choroid 46
ciliary body 46, 48
ciliary muscle 47
ciliary processes 48
circumflex branch of left coronary artery 87
cisterna chyli 79
clavicular intersection 50
cleidobrachialis muscle 53, 186, 187
cleidocephalicus muscle 186, 187
cleidomastoideus muscle 51, 186, 187
cleidooccipitalis muscle 51, 186
clitoral fossa 166
cochlea 223
coffin bone 184
coffin joint 184
colon 126
common calcanean (Achilles) tendon 238, 239
common carotid artery 30, 55, 77
common digital extensor muscle 197
common extensor tendon of digits III and IV 197
common fibular (peroneal) nerve 245, 247
conjunctiva 46
conjunctival sac 45
connecting pleura 71
constrictor pupillae 47
conus arteriosus 85
coracobrachialis muscle 195
cornea 46
cornual artery 5, 30
cornual diverticulum 9, 13
cornual nerve 5, 35, 37
cornual process 2, 3
coronary circulation 75
coronary groove 85, 87, 118
coronary sinus 75, 77, 86
coronoid process 9
corpora nigra 47
corpus cavernosum penis 144
costal cartilage 65
costocervical trunk 77
costochondral junction 65
costodiaphragmatic recess 68
cotyledonary 163
cranial flexure 125
cranial gluteal artery 141, 240, 245
cranial groove 115
cranial laryngeal nerve 37, 55
cranial lung lobe 74
cranial mediastinum 74
cranial mesenteric artery 135
 lymphocenter 136
cranial mesenteric vein 136
cranial nerves 35
cranial part of the duodenum 123
cranial pillar 120
cranial sac 116, 120
cranial superficial epigastric vein 78
cranial tibial artery 241
cranial tibial muscle 233, 237
cranial vena cava 76, 77
cremaster muscle 157
cricoarytenoideus dorsalis muscle 29
cricoid 42
cricopharyngeus 29
crown 17
crura 145
 retinacula 237
crural extensor retinacula 237
crus 145
cusps 87
cutaneus colli muscle 98
cutaneus faciei muscle 25, 26, 27, 98
cutaneus omobrachialis muscle 69, 98, 185
cutaneus trunci muscle 68, 98, 185

d

deciduous incisors   22
deep antebrachial fascia   196
deep artery of the penis   154
deep cervical lymph nodes   34
deep circumflex artery   135
deep digital flexor muscle   201, 239
deep gluteal muscle   226, 230
deep leaf of the greater omentum   107, 109
deep pectoral muscle   186
deep peroneal nerve   241, 245
deltoideus muscle   194
deltoid tuberosity   180
dens   50
dental pad   3, 17, 19
dentin   17
depressor labii inferioris muscle   28
descending aorta   76
descending colon   123, 129
descending duodenum   123
descending pectoral muscle   188
dewclaws   184, 225
diaphragmatic line of pleural reflection   64, 65
diastema   17, 21
digastricus muscle   28
digital joints (fetlock, pastern, and coffin)   250
dilator pupillae muscle   47
distal bend of the sigmoid flexure   151
distal digital annular ligament   204
distal (metatarsal) extensor retinaculum   237
distal interdigital ligament   204
distal intertarsal joint   250
distal loop   126, 129
distal paravertebral nerve blocks   96, 97
distal sesamoid bone   184
dorsal artery of the penis   154
dorsal axial longitudinal groove   183
dorsal axial proper digital nerves III and IV   212
dorsal branch of the accessory nerve   37
dorsal buccal branches (facial nerve)   30, 36, 37
dorsal commissure   167
dorsal common digital nerve III   212, 245, 249
dorsal common digital nerves II and III   212
dorsal common digital nerves II, III, and IV   249
dorsal common digital vein III   209, 242
dorsal (right and left) coronary pillars   116, 118, 120
dorsal mesogastrium   107
dorsal metatarsal artery III   241
dorsal metatarsal nerve III   249
dorsal nerve of the penis   150
dorsal pedal artery   241
dorsal sac   116
dorsal vagal trunk   81
ductus deferens   157
duodenocolic fold   123, 125
duodenojejunal flexure   123, 125
duodenum   123

e

elbow joint   180, 181
enamel   17
endothoracic fascia   71
epaxial muscles   70
epicardium   82
epiceras gland   38
epidural   98
epiglottis   42
epihyoid bone   43
epiploic foramen   110, 111
esophageal hiatus   81
ethmoid meatuses   10
extensor carpi obliquus muscle   199
extensor carpi radialis muscle   196
extensor groove   223
extensor process   184
extensor retinaculum   203
external abdominal oblique   98
external carotid artery   30
external iliac artery   154, 240
external intercostal muscles   68
external jugular vein   32, 55
external lamina of the prepuce   152
external (outer or superficial) lamina of rectus sheath   101
external occipital protuberance   7
external pudendal artery   170, 270
external pudendal vein   170
external urethral orifice   146
external uterine (or cervical) ostium   164, 165
extraocular muscles   27
extrinsic laryngeal muscles   29
extrinsic lingual muscles   29

f

facial artery   30, 39
facial nerve (CN VII)   27, 36
facial tuberosity   3, 4
facial vein   32, 39
fascia lata   226, 229
fat pad   44
femoral artery   240
femoral nerve   245, 246
fetal cotyledon   163
fetlock joint   184
fibrocartilaginous joint   25
fibroelastic type   144
fibrous pericardium   82
fibrous tunic   46
fibula   223
fibularis (peroneus) longus muscle   234, 235
fibularis (peroneus) tertius muscle   234, 235
flexor carpi radialis muscle   200
flexor carpi ulnaris muscle   199
flexor manica   201, 205
flexor retinaculum   203
fold of the flank   185
foramen magnum   7
foramen orbitorotundum   6, 36, 39
forestomach   112
fornix   45
fossa   41
fossa linguae   41
fossa ovalis   86
fourth carpal bone   182
fourth digit   184

fourth tarsal bone   224
fovea capitis femoris   220
freemartin   164
free part of the penis   148, 153
frontal bone   3
frontalis   27
frontal process of the zygomatic bone   5
frontal sinus   9, 13
frontal vein   4, 32
fundus   48
fundus of the abomasum   112
Furstenberg's rosette   170
fused interosseus III and IV   201
fused second and third carpal bones   182

g

gallbladder   130
gastric (or esophageal) groove   115, 119, 123
gastric lymph nodes   136
gastrocnemius muscle   238, 239
gastroduodenal vein   136
geniohyoideus muscle   29
genital fold   142
genitofemoral nerve   157, 172
gland of the third eyelid   46
gland sinus   170
glans clitoris   166
glenoid cavity   179
glossopharyngeal nerve   28
glottis   43
gluteal muscles   226
gluteobiceps muscle   229, 230
gonadal (testicular or ovarian) artery   135
gonitis   250
gracilis muscle   231
great auricular nerve   37, 54
great cardiac vein   86
great mesentery   125
greater ischiatic foramen   141, 240, 246
greater omentum   106, 107
greater trochanter   220
greater tubercle   180
gubernaculum testis   157

h

hamstring muscles   226
hardware disease   119
hepatic artery   135
hepatic lymph nodes   136
hepatic veins   136
hilus   133
hip (or coxofemoral) joint   220, 250
hock joints   250
honeycomb appearance   115
hook   140
horn buds   5
horn sheath   4
humeral crest   180
humeral head   200, 201
hump   54, 187
hyoid muscles   27
hyopharyngeus muscle   28
hypoglossal canal   37
hypoglossal nerve (CN XII)   29, 37

i

I1 (central or pincher)   17, 24
I2 (first intermediate)   17, 24
I3 (second intermediate)   17, 24
I4   17, 24
ileal orifice   123, 126
ileocecal fold   123, 126
ileum   123, 126
iliacus muscle   226
iliocostalis thoracis muscle   68
iliopsoas muscle   226
ilium   140
incisive bone   4
incisors   16
infraorbital foramen   4, 5
infraorbital nerve   36, 37
infraspinatus muscle   193
infraspinatus subtendinous bursa   194
infraspinous fossa   178
infratrochlear nerve   5, 37
infundibulum   161
inguinal canal   101
inguinal ligament   99
intercapital notch   225
intercondylar fossa   221
intercornual ligament(s)   162

intercornual protuberance   4, 7
intercostal arteries   71
intercostal lymph node   79
intercostal nerves   70, 71
intercostal veins   71
interdigital fat pad   217
intermammary groove   169
intermediate carpal bone   181
internal iliac arteries   155, 240
internal intercostal muscles   68
internal lamina of the rectus sheath   102
internal preputial lamina   153
internal pudendal artery   153
internal thoracic artery   77, 78
internal uterine (or cervical) ostium   164
interosseus muscle   239
intertrochanteric crest   221
intertrochlear notch   183
intertubercular bursa   196
intertubercular groove   180
intervenous tubercle   86
interventricular septum   86
intestinal trunk   136
intrasinual lamellae   13
intrinsic laryngeal muscles   29
intrinsic lingual muscles   29
inverted L-nerve block   97, 98
iridic granules   47
iridocorneal angle   48
iris   46
ischiatic arch   140
ischiatic tuberosities (pins)   145
ischiocavernosus muscle   145
ischium   140
isthmus   161

j

jejunal (mesenteric) lymph nodes   125, 129, 135
jejunum   123, 125
jugular foramen   36
jugular furrow   50

l

L1 (iliohypogastric)   95, 96
L2 (ilioinguinal)   95, 96

labial surface   17
lacrimal bone   4
lacrimal bulla   6
lacrimal gland   46
lacrimal sac   45
lactiferous sinus   170
laminae of the prepuce   153
large intestines   123
large metacarpal bone   183
laryngeal muscles   27
laryngopharynx   40
lateral branch of the median nerve   212
lateral digital extensor muscle   198, 234, 235, 236, 239
lateral epicondyle (humerus)   180, 222
lateral head of deep digital flexor muscle   239
lateral malleolus   223
lateral plantar artery   244, 250
lateral pterygoid muscle   28
lateral retropharyngeal lymph node   34
lateral saphenous vein   242
lateral trochlear ridge   222
latissimus dorsi muscle   68, 186
left atrioventricular (mitral) valve   76, 87
left azygos vein   77, 79, 86
left coronary artery   87
left gastric artery   135
left longitudinal groove   106, 109, 113
left recurrent laryngeal nerve   81
left subclavian artery   77
lesser ischiatic foramen   141, 240
lesser omentum   106, 107, 110, 120
lesser trochanter   220
lesser tubercle   180
levator labii superioris muscle   28
levator nasolabialis muscle   28
levator palpebrae superioris muscle   29
ligament of the head of the femur   220, 250, 256

ligament of the tail of the epididymis   155
ligamentum arteriosum   85
limbus   46
lingual artery   30
lingual fossa   40, 42
lingual muscles   27
lingual process of the basihyoid bone   43
lingual surface   17, 21
lingual torus   41
linguofacial trunk   30
long and (short) digital extensor muscles   235, 236
longissimus thoracis muscle   68
long thoracic nerve   70
longus colli muscle   71
lower incisor teeth   19
lumbosacral plexus   245
lymphocenters   34, 136

m

major duodenal papilla   130
malaris muscle   28
mammary artery   170
mammary glands   169
mammary lymph nodes   34, 153
mandibular ducts   40
mandibular foramen   9
mandibular fossa   24
mandibular nerve   28, 36
mandibular notch   9
mandibular salivary gland   39
mandibular sublingual gland   39
manus   181
masseter muscle   25, 28
maternal caruncle   163
maxilla   4
maxillary artery   30
maxillary nerve   36
maxillary sinus   10, 14
medial and lateral femoral condyles   221
medial and lateral tibial condyles   223
medial branch of the median nerve   212
medial canthus   45

medial digital extensor tendon   197, 235
medial digital flexor muscle   239
medial femoral epicondyle   222
medial head of the deep digital flexor muscle   239
medial malleolus   223
medial plantar artery   241
medial plantar nerve   245, 250
medial retropharyngeal lymph nodes   34
medial saphenous vein   240, 242
medial tendon of the common digital extensor muscle   198
medial trochlear ridge   222
median artery   206
median caudal artery   60
median caudal vein   60
median artery Palmar common digital artery III   207
median cubital vein   209
median ligament of the bladder   143
median nerve   207, 209, 211, 216
mediastinal lymph nodes   79
mediastinal pleura   82
mental foramen   9
mental nerve   36, 37
mesial surface   17
mesoductus deferens   157, 158
mesoduodenum   111, 125
mesojejunum   123, 125
mesorchium   157, 158
mesosalpinx   161
mesovarium   161
metacarpal tuberosity   183
metatarsal (distal) extensor retinaculum   237, 238
metatarsal sesamoid   225
midcarpal joint   13
middle cervical ganglion   82
middle gluteal muscle   229, 230
middle mediastinum   74
middle nasal meatus   10, 14
middle (P2) phalanges   184, 226
milk teeth   16
milk vein   78, 172
milk well   78, 172

minor duodenal papilla   130
mitral valve   76, 87
molar teeth   16
monostomatic sublingual gland   39
multi-pyramidal kidney   130
muscles of facial expression   27
muscles of mastication   27
musculocutaneous nerve   211
mylohyoideus   29

n

nasal bone   4
nasoincisive notch   4
nasolacrimal duct   45
nasopharynx   40
navicular bone   184
neck   17, 65
nervous tunic   46
nuchal diverticulum   13
nuchal ligament   56
nucleus pulpous   25

o

oblique eye muscles   29
oblique transverse septum   13
obturator foramen   140
obturator nerve   245, 246
occipital condyles   7, 24
occlusal surface   17
oculomotor nerve (CN III)   29, 36
odontoid process   50
olecranon fossa   180
olecranon tuber   181
olfactory nerve (CN I)   36
omasal groove   120, 121, 123
omasal laminae   120, 121
omasoabomasal orifice   120
omasum   105, 111, 120
omental bursa   105, 109
omohyoideus muscle   29
omotransversarius muscle   53, 55, 186
ophthalmic nerve   36
optic canal   36
optic disc   48
orbicularis oculi muscle   27
orbicularis oris muscle   28
oropharynx   40
ossa cordis   87
ovarian artery   167
ovarian bursa   159
ovarian tube   159
ovary   158

p

palatine tonsil   40
palatoglossal arch   40
palatopharyngeal arch   40
palmar annular ligament   204
palmar axial longitudinal groove   183
palmar carpal ligament   203
palmar common digital artery III   206, 207
palmar common digital nerve III   212
palmar common digital nerves III and II   212
palpebrae   44
palpebral conjunctiva   44
pampiniform plexus   157
pancreatic duct   130
pancreaticoduodenal lymph nodes   136
papillary muscles   86, 87
paraconal interventricular groove   85
paracondylar processes   7
pararectal fossae   142
parasympathetic fibers   35
parietal layer of the serous pericardium   82
parietal peritoneum   105
parietal vaginal tunic   155
parotid duct   39
parotid lymph node   34, 35
parotid salivary gland   39
pastern joint   184
patella   222
patellar ligaments   233
pecten   140
pectinate muscles   86
pectineus muscle   232
pegs   22
pelvic canal   141
pelvic diaphragm   234
pelvic inlet   140
pelvic symphysis   140
pelvic tendon   99
pelvic urethra   150
penile urethra   150
penis   144
pericardial cavity   82
pericardium   82
periorbita   29
peritoneal cavity   107
permanent incisors   22
persistent frenulum   153
pes   220
pharyngeal muscles   27
pharyngeus (suffix)   28
phrenicoabdominal artery   135
phrenicopericardial ligament   82
pillars   116, 120
pin   140
piriformis muscle   229
placentome   163
plane (flat) synovial joint   25
plantar common digital artery III   241
plantar common digital nerve III   250
plantar common digital nerve IV   250
plantar common digital nerves II and III   250
plantar longitudinal groove   225
platysma   27
pleura   71
plica vena cava   72
point of the hock   224
points for puncta maxima   64
popliteal artery   241
popliteal lymph node   244
popliteus muscle   238, 239
portal vein   136
posterior chamber   48
postorbital diverticulum   9, 13
premolars   16
prepubic tendon   102
prepuce   144
prepuce (external lamina)   152
preputial cavity   148, 153
preputial hair ring   152

preputial orifice   152, 153
promontory   140
pronator teres muscle   201
proper extensor tendon of digit III   197
proper gastric glands   122
proper ligament of the ovary   161
proper ligament of the testis   157
prostate gland   158
proximal digital annular ligament   204
proximal (crural) extensor retinaculum   237
proximal intertarsal joint   224, 251
proximal loop of the ascending colon   126
proximal (dorsal) paravertebral nerve block   96, 97
proximal (P1) phalanges   184, 226
proximal sesamoid bones   184
pseudo-unipyramidal   130
psoas major muscle   226
psoas minor muscle   226
pubovesical pouch   142
pudendal nerve   150, 154, 155
pudendoepigastric trunk   170
pulmonary arteries   85
pulmonary circulation   75
pulmonary ligament   72
pulmonary pleura   72
pulmonary semilunar valves   75, 88
pulmonary trunk   75, 85
pulmonary valve   88
pulmonary veins   76
puncta maxima   64
pyloric glands   122
pyloric region   121
pylorus   121

q

quadrate liver lobes   130

r

radial carpal bone   181
radial fossa   180
radial head   201
radial nerve   209
radial tuberosity   181

radiocarpal joint   181
ramus   9
rectogenital pouch   142
rectus eye muscles   29
rectus femoris muscle   233
rectus sheath   101
rectus thoracis muscle   68
recurrent laryngeal nerve   37, 54, 55
renal arteries   135
renal cortex   133
renal crest   133
renal medulla   133
renal pelvis   133
renal sinus   133
rete mirabile   30
reticular groove   112, 115, 119, 123
reticular mucosa   111
reticulo-omasal orifice   112, 115, 120
reticulum   105, 111, 112
retina   48
retractor bulbi muscle   29
retractor penis muscle   146
rhomboideus muscle   186
ribs   2, 64
right atrioventricular valve   77, 86
right azygos vein   77
right longitudinal groove of the rumen   109
right longitudinal pillar   118
rima glottidis   43
rods   22
round ligament(s) of the bladder   143
round ligament of the liver   130
rudimentary teats   152
rumen   105, 111, 112
ruminal atrium   120
ruminal pillars   120
ruminal recess   120
ruminoreticular compartment   115
ruminoreticular fold   112, 118, 120

s

sacrosciatic ligament   141
saphenous artery   232, 240, 241
saphenous nerve   240, 246

sartorius muscle   226, 231
scalenus muscle   68
scapular cartilage   180
scent gland   38
sciatic (or ischiatic) nerve   141, 233, 244, 245, 246
sclera   46
scrotal (spermatic) fascia   155
scrotal lymph nodes   153
semimembranosus muscle   230, 232
semitendinosus muscle   230
serrated face   179, 189
serratus dorsalis muscle   68
serratus ventralis muscle   68, 186
sheath   153
short (brevis) digital extensor muscle   236
short mouth   22, 24
shoulder joint   179
sigmoid flexure   123, 125, 126, 144, 146
small intestine   123
smooth mouth   22
soft palate   40
soleus muscle   238
solid mouth   22
spermatic cord   157
spinalis et semispinalis thoracis muscle   68
spine of the scapula   178
spiral loop   129
spleen   112
splenic artery   135
splenic lymph nodes   136
splenic vein   136
sternal lymph node   79
sternohyoideus muscle   29, 54
sternomandibularis muscle   25, 53, 55
sternomastoideus muscle   53
sternopericardial ligament   82, 83
sternothyroideus muscle   29, 54
sternozygomaticus muscle   25, 53
sternum   2, 64
stifle joint   220, 223, 250
stylohyoid bone   43
styloid process of the radius   181

styloid process of the ulna   181
stylomastoid foramen   36
stylopharyngeus muscle   28
subclavian artery   77
subclavius muscle   186
subcutaneous abdominal vein   172
sublingual caruncle   40
sublingual salivary gland   39
subscapular fossa   179
subscapularis muscle   194
subsinuosal interventricular groove   85, 87
subtendinous bursa of the triceps brachii   195
subtendinous calcanean bursa   239
suburethral diverticulum   166
superficial branch of the radial nerve   212
superficial cervical artery   77, 78
superficial cervical lymph nodes   53, 188
superficial digital flexor muscle   201, 238
   flexor manica   201
superficial gluteal muscle   229
superficial inguinal lymph nodes   153, 172
superficial inguinal ring   99
superficial layer of the greater omentum   106, 107, 109
superficial pectoral muscle   186
superficial peroneal nerve   249
superficial temporal artery   30
supracondylar fossa   223
supracondylar tuberosities   238
supraomental recess   105, 109, 123, 125
supraorbital canal   13
supraorbital foramen   4
supraorbital groove   4
supraorbital nerve   36
supraspinatus muscle   193
supraspinous bursa   56
supraspinous fossa   178
suspensory apparatus   169
sustentaculum tali   224
synsarcosis   189
systemic circulation   75

t

T13 (costoabdominal)   95, 96
tail vein   15
talus   224
tapetum lucidum   48
tarsocrural joint   223
tarsometatarsal joint   250, 251
teat   169
teat canal   170
teat orifice   169
teat sinus   170
temporal line   4, 5, 6
temporal muscle   28
temporal process of the zygomatic bone   4
temporomandibular joint   9
tensor fasciae antebrachii muscle   195
tensor fasciae latae muscle   226
teres major muscle   194
teres minor muscle   194
testicular vein   157
third metacarpal bone   183
thoracic inlet   65
thyroarytenoideus muscle   29
thyrohyoid bone   43
thyrohyoideus muscle   29
thyroid gland   55
thyropharyngeus muscle   28
tibia   223
tibial nerve   238, 245
tibial tuberosity   223, 233
tibiotarsal joint   250, 251
torus linguae   40, 41, 42
torus pyloricus   121, 122
trabeculae carneae   86
trabecula septomarginalis   86
tracheal bronchus   74
tracheobronchial lymph node   79
transverse colon   123, 129
transverse facial artery   30
transverse humeral retinaculum   196, 203
transverse pectoral muscle   188
trapezius muscle   37, 186
triceps brachii muscle   194
tricuspid valve   87
trigeminal nerve   36
trigone of the bladder   151, 152
trochanteric bursa   229
trochanteric fossa   221
trochlea of the femur   222
trochlear nerve (CN IV)   29, 36
trochlear notch   181
tuber calcaneus   224
tunica albuginea penis   144
tunica dartos   155
tunica flava abdominis   98

u

ulnar carpal bone   181
ulnar nerve   209, 212
ulnaris lateralis muscle   199
umbilical artery   155
umbilicus   152
ureters   142
urethral process (vermiform appendage)   146, 148
uterine artery   155, 167
uterine tube   159
uterus   159
uvea   46

v

vagina   159
vaginal artery   167
vaginal fornix   164
vaginal tunic   101, 157
vagosympathetic trunk   37, 54, 55, 82
vagus nerve   29, 36
vastus intermedius muscle   233
vastus lateralis muscle   233
vastus medialis muscle   233
vela abomascia   120, 121
ventral branch of the accessory nerve   37
ventral buccal branches of the facial nerve   37
ventral commissure   167
ventral (right and left) coronary pillars   118, 120
ventral mesogastrium   107
ventral sac of the rumen   118
ventral vagal trunk   81
vertebral artery   78
vertebral column   2

vertebral formula   14
vesicogenital pouch   142
vesicular glands   158
vestibule   159
vestibulocochlear nerve   36
visceral layer of the serous pericardium   82
visceral peritoneum   107
visceral (pulmonary) pleura   72
vitreous body   48
vitreous chamber   48
vocal fold   43
vulva   159

W

wings of the atlas   49

Z

zonular fibers   48
zygomatic arch   4
zygomatic bone   4
zygomatic process of the frontal bone   5
zygomatic process of the temporal bone   4